Vitamins
Nutrition
and Cancer

Vitamins
Nutrition
and Cancer

Editor: K.N. Prasad, Denver, Colo.

42 figures and 90 tables, 1984

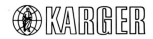

KARGER

S. Karger · Basel · München · Paris · London · New York · Tokyo · Sydney

National Library of Medicine, Cataloging in Publication
Vitamins, nutrition, and cancer
Editor, K.N. Prasad. – Basel; New York: Karger, 1984.
Includes index.
'Based on papers presented at the International Symposium on Vitamins, Nutrition, and
Cancer, held in Denver, Colorado, June 20–22, 1983' – P. x.
1. Neoplasms – congresses   2. Nutrition – congresses   3. Vitamins – congresses
I. Prasad, Kedar N.   II. International Symposium on Vitamins, Nutrition, and Cancer
(1983: Denver, Colo.)
QZ 202 V837 1983
ISBN 3-8055-3846-4

Drug Dosage
The authors and the publisher have exerted every effort to ensure that drug selection and dosage
set forth in this text are in accord with current recommendations and practice at the time of
publication. However, in view of ongoing research, changes in government regulations, and the
constant flow of information relating to drug therapy and drug reactions, the reader is urged to
check the package insert for each drug for any change in indications and dosage and for added
warnings and precautions. This is particularly important when the recommended agent is a new
and/or infrequently employed drug.

©   Copyright 1984 by S. Karger AG, P.O. Box, CH–4009 Basel (Switzerland)
Printed in Switzerland by Thür AG Offsetdruck, Pratteln
ISBN 3-8055-3846-4

Contents

Contents

Other Vitamins and Nutrients

Clinical Trials

Chemoprevention Program at NCI

Abstracts

Contents

Preface

The role of vitamins and other nutrients in prevention and treatment is becoming increasingly evident. I personally consider this as the 'new frontier' of cancer research. Several experimental and human epidemiological studies have already suggested that the high levels of vitamins may be of protective value against cancer. In addition, diet enriched in fibre, fruits, and vegetables appear to be associated with a low risk of cancer, whereas diets containing excess of fat and meat are associated with a high risk of cancer. However, at this time, we have no data in humans to evaluate the extent of the involvement of these nutrients in the reduction or the enhancement of cancer incidence. It must be shown by an intervention trial that the supplemental vitamins and other nutritional elements, indeed, reduce the incidence of cancer in humans. It is only then that we can be sure of the protective value of these nutrients against human cancer. Vitamins could reduce the incidence of cancer by more than one mechanism: (1) they can directly kill the newly transformed cells; (2) they can reverse the newly transformed cells back to normal cells; (3) they can indirectly kill the newly transformed cells by stimulating the host's immune system, and (4) they can prevent the action of tumor-promoting as well as tumor-initiating agents. Some intervention trials are in progress and some are planned using mostly one vitamin at a time. It is very important that we initiate an intervention trial in humans systematically and carefully using only one agent at a time. From intervention studies we would like to answer the following questions: (a) How much vitamin is needed for protection? (b) Do we need one or more vitamins for a maximal protection? (c) Is one type of vitamin more effective than another against certain tumors? (d) Are vitamins by themselves sufficient or do they need the presence of other dietary factors for a maximal protection, and what are the long-term effects of these vitamins and nutrients? It is very encouraging to note that the National Cancer Institute (Division of Chemoprevention Program) is initiating several intervention trials among the high risk population using the individual nutrients. I believe that, during the next 10 years, we will be able to answer some of the above questions in a definitive manner.

This volume deals with basic mechanisms of carcinogenesis as well as those factors which modify the biochemical steps involved in the processes of cancer formation. The two-step theory of carcinogenesis involving initiation and promotion has helped a great deal in identifying carcinogenic and anticarcinogenic substances. However, the crucial biochemical events associated with the promotion stage of carcinogenesis remains to be elucidated. The knowledge of these events is important for developing a biochemical strategy for the prevention of tumor.

In addition to having a preventive role, vitamins (primarily A, C and E) and certain nutrients may markedly improve the current management of tumor by several mechanisms. Vitamins alone may induce differentiation associated with or without growth inhibition. The extent and the type of effect depend upon the form of vitamin and the type of tumor. Vitamins may enhance the growth inhibitory effect of tumor therapeutic agents (chemical, radiation, and hyperthermia). The extent of enhancement depends upon the form of vitamin, the type of tumor and the form of tumor therapeutic agent. Vitamins may reduce some of the side toxic effects of certain chemotherapeutic agents, and they may also increase the humoral and cellular immunity. This monograph describes these functions of vitamins in the treatment of tumor. In addition, it contains recent clinical data on the role of retinoids and vitamin E in the treatment of human tumor.

This book will be valuable to cell biologists, epidemiologists, nutritionists, oncologists (basic and clinical), and pharmacologists.

Kedar N. Prasad, PhD

Acknowledgement

This monograph is based on papers presented at the International Symposium on Vitamins, Nutrition, and Cancer, held in Denver, Colorado, June 20–22, 1983. The financial support of the symposium by the following institutions and companies is highly appreciated: Cancer Research Institute, Hoffmann-La Roche, Henkel Corporation, American Cancer Society (Colorado Division), and Campbell Soup Company.

Vitamin A

Prasad (ed.), Vitamins, Nutrition, and Cancer, pp. 1–19 (Karger, Basel 1984)

Vitamin A and Beta-Carotene as Adjunctive Therapy to Tumor Excision, Radiation Therapy, and Chemotherapy

Eli Seifter[a,b]*, Giuseppe Rettura*[a]*, Jacques Padawer*[c]*,*
Stanley M. Levenson[a]

[a] Department of Surgery, [b] Department of Biochemistry, [c] Department of Anatomy,
Albert Einstein College of Medicine, Yeshiva University, Bronx, N.Y., USA

Introduction

Previous work from our laboratory [1–3] showed that supplemental vitamin A fed to C3H or CBA mice inoculated with 1×10^4 C3HBA (breast adenocarcinoma) tumor cells protected them in the following ways: it reduced tumor incidence, in both males and females, from 50 to 10%. For those vitamin A-supplemented animals exhibiting tumor development, the latent period for tumor development was prolonged considerably, tumor growth was slowed, and metastasis (as determined by gross examination at autopsy) occurred more rarely. As a result, tumor-bearing mice receiving supplemental vitamin A survived more than twice as long as those not receiving the supplement. All mice, including those fed supplemental vitamin A, developed tumors after they were inoculated with 1×10^5 C3HBA cells; however, supplementation with vitamin A increased the latent period, slowed tumor growth and increased survival time. Vitamin A supplementation also slowed both time of tumor appearance and growth and increased survival time in mice inoculated with 1×10^6 C3HBA tumor cells [4].

In each of the above cases supplemental vitamin A inhibited the growth of a tumor transplant. The purpose of the studies reported in this paper was to determine how supplemental vitamin A affects the *regrowth* of C3HBA tumor after the transplanted tumor was reduced by *local tumor excision, irradiation,* or *systemic tumor chemotherapy.* We hypothesized that if these treatments reduced tumor cell numbers sufficiently, e.g., to a level of 1×10^4 or fewer, supplemental vitamin A would inhibit tumor *recurrence* and tumor growth in those mice with recurrent tumors. Another purpose was to compare the actions of supplemental vitamin A with those of β-carotene in some *combination therapies.*

Materials and Methods

6 experiments were carried out to study the effect of supplemental vitamin A on tumor regrowth following tumor excision (experiments 1 and 2), radiation (experiments 3 and 4), or chemotherapy (experiments 5 and 6).

Mice
All mice used were obtained from the Jackson Laboratory, Bar Harbor, Me. 5-week-old female C3H mice were used in experiments 1 and 2; 5-week-old male CBA mice were used in the other studies. C3HBA tumor growth in CBA mice is similar to growth in C3H mice [2].

Housing, Husbandry
On arrival in our laboratory, mice were distributed randomly into plastic shoe box-type cages, $11 \times 6.5 \times 5$ in, 5 per cage (6 in experiments 3 and 4) and were fed ad libitum a commercial powdered laboratory chow, hereafter called the basal or control chow. Before being used in any experiment, the mice were kept in these groups for a minimum of 1 week and maintained in a windowless room with a 12-hour light, 12-hour dark cycle (0700–1900 light). Temperature was maintained at 20 °C during the dark cycle and 25 °C during the light cycle. Relative humidity was approximately 37 % at all times.

Diets
The basal or control diet used in experiments 1 and 2 was a powdered laboratory rodent chow (Teklad, Monmouth, Ill.). It contains 6,190 IU vitamin A palmitate/kg diet in addition to 4.3 mg carotene (equivalent to 7,167 IU vitamin A). The total vitamin A equivalent of this diet is 13,357 IU/kg diet. This diet supports normal growth, reproduction, lactation, and longevity of normal mice and is well above the NRC recommended daily requirement for normal rodents, which averages 6,000 IU/kg diet for growth, pregnancy, and lactation. In the succeeding experiments, ground Purina Laboratory Chow (No. 5001, Ralston Purina Co., St. Louis, Mo.) was used as the basal or control chow. It contains 15,000 IU vitamin A and 6.4 mg β-carotene/kg diet (total = 18,000 IU vitamin A/kg diet), about 35 % more than the amount present in the basal diets for experiments 1 and 2, and 3 times as much as the NRC recommended dietary allowances (RDA). Therefore, the experimental results are not attributable to supplementation of a vitamin A-inadequate diet. Supplemented diets were made by the addition of ethanolic solutions of vitamin A palmi-

tate (1,000 IU/mg; ICN Pharmaceuticals, Inc., Cleveland, Ohio) or β-carotene (Eastman Kodak, Rochester, N.Y.). Diets were supplemented with either 150,000 IU vitamin A or 90 mg of β-carotene/kg. All mice had food and tap water ad libitum.

Tumors, Inoculation, Measurements

Adenocarcinoma C3HBA [4] was obtained from The Jackson Laboratory as a transplant in young C3H/HeJ mice. For use in experiments 1 and 2, the tumors were passed into C3H mice. For inocula used in the other experiments, tumor cells were passed into CBA mice. Preparation of inocula have been described previously [1]. In experiments 4 and 5, the inoculum consisted of 7.5×10^5 cells injected subcutaneously in an area of the nipple line, approximately 1.3 cm above the right inguinal lymph node. In the other experiments, CBA mice were inoculated with 2×10^5 tumor cells subcutaneously in the outer aspect of the right thigh.

Tumor size was recorded as the mean of the major and minor diameters of the tumors. Measurements were made to the nearest millimeter. Recorded values are the means of measurements and are derived values taken to tenths of millimeters.

Tumor Excision

In experiments 1 and 2, tumor excision was carried out under light pentobarbital anesthesia. The operation consisted of removing all macroscopically visible tumor nodule(s) without an attempt to excise healthy surrounding tissue. In cases where the tumor was fixed to the abdominal muscles, the tumor excision included a limited en bloc resection of the immediate underlying muscle wall. Half the chow-fed and half the vitamin A-supplemented mice were anesthetized but not operated.

Tumor X-Irradiation

In experiments 3 and 4, mice were anesthetized lightly with sodium pentobarbital (1 mg/20 g body weight, i.p.) and were then irradiated with a Picker-Vanguard 280 kVp X-ray therapy unit, half value layer (HVL) = 0.5 mm copper. The unit was calibrated to deliver 450 R/min and was timed to deliver a single dose of 30 Gy (3,000 rad) to the hind leg bearing the tumor. The rest of the body, including the other hind limb, was covered by a 2-mm thick lead shield.

Cyclophosphamide Chemotherapy

Cyclophosphamide chemotherapy was used in experiments 5 and 6. In experiment 5, cyclophosphamide (Mead Johnson Laboratories, Evansville, Ind.) was administered intraperitoneally at a dosage of 24 mg/kg body weight starting 2 weeks after tumor inoculation, when tumors averaged 6.2 ± 0.3 mm in diameter. There were 7 injections, 1 given every other day. In experiment 6, cyclophosphamide treatment was begun when the tumors averaged 5.3 ± 0.5 mm. At that time, cyclophosphamide (36 mg/kg body weight) was administered. 6 days later, a similar dose was given. After a 2-week interval, a single dose of 24 mg/kg was injected. Although the purpose of the study was to gauge the action of cyclophosphamide at a higher dose than was employed in experiment 5, serious toxicity was evident after the first treatment, and the treatment regimen was therefore modified. In fact, the cumulative amount of cyclophosphamide administered in experiment 6 was less than in experiment 5.

Experimental Design

Experiments 1 and 2

Experiment 1 was started in December 1977, and experiment 2 in March 1978. For each experiment, 8 groups of 10 mice each were inoculated with aliquots of 7.5×10^5 C3HBA cells from a single inoculation pool. 2 groups served as unoperated controls and 1 of them was started on the supplemental vitamin A feeding immediately after inoculation. Mice of 2 other groups underwent local tumor excision on either day 9, 13, or 16 after inoculation. At these times, tumor scores were 4.6, 7.2, and 9.4 mm, respectively, and the average weights of the excised tumors were 7.7, 64.3, and 187 mg, respectively. Immediately after excision, 1 subgroup was started on the vitamin A-supplemented diet while the other subgroup served as chow-fed control. Experiment 2 was a repeat of experiment 1, using the same experimental design and numbers of animals, but it was carried out on a different shipment of mice and begun after experiment 1 was completed.

Experiments 3 and 4

2 similarly designed experiments, separated by a 9-week interval, were carried out; the first (experiment 3) was started in November 1980, the second in January 1981. 13 days after they were inoculated, when tumors had a mean diameter of 6.2 mm in experiment 3 and 5.3 mm in experiment 4, mice in each experiment were distributed randomly into 3 groups of 10 each and housed 5/cage. These 3 groups were not irradiated. Group 1 was continued on the control chow, while groups 2 and 3 were started on chows supplemented with vitamin A or β-carotene, respectively. 36 additional tumor-bearing mice were subjected to local tumor irradiation as described. Following this, they were divided randomly into 3 groups of 12 mice each, housed 6/cage. Group 4 was continued on the control chow for the postradiation period. Mice of groups 5 and 6 were given the vitamin A- or β-carotene-supplemented chow, respectively, starting immediately after irradiation.

1 year after radiation in experiment 3, the diet of some of the surviving mice was altered. 5 of the 11 mice from group 5 were continued on that same vitamin A-supplemented diet, whereas 6 mice were switched back to the unsupplemented control chow. Similarly, 5 mice from group 6 were continued on their β-carotene-supplemented diet, and the remaining 5 animals were switched back to the unsupplemented control ration. In the

fourth experiment, similar dietary changes were made 13.5 months after irradiation and the start of the supplemented diets. In both experiments, survival studies were continued for 24 months from the day of radiation therapy, at which time survivors were killed and autopsied.

Experiments 5 and 6

2 experiments using cyclophosphamide were carried out in parallel with experiments 3 and 4. There were 6 groups (10 mice each) in experiment 3, and 6 groups in experiment 4. All of the mice were inoculated as previously described. In experiment 5, chemotherapy and dietary supplementation were started when tumors had mean diameters of 6.2 ± 0.3 mm. In experiment 4, treatments were begun when tumor diameters averaged 5.3 ± 0.2 mm.

Statistical Analyses

Tumor size and latent period for tumor reappearance were analyzed by Student's t test, and survival time by Anova. Where warranted by the F ratio, the data were further examined by the Newman-Keuls test to establish allowable comparisons and their p values. Tumor incidence (frequency of tumor recurrence) was evaluated by a χ^2 method.

Results

Surgical Excision (Experiments 1 and 2)

Among unoperated mice in experiment 1 (table I), those given supplemental vitamin A starting on the day of inoculation developed smaller tumors (0.5 ± 0.2 vs 3.7 ± 0.3 mm, $p < 0.001$, at day 6 postinoculation; 3.0 ± 0.7 vs 6.8 ± 0.6 mm at day 13, $p < 0.005$) and survived longer (72.1 ± 13.3 vs 32.3 ± 1.7 days, $p < 0.001$). Among mice not receiving supplemental vitamin A, those whose tumors were excised survived significantly longer than unoperated groups (43.9 ± 3.8 days for mice operated on day 9 postinoculation, $p < 0.01$; 45.6 ± 4.6 days for mice operated on day 13, $p < 0.01$; 48.7 ± 3.9 days for mice operated on day 16, $p < 0.001$). These data must be compared with a survival time of 32.3 ± 1.7 days for unoperated mice (tables I, III).

Mice subjected to both local tumor excision plus supplemental vitamin A (starting right after excision) survived significantly longer than those only subjected to tumor excision (63.2 ± 5.6 vs 43.9 ± 3.8 days for mice oper-

Table I. Effects of supplemental vitamin A on tumor growth and survival time in mice inoculated with C3HBA cells[1]

Treatment	Experiment No.	Number of mice	Latency period days	Tumor size (mm) at different days postinoculum				Survival time days
				6	9	13	16	
Control	1	10	3.4 ± 0.2[2]	3.7 ± 0.3	4.4 ± 0.2	6.8 ± 0.6	7.7 ± 0.8	32.3 ± 1.7
Vitamin A		10	7.8 ± 0.7	0.5 ± 0.2	1.6 ± 0.5	3.0 ± 1.3	4.5 ± 1.3	72.1 ± 13.3
p value[3]			<0.001	<0.001	<0.001	<0.005	<0.05	<0.001
Control	2	10	4.5 ± 0.8	3.6 ± 0.5	4.6 ± 0.7	7.3 ± 0.8	9.8 ± 1.5	38.9 ± 2.9
Vitamin A		10	10.6 ± 1.9	1.1 ± 0.3	2.2 ± 0.7	3.9 ± 1.1	5.6 ± 1.0	63.7 ± 6.7
p value			<0.01	<0.003	<0.05	<0.05	<0.5	<0.005

[1] These are the unoperated tumor-bearing mice.
[2] Mean ± standard error of the mean.
[3] Analyzed by Student's t test for small unpaired samples.

Table II. Effect of supplemental vitamin A on tumor regrowth following limited local tumor excision

	Days between inoculation[1] and excision					
	9		13		16	
Days post excision:	10	12	8	12	8	15
Experiment 1						
Control	6.8 ± 0.6[2]	9.8 ± 1.1	10.1 ± 1.1	13.1 ± 1.8	9.2 ± 1.9	11.9 ± 1.6
Vitamin A	4.9 ± 0.5	6.7 ± 1.0	5.5 ± 1.2	8.3 ± 1.1	7.8 ± 1.2	10.7 ± 1.7
p value[3]	<0.01	<0.05	<0.02	<0.05	NS	NS
Experiment 2						
Control	7.6 ± 1.0	9.2 ± 1.1	8.2 ± 1.5	12.6 ± 0.9	7.0 ± 0.6	13.3 ± 2.7
Vitamin A	4.0 ± 1.1	5.6 ± 1.1	3.0 ± 0.3	8.8 ± 0.9	3.8 ± 0.9	13.0 ± 1.8
p value	<0.02	<0.05	<0.01	<0.01	<0.01	NS

[1] C3HBA cells.
[2] Tumor size (mm): mean ± standard error of the mean. NS = Not statistically significant ($p > 0.05$).
[3] Analyzed by Student's t test for small unpaired samples.

ated on day 9 postinoculation, p <0.001; 59.8 ± 2.2 vs 45.6 ± 4.6 days for mice operated on day 13, p <0.02; 75.4 ± 3.4 vs 48.7 ± 3.9 days for mice operated on day 16, p <0.05). These data are summarized in table III.

The data obtained in experiment 2 are similar to those obtained in experiment 1. For those mice not undergoing excision, supplemental vitamin A increased the latency period (10.6 ± 1.9 vs 4.5 ± 0.8 days, p <0.01) and the vitamin A-supplemented mice had smaller tumors at days 6, 9, 13, and 16, p <0.003, <0.05, <0.05, and <0.05, respectively. Supplemental vitamin A also increased survival time (63.7 ± 6.7 vs 38.9 ± 2.9 days, p <0.005). The data are summarized in table I.

Tumor excision at day 9 prolonged survival of mice not receiving supplemental vitamin A (52.8 ± 7.2 vs 38.9± 2.9 days, p <0.08; table II, III), as was also found in experiment 1. Similarly, the latency period for tumor regrowth was found not to be related to the time of tumor excision. As in experiment 1, supplemental vitamin A increased the latency period for tumor regrowth following excision, especially for mice undergoing excision before day 16. Supplemental vitamin A also inhibited regrowth of tumors.

Table III. Effects of supplemental vitamin A on latency period and survival of mice subjected to local tumor excision (in days)

| | Days between inoculation[1] and excision | | | | | |
| | 9 | | 13 | | 16 | |
	latency period	survival time	latency period	survival time	latency period	survival time
Experiment 1						
Control	6.8±0.8[2]	43.9±3.8	7.6±0.8	45.6±4.6	7.7±0.7	48.7±3.9
Vitamin A	12.8±1.3	63.2±5.6	8.6±0.7	59.8±2.2	8.0±0.8	75.4±3.4
p value[3]	<0.02	<0.01	NS	<0.02	NS	<0.05
Experiment 2						
Control	7.0±0.7	52.8±7.2	8.9±0.5	50.3±6.9	9.6±1.2	54.5±3.7
Vitamin A	11.0±1.7	76.4±3.3	13.8±2.4	78.8±6.6	11.0±1.2	67.8±4.5
p value	<0.05	<0.01	<0.05	<0.01	NS	<0.05

[1] C3HBA cells.
[2] Mean ± standard error of the mean. NS = Not statistically significant (p >0.05).
[3] Analyzed by Student's t test for small unpaired samples.

Table IV. Experiment 3. Influence of supplemental vitamin A, β-carotene, and local X-irradiation on C3HBA tumor size (mm)

Treatment	Days post-treatment					
	0	4	8	11	14	18
None	6.2±0.3	10.1±0.8	14.4±0.8	16.8±0.9	18.0±0.8	20.4±0.9
X-ray	6.2±0.3	5.5±0.3[1]	5.2±0.2[1]	4.8±0.2[1]	4.0±0.1[1]	4.0±0.1[1]
Vitamin A	6.2±0.2	9.4±0.6	10.1±0.3	11.4±0.8[1]	13.7±0.8[1]	15.8±0.5[1]
X-ray + vitamin A	6.2±0.3	4.3±0.2[1]	2.6±0.1[1,2]	0.5±0.1[1]	0.2±0.1[1,2]	0.0
β-Carotene	6.2±0.2	9.5±0.5	7.8±0.3	8.5±0.4[1]	10.0±0.8[1]	12.7±0.4[1]
X-ray + β-carotene	6.2±0.3	4.3±0.2[1]	2.4±0.2[1,2]	0.9±0.1[1]	0.2±0.1[1,2]	0.0

[1] $p < 0.001$, compared to untreated group.
[2] $p < 0.001$ compared to X-ray group.

For animals whose tumors were excised on day 9, tumor scores were 4.0 ± 1.1 vs 7.6 ± 1.0 mm, $p < 0.02$ on day 19 and 5.6 ± 1.1 vs 9.2 ± 1.1 mm, $p < 0.05$, on day 21. For animals operated on day 13, the scores were 3.0 ± 0.3 vs 8.2 ± 1.5 mm, $p < 0.01$, on day 21 and 8.8 ± 0.9 vs 12.6 ± 0.9 mm, $p < 0.01$, on day 25. Lastly, for those operated on day 16, the tumor scores were 3.8 ± 0.9 vs 7.0 ± 0.6 mm on day 24, $p < 0.01$ (table II). Supplemental vitamin A also prolonged the survival of mice: 76.4 ± 3.3 vs 52.8 ± 7.2 days, $p < 0.01$, for those operated on day 9, 78.8 ± 6.6 vs 50.3 ± 6.9 days, $p < 0.01$, for those operated on day 13, and 67.8 ± 4.5 vs 54.5 ± 3.7 days, $p < 0.05$, for those operated on day 16 (table III).

Local Tumor Irradiation (Experiments 3 and 4)
The following data pertain to the first year of the experiments.

Effects of Local Tumor Irradiation, Supplemental Vitamin A, or Supplemental β-Carotene, Each Used Singly. As shown in table IV, supplemental vitamin A or β-carotene each slowed tumor growth, and there were no significant differences between the effects of vitamin A or β-carotene. On the other hand, local radiation, of itself, caused tumor regression. In experiment 3, local irradiation caused partial tumor regression in all mice, but tumor growth resumed after a few weeks. Similarly, in experiment 4, local

Table V. Experiment 4. Influence of supplemental vitamin A or β-carotene, and local X-irradiation on C3HBA tumor size (mm)

Treatment	Days post-treatment						
	0	3	5	7	10	14	18
None	5.6±0.2	7.4±0.4	8.9±0.4	10.0±0.6	11.7±0.8	12.8±0.7	16.4±0.6
X-ray	5.6±0.2	5.3±0.2[1]	4.9±0.1[1]	4.0±0.2[1]	3.3±0.1[1]	3.1±0.1[1]	3.2±0.1[1]
Vitamin A	5.6±0.2	6.4±0.2	7.5±0.4	8.9±0.4[2]	9.2±0.4[1]	10.0±0.4[1]	13.1±0.7[1]
X-ray + vitamin A	5.6±0.1	4.5±0.1[1]	2.4±0.1[1,3]	1.5±0.1[1,3]	0.3±0.1[1,3]	0.0	0.0
β-Carotene	5.6±0.2	6.7±0.3	7.5±0.3	8.3±0.3[2]	9.1±0.3[1]	10.0±0.3[1]	12.9±0.6[1]
X-ray + β-carotene	5.6±0.1	4.3±0.3[1]	2.6±0.1[1,3]	1.7±0.1[1,3]	0.5±0.1[1,3]	0.0	0.0

[1] $p < 0.001$, compared to untreated group.
[2] $p < 0.02$, compared to untreated group.
[3] $p < 0.001$, compared to X-ray group.

radiation caused partial regression in 11 or 12 mice and temporary 'complete' regression in one (table V). Mice receiving neither dietary supplementation nor radiation survived an average of 41.2 days (in all cases, the word 'day' refers to days after inoculation) in experiment 3 and 43.3 days in experiment 4. Supplemental vitamin A or β-carotene increased survival time to an average of 60.2 and 61.2 days, respectively, in experiment 3, and of 64.2 and 63.3 days, respectively, in experiment 4 (p < 0.001 in each case). Local radiation increased survival time even longer, to 84.4 days (p < 0.001) in experiment 3 and 99.1 days (p < 0.001) in experiment 4 (table VI).

Effects of Local Tumor Irradiation Together with Supplemental Vitamin A or β-Carotene. The results from experiments 3 and 4 were similar, and therefore combined results are described. All mice receiving both radiation and supplemental vitamin A (24/24) showed complete tumor regression. However, in 2 cases (1 in each experiment), the regression was temporary; a tumor reappeared although only after several months, followed by death several months after tumor regrowth. The remaining animals (22/24) survived without palpable tumor during the *first year*. Irradiated mice receiving supplemental β-carotene responded in a similar way (table V). In experiment 3, there were 2 deaths in β-carotene-supplemented mice during

Table VI. Effect of supplemental vitamin A, β-carotene, or 30 Gy local X-irradiation on survival of CBA/J mice with C3HBA tumors

	Group					
	1	2	3	4	5	6
Supplement	0	Vit A[1]	β-car	0	Vit A	β-car
X-ray	0	0	0	+	+	+
Number of mice with complete tumor regression						
Experiment 3	0	0	0	0	12	12
Experiment 4	0	0	0	0	12	12
Number of mice surviving 1 year or longer						
Experiment 3	0	0	0	0	11	11
Experiment 4	0	0	0	0	11	11
Survival time of nonsurvivors						
Experiment 3	41.2 ± 2.5[2]	60.2 ± 3.0	61.2 ± 2.1	84.4 ± 5.4	142	136
Experiment 4	43.3 ± 0.8	63.3 ± 1.8	64.2 ± 1.9	99.1 ± 5.9	182	199

p values[3], Gp:	1 vs 2	1 vs 3	1 vs 4	2 vs 3	2 vs 4
Experiment 3	<0.001	<0.001	<0.001	NS[4]	<0.001
Experiment 4	<0.001	<0.001	<0.001	NS	<0.001

[1] Vit A = vitamin A; β-car = β-carotene.
[2] Mean ± standard error of mean, in days.
[3] By analysis of variance and Neuman-Keuls test.
[4] Not statistically significant.

the first year. In 1 of these mice, tumor recurred 45 days after initial regression and death followed 75 days later. The other death was accidental and not tumor-related. For the surviving mice, the following findings pertain to the second year.

Mice Treated by Local Tumor Irradiation and Then Supplemented with Vitamin A or β-Carotene: Effects of Continuing or Withdrawing Supplementation on Tumor Recurrence. Because results obtained in experiments 3 and 4 were similar, the data from both have been combined in table VII.

Table VII. Influence of continuing or discontinuing supplements on tumor regrowth[1]

	Vitamin A		β-Carotene	
	maintained on supplement	supplement discontinued	maintained on supplement	supplement discontinued
Number of mice/group	10	12	11	10
Number of mice with tumor recurrence	0	8[2]	0	2
Number of deaths with tumor	0	8	0	2
Number of deaths without tumor	8	3	4	6
Survival time (days) for tumor-bearing mice	–	514 ± 2	–	654 ± 21
Survival time (days) for nontumor-bearing mice	642 ± 13	546 ± 10	682 ± 4	618 ± 12

[1] Table includes data combined from experiments 3 and 4 which pertain to events occurring during the second year of experiments.
[2] $p < 0.001$ (χ^2) for comparing the effect of continuing or discontinuing supplemental vitamin A on subsequent tumor recurrence.

Vitamin A Supplementation

In experiment 3, of the 5 mice that continued to receive vitamin A, none redeveloped tumors. 4 of these died after surviving a normal life span. Of the 6 mice switched to unsupplemented chow, 5 redeveloped tumors and died of tumor disease. The remaining mouse died 140 days before death occurred in nontumor-bearing mice receiving vitamin A.

In experiment 4, of the 5 mice continued on supplemental vitamin A, none redeveloped tumors. 4 of these mice died after surviving a normal life span [7]; the remaining mouse was killed at the termination of the experiment (730 days after inoculation). Of the 6 mice switched from supplemental vitamin A to unsupplemented control chow, 3 redeveloped tumors and died of tumor disease. 2 or the mice not showing tumor development died prematurely (548 days), 1 survived a normal life span of approximately 600 days [5], and 1 was killed at the termination of the experiment.

β-Carotene Supplementation

In experiment 3, of the 5 mice continued on supplemental β-carotene, none redeveloped tumors. However, 3 mice died of nontumor causes after having survived for a normal life span, while the other 2 mice survived the

Table VIII. Experiment 5. Effects of supplemental vitamin A, supplemental β-carotene, and/or cyclophosphamide on tumor growth and survival time of mice bearing C3HBA tumors

Day post-treatment	Tumor size[1]				Survival time days
	0	8	12	20	
Control	6.2±0.2	13.1±0.4	15.9±0.6	20.2±0.7	40±3
Vitamin A	6.2±0.3	9.0±0.3[2]	10.4±0.5[2]	14.8±0.3[2]	58±3[2]
β-Carotene	6.3±0.2	9.6±0.4[2]	10.5±0.4[2]	14.0±0.5[2]	59±3[2]
CY[3]	6.2±0.2	10.5±0.4[2]	12.3±0.4[2]	14.7±0.5[2]	61±2[2]
CY + vitamin A	6.2±0.2	8.2±0.3[2,4]	9.4±0.3[2,4]	12.1±0.4[2,4]	82±6[2,4]
CY + β-carotene	6.3±0.2	7.9±0.4[2,4]	8.8±0.3[2,4]	11.0±0.3[2,4]	89±5[2,4]

[1] Mean ± SEM, in millimeters.
[2] $p < 0.001$ compared to control group.
[3] Cyclophosphamide.
[4] $p < 0.001$ compared to cyclophosphamide group.

second year and were killed 730 days after inoculation. Of the 5 mice switched back to the control chow, 2 redeveloped tumors 133 and 275 days, respectively, after the β-carotene supplementation was discontinued, and they died about 52 days later. 3 mice died without gross evidence of tumor, having survived for a normal life span.

In experiment 4, of the 6 mice continued on their β-carotene supplements, none redeveloped tumors; however, 1 died of nontumor causes 195 days after the dietary change while 5 mice survived to the end of the experiment. Of the 5 β-carotene-supplemented mice switched back to the control chow, none redeveloped tumors. 3 of these mice died, having survived for a normal life span, while the other 2 survived to the end of the experiment.

Cyclophosphamide Chemotherapy (Experiments 5 and 6)

In experiment 5 (table VIII) each of the individual treatments (cyclophosphamide, supplemental vitamin A, supplemental β-carotene) slowed tumor growth and increased survival times. Combined treatments were additive with regard to tumor growth and survival times; however, neither single nor combined therapies caused tumor regression. In experiment 6 (table IX) the individual treatments had the following effects: supplemental

Table IX. Experiment 6. Effects of supplemental vitamin A, supplemental β-carotene, and/or cyclophosphamide on tumor growth and survival time of mice bearing C3HBA tumors

Day post-treatment	Tumor size[1]				Survival time days
	0	8	12	20	
Control	5.4 ± 0.2	10.2 ± 0.4	12.7 ± 0.4	18.4 ± 0.3	42 ± 2
Vitamin A	5.4 ± 0.2	7.8 ± 0.4^2	9.2 ± 0.3^2	14.1 ± 0.3^2	65 ± 2^2
β-Carotene	5.4 ± 0.3	8.0 ± 0.3^2	9.8 ± 0.4^2	14.6 ± 0.4^2	63 ± 3^2
CY[3]	5.3 ± 0.2	4.6 ± 0.2^2	5.0 ± 0.2^2	6.5 ± 0.2^2	65 ± 3^2
CY + vitamin A	5.4 ± 0.3	$2.6 \pm 0.2^{2,4}$	$1.7 \pm 0.1^{2,4}$	$2.7 \pm 0.3^{2,4}$	$85 \pm 5^{2,4}$
CY + β-carotene	5.4 ± 0.2	$2.5 \pm 0.2^{2,4}$	$1.9 \pm 0.1^{2,4}$	$2.7 \pm 0.2^{2,4}$	$83 \pm 2^{2,4}$

[1] Mean ± SEM, in millimeters.
[2] $p < 0.001$ compared to control group.
[3] Cyclophosphamide.
[4] $p < 0.001$ compared to cyclophosphamide group.

vitamin A or β-carotene each slowed tumor growth and increased survival times. Cyclophosphamide (36 mg/kg) produced slight and significant tumor regression, but some mice in this treatment group died of drug toxicity. The combined therapies (cyclophosphamide + vitamin A, cyclophosphamide + β-carotene) produced quantitatively greater tumor regression than did the cyclophosphamide alone. Additionally, mice receiving the combined therapy did not evidence overt cyclophosphamide toxicity and they all survived longer than animals receiving only one of the therapeutic agents.

Discussion

Excisional Tumor Surgery (Experiments 1 and 2)

From the quantitative and perhaps qualitative standpoints, excisional surgery is one of the most important procedures performed on tumor patients. The surgery may be performed for diagnostic and therapeutic reasons, including operations for curative or palliative purposes. Excisional tumor debulking in conjunction with other forms of therapy, e.g. chemotherapy and radiation, may improve the efficacy of the nonsurgical therapy. In addition, surgery may be employed to obtain tumor to be used for preparation of autochthonous vaccines or other immune procedures, such as the isolation of cytotoxic or blocking antibodies that may be converted to cytotoxic agents.

Positive Effects of Surgical Excision. Surgical excision of tumors has both *positive* and *negative* effects on tumor regrowth and the morbidity and survival of the affected individual. The positive features predominate when surgical excision of some tumors is curative, i.e. the tumor is still 'local', the tumor cell population is reduced below some critical value (perhaps 10^8 cell/human or 10^{4-5} cells/mouse), and host defenses are able to prevent regrowth of the tumor. However, for some tumor types even 10^8 tumor cells are more than the patient can contain, and there are strong variations in the ability of different individuals to prevent tumor growth after challenges with 'identical' tumor loads. Also, the tumor is frequently no longer only local at the time of operation. Thus, for a large number of tumor-bearing individuals, excisional surgery is not curative, though it may produce useful responses, such as improved general feeling, weight gain, increased immune competence, increased physical activity, and prolongation of life. In this regard, much of the positive response to surgery is due to removal of some of the negative catabolic effects of the tumor.

Negative Aspects of Surgical Excision. In addition to the positive anti-tumor effects of tumor excision described above, there are negative aspects to such surgery. *Oberling* [20] pointed out that the removal of a malignant neoplasm may be followed after a brief interval by the sudden and fatal eruption of metastases. *Roberto* et al. [6] were concerned with the role that operative techniques play on enhancing metastatic tumor development by increasing the numbers of blood-borne tumor cells and thin seeding in lymph nodes. *Buinauskas* et al. [7] demonstrated that laparotomy of experimental animals increased tumor incidence and the numbers of 'takes/animal' following inoculation with cells of various tumor lines. They thought that this was due to an impairment of the host's ability to destroy circulating cancer cells because of 'operative stress'. In our experiments, we saw to a modest extent the negative effects of minor sham operation: increased tumor growth, depressed weight and lymphocyte content of the thymus glands in agreement with the work of others who have observed comparable effects of anesthesia on circulating lymphocytes.

Scovill and Saba [8] have reviewed the problem of operative stress and host defense. They demonstrated, as have others, a pronounced depression of phagocytic activity during and after major abdominal surgery, as judged, for example, by the clearance of bacteria. The depressed activity was thought by them to be related to either loss or inactivation of humoral recognition factors, and they suggested a role for the pituitary-adrenal axis in the response.

The impaired phagocytic activity reported above is closely related to the findings of *Donovan* [9] and *Fisher and Fisher* [10] who have considered the special problem of depression of reticuloendothelial activity due to surgery for cancer and the implications this has for development of metastases and/or infection. Interference with neutrophil and macrophage function are also associated with injury. These factors, along with the consideration that many tumors are no longer localized at the time of operation, have led to use of chemotherapeutic and/or radiation treatment in combination with surgery.

Limited Excision of Tumors. The technique for excision of tumors practiced in the experiments reported in this paper was of a limited nature, and not in any sense a cancer therapeutic operation. Under this circumstance, the initial experiments demonstrated clearly the antitumor efficacy (decreased tumor growth, increased survival times) of supplemental vitamin A in both operated and unoperated mice. The data do not allow for a comparison of the effectiveness of supplemental vitamin A in combination with excision with that of supplemental vitamin A alone, because in the latter instance supplemental vitamin A was started sooner after tumor inoculation than in the latter cases. The combination of limited local excision and supplemental vitamin A did not produce sustained tumor regression.

Radiation (Experiments 3 and 4)
The present studies confirm earlier reports of the additive antitumor therapeutic actions of radiation and supplemental dietary vitamin A in mice with C3HBA tumors [11–13] and, in contrast to the previously cited works, show that this added therapeutic effect can be accomplished in a remarkable way without inducing toxicity even when the supplemental vitamin A is fed for a very extended period of time. Moreover, under these conditions, protection against tumor regrowth persists for several months after dietary supplementation is discontinued. We think that incorporating supplemental vitamin A into the diet (analogous in humans to giving a vitamin A supplement at mealtime) is more efficacious and less toxic than is intraperitoneal injection, the route most frequently employed by others.

Additionally, the present studies demonstrate that supplemental dietary β-carotene, a vitamin A precursor, contributes additively to the antitumor action of X-irradiation in a manner similar to that of vitamin A, but exerts an even more pronounced dramatic protective action against tumor regrowth even after feeding of the β-carotene is discontinued. This finding may be of major importance in the prevention and treatment of tumors in humans.

Radiation Dosage

Previously, we confirmed [14] the finding of *Fisher* et al. [15] that 30 Gy causes partial regression of C3HBA tumors. We employed 30 Gy in the present study to determine if supplemental vitamin A or β-carotene would further enhance radiation-induced tumor regression. In these experiments we have not used β-carotene or vitamin A supplements as primary agents to obtain tumor regression; rather, we have used these compounds to: (a) slow C3HBA tumor growth; (b) ameliorate X-radiation toxicity [16], and (c) prevent the thymic involution, adrenal enlargement, and weight loss caused by C3HBA tumor growth. We are aware that single-dose local radiation is not used clinically for tumor therapy; however, we have employed it in these experiments to test our hypothesis that supplemental vitamin A or β-carotene would each enhance the therapeutic effectiveness of radiotherapy. The results of our experiments show this to be the case.

Cyclophosphamide Therapy (Experiments 5 and 6)

The present studies confirm earlier reports of the additive antitumor effects of supplemental vitamin A and cyclophosphamide [14]; in the present studies, however, the additive antitumor effects are accompanied by decreased toxicity, as compared to the increase in toxicity observed previously by other workers. We believe that this discrepancy is due to the different amounts and routes of administration of vitamin A employed in our studies.

Although the cyclophosphamide experiments reported in the present work are less dramatic than the radiation experiments, they may have even greater implications for tumor therapy. We believe it probable that combination of high level cyclophosphamide administration (in experiment 6) would have caused complete tumor regression without deaths in animals receiving either vitamin A or β-carotene. Theoretical treatment of these interactions between vitamin A and toxic tumor therapies leading to sustained tumor regression is discussed elsewhere [17].

Conclusions

General Role for Vitamin A and β-Carotene in Tumor Therapy
The finding that supplemental vitamin A or β-carotene reduce the toxicity (in both healthy and tumor-bearing rodents) of excision, radiation, or chemotherapy, is an important contribution to tumor therapy. It makes possible more extensive and intensive therapy without an increase in morbidity or mortality; in fact, because the therapy also decreases tumor-induced stress, vitamin A and β-carotene increase the efficacy of the therapy. These findings support the concept that vitamin A and one of its biologic precursors, β-carotene, will have a general role in tumor therapy.

In addition to inhibiting tumor growth moderately and ameliorating radiation toxicity, cyclophosphamide toxicity, and important adverse effects of surgical trauma, supplemental vitamin A or β-carotene have an additional and important action in tumor-bearing animals. Like many other tumors, C3HBA induces some responses in the host that mitigate against survival and enhance further tumor growth. The progressive and often accelerating course of many malignant tumors is associated with immune depression and alterations in metabolism of nontumor host tissues. Because of these events, the host's ability to contain or limit the growth of even a small tumor burden is diminished, and tumor growth progresses. Catabolic responses occur which are similar to those described by *Selye* [18] as stress and by *Cuthbertson* [19] as the metabolic response to injury. These derive in part from intensified pituitary-adrenal medullary and cortical activities that ultimately subserve tumor growth by thymolytic and lympholytic activities and by stimulating host proteolysis and gluconeogenesis. A major finding of previous work from this laboratory is the observation that supplemental vitamin A or β-carotene inhibit some of the most negative aspects of tumor-induced metabolism, such as weight loss, adrenal enlargement, thymic involution and lymphopenia (and the associated immune depression), and bleeding associated with thrombocytopenia. This moderation of tumor-induced stress responses and enhancement of host resistance to tumor regrowth are important properties of supplemental vitamin A or β-carotene.

Surgery, radiation, and chemotherapy remain the major approaches for tumor therapy. Because supplemental vitamin A and β-carotene add to the effectiveness of each of the therapies with experimental animals, we anticipate that these specific nutrients will play an analogous and important role in clinical tumor therapy.

References

1   Seifter, E.; Rettura, G.; Levenson, S.: Decreased resistance of C3H/HeHa mice to C3HBA tumor transplants: increased resistance due to supplemental vitamin A. J. natn. Cancer Inst. *67:* 467–472 (1981).

2   Seifter, E.; Rettura, G.; Levenson, S.; Critselis, A.: Mechanisms of action of vitamin A in immunogenic tumor systems; in Steegenthaler; Luthy, 10th Int. Congr. Chemo., Zürich 1977. Current Chemother., pp. 1290–1292 (Am. Soc. Microbiol., Washington 1978).

3   Seifter, E.; Rettura, G.: Vitamin A in animal tumor therapy: adrenolytic, thymotropic, and lymphopoietic actions; in 6th Pan Am. Canc. Cytol. Congr., Las Vegas 1978. Canc. Cytol., No. 17, pp. 21–22 (1978).

4   Rettura, G.; Schittek, A.; Hardy, M.; Levenson, S.M.; Demetriou, A.; Seifter, E.: Antitumor action of vitamin A in mice inoculated with adenocarcinoma cells. J. natn. Cancer Inst. *54:* 1489–1491 (1975).

5   Storer, J.B.: Longevity and gross pathology of death in 22 inbred mouse strains. J. Geront. *21:* 404–409 (1966).

6   Roberto, S.; Johansson, O.; Long, L.; McGrath, R.; McGrew, E.; Cole, W.: Clinical significance of cancer cells in circulating blood. Ann. Surg. *154:* 362–371 (1961).

7   Buinauskas, P.; McDonald, G.; Cole, W.: Role of operative stress on the resistance of the experimental animal to inoculated cancer cells. Ann. Surg. *148:* 642–648 (1958).

8   Scovill, W.A.; Saba, T.M.: Humoral recognition deficiency in the etiology of the reticuloendothelial depression induced by surgery. Ann. Surg. *178:* 59–64 (1973).

9   Donovan, A.J.: The effect of surgery on reticuloendothelial function. Archs Surg. *94:* 247–250 (1967).

10 Fisher, B.; Fisher, E.: Host factors influencing the development of metastases. Surg. Clins N. Am. *42:* 335–351 (1962).

11 Brandes, D.; Anton, E.: The role of lysosomes in cellular lytic processes. III. Electron histochemical changes in mammary tumor after treatment with cytoxan and vitamin A. Lab. Invest. *15:* 987–1006 (1966).

12 Brandes, D.; Sloan, K.W.; Anton, E.; Bloedorn, F.: The effect of X-irradiation on lysosomes of mouse mammary gland carcinomas. Cancer Res. *27:* 731–746 (1967).

13 Tannock, I.F.; Suit, H.D.; Marshall, N.: Vitamin A and the radiation response of experimental tumors: an immune-mediated effect. J. natn. Cancer Inst. *48:* 731–741 (1972).

14 Zaravinos, T.; Vogel, S.; Rettura, G.; Seifter, E.: Intermittent combined radiation (RT) and chemotherapy (CT) in a murine mammary cancer. Suboptimal RT plus CT improves local tumor control with acceptable toxicity. The 16th Ann. Meet. Am. Soc. Clin. Onc., San Diego, Abstract (1980).

15 Fisher, B.; Gebhardt, M.C.; Saffer, E.A.: Further observations on the inhibition of tumor growth by *Corynebacterium parvum* with cyclophosphamide. VII. Effect of tumor radiation prior to therapy. Int. J. Radiat. Oncol. Biol. Phys. *4:* 975–982 (1978).

16 Seifter, E.; Rettura, G.; Stratford, F.; Yee, C.; Weinzweig, J.; Jacobson, N.; Levenson, S.M.: Vitamin A inhibits some aspects of systemic disease due to local X-radiation. J. Parenteral Enteral Nutr. *5:* 288–294 (1981).

17   Seifter, E.; Rettura, G.; Padawer, J.; Stratford, F.; Goodwin, P.: Levenson, S.M.:
      Regression of C3HBA mouse tumor due to X-ray therapy combined with supplemen-
      tal β-carotene or vitamin A. J. natn. Cancer Inst. *71:* 409–417 (1983).
18   Selye, H.: Thymus and adrenals in the response of the organism to injuries and
      intoxications. Br. J. exp. Path. *17:* 234–248 (1936).
19   Cuthbertson, D.P.: The disturbance of metabolism produced by bony and non-bony
      injury with notes on certain abnormal conditions of bone. Biochem. J. *24:* 1244–1263
      (1930).
20   Oberling, C.: Le problème du cancer (Yale University Press, New Haven 1952).

Dr. E. Seifter, Department of Surgery, Albert Einstein College of Medicine,
1300 Morris Park Avenue, Bronx, NY 10461 (USA)

Prasad (ed.), Vitamins, Nutrition, and Cancer, pp. 20–32 (Karger, Basel 1984)

Modulation of Mammary Carcinogenesis by Retinoids

Richard C. Moon, Rajendra G. Mehta, David L. McCormick

Laboratory of Pathophysiology, Life Sciences Division, IIT Research Institute, Chicago, Ill., USA

Introduction

The lack of dietary vitamin A leads to clinical deficiency symptoms manifested in growth retardation, degeneration of reproductive organs, metaplasia and hyperkeratinization of epithelial tissues [1]. Additionally, animals deficient in vitamin A are more susceptible to chemical carcinogens than are nondeficient animals [2, 3]. It is also well documented that the exogenous administration of retinoids (natural and synthetic analogs of vitamin A) to experimental animals suppresses epithelial carcinogenesis in several organs [4, 5]. Similarly, in vitro studies have shown that the expression of malignant phenotype is also suppressed by the certain retinoids [6].

Over the past few years, several retinoids have been evaluated in our laboratory for their efficacy against bladder [7, 8], tracheal [9], esophageal [10] and mammary carcinogenesis [11–14] induced by chemical carcinogens. The results from these studies indicate clearly that an order of specificity exists in the responsiveness of each organ to a retinoid. For example, 13-*cis*-retinoic acid is highly effective against bladder cancer [7] but exerts little effect against mammary carcinogenesis. Although several examples may be cited relative to the efficacy of retinoids against epithelial carcinogenesis, we shall limit our discussion in this report to carcinogenesis of the mammary gland.

Suppression of Mammary Carcinogenesis by Retinoids

The initial study demonstrating the effectiveness of retinoids as chemopreventive agents in chemically induced mammary carcinogenesis was conducted in our laboratory using 7,12-dimethylbenz[a]anthracene (DMBA)-treated Sprague-Dawley female rats and retinyl acetate [11]; DMBA-treated animals receiving a diet supplemented with the retinoid exhibited a significant reduction in mammary cancer incidence and multiplicity from that of control rats fed a placebo diet. Since then a number of retinoids have been evaluated for chemopreventive activity against both DMBA and N-methyl-N-nitrosourea (MNU)-induced mammary carcinogenesis as well as against mammary cancer development in both mammary tumor virus-positive and mammary tumor virus-negative mice [15, 16]. All the active compounds listed in table I are effective in decreasing the tumor multiplicity and increasing latency at retinoid concentrations which are nontoxic. Since N-(4-hydroxyphenyl)retinamide (HPR) has been found to be the most effective retinoid against mammary carcinogenesis, when both toxicity and efficacy are taken into consideration, it has been used as the retinoid of choice in a majority of such experiments.

Subsequent studies by *McCormick* et al. [17] have shown that a significant inhibition of carcinogenesis may be obtained if the retinoid is

Table I. Retinoids evaluated for cancer chemopreventive activity against experimental mammary cancer in rats

Active	Inactive
Axerophthene[1]	13-*cis*-retinoic acid
Retinyl acetate	retinyl butyl ether
Retinyl methyl ether	N-ethyl retinamide
N-4-Hydroxyphenyl retinamide	N-2-hydroxyethyl retinamide
N-4-Hydroxyphenyl-13-*cis*-retinamide	N-4-pivaloyloxyphenyl retinamide
	N-4-proprionoxyphenyl retinamide
	retinylidene dimedone
	retinylidene acetylacetone
	TMMP analog of retinoic acid ethyl ester
	TMMP analog of ethyl retinamide
	TMMP analog of retinyl methyl ether

[1] TMMP = 4-Methoxy-2,3,6-trimethylphenyl.

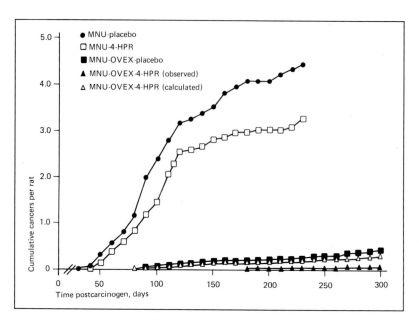

Fig. 1. Influence of ovariectomy and HPR on the multiplicity of mammary adenocarcinoma in rats treated with MNU. Sprague-Dawley female rats were injected i.v. with MNU (50 mg/kg) at 50 days of age. Animals received either placebo or HPR (2 mmol/kg) supplemented diet at 7 days postcarcinogen, and 2 groups of the animals were bilaterally ovariectomized at 14 days postcarcinogen [from ref. 23, with permission].

included in the diet for only a limited period, 2 weeks before until 1 week after carcinogen administration. Although a continuous treatment with the retinoid is necessary if retinoid supplementation begins after treatment with a carcinogen, it has been recently observed that the retinoid treatment may be delayed for up to 16 weeks postcarcinogen and still retain its protective effect [18]. Delaying retinoid administration for 20 weeks, however, resulted in a loss of chemopreventive activity of the retinoid [18].

Combination Chemoprevention: Hormones and Retinoids

Modulation of mammary carcinogenesis by hormonal alteration is well established [19, 20]. Surgical ablation of the ovaries [20] or the use of anti-hormones, such as the anti-estrogen, tamoxifen [21], inhibit the appearance of mammary cancers in carcinogen-treated animals. Similarly, treatment of

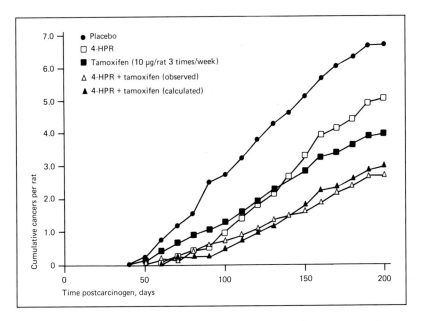

Fig. 2. Influence of HPR and tamoxifen on the multiplicity of mammary carcinoma in rats treated with MNU. Sprague-Dawley female rats were injected i.v. with MNU (50 mg/kg) at 50 days of age. At 7 days postcarcinogen the animals received either placebo diet or diet supplemented with 2 mmol/kg HPR. Tamoxifen citrate treatment (10 µg, 3 times each week, s.c.) was also started 7 days postcarcinogen until the end of the study.

carcinogen-treated rats with inhibitors of prolactin secretion (e.g. 2-bromo-α-ergocryptine) also results in a suppression of carcinogenesis [22]. Experiments, therefore, were undertaken to determine if combination treatment of either ovariectomy and retinoid or tamoxifen and retinoid would provide a synergistic inhibition of the MNU-induced mammary carcinogenesis. As indicated in figure 1, both HPR and ovariectomy effectively inhibit mammary cancer induced by MNU; however, the combination of ovariectomy and HPR is significantly more effective than either treatment alone [23]. Figure 1 also shows that the observed inhibition resulting from this combination treatment is significantly greater than that which would be expected if the combined treatment was simply additive (calculated line). Similarly, in studies in which carcinogen-treated animals received either HPR in the diet or subcutaneous injections of tamoxifen, tumor incidence was reduced. However, as shown in figure 2, HPR and tamoxifen when given in combination resulted in an additive effect on tumor multiplicity (calculated line).

In addition to the effect on tumor multiplicity, HPR + tamoxifen treatment increased the time to 50% tumor incidence from 63 days in control rats to 183 days in those receiving the retinoid and anti-estrogen. Thus, these results indicate that the combined effect of tamoxifen + HPR does not mimic the synergistic inhibition observed by the combination of ovariectomy + HPR and that the deprivation of ovarian hormones other than estradiol may be of significance in retinoid combination chemoprevention of mammary carcinogenesis.

Mechanism of Retinoid Action

Although the precise mechanism of retinoid action in epithelial differentiation and in cancer prevention remains to be unraveled, several hypotheses have been proposed, each with some supporting data. Retinoids exert an influence on DNA synthesis [24, 25], cell division [26], RNA synthesis [27], protein synthesis [28], post-translation glycosylation of proteins [29], lysosomal membrane stability [30], agglutination and adhesive properties of transformed cells [31], and stimulation of gap junctions [32]. However, which of the above-mentioned effects or combination of effects may provide a key to the elucidation of retinoid action remains to be seen. Retinoids control the expression of several proteins, such as ornithine decarboxylase [33], plasminogen activator [34], and alkaline phosphatase [34]. More recently, evidence has been presented indicating that all-trans-retinoic acid suppresses the expression of the myc oncogene [35], and it has been suggested that such control of gene expression may be mediated by retinoid receptors [36]. Data both in support of [37, 38] and in opposition to [39, 40] receptor-mediated action of the retinoids have been reported.

Upon the assumption that the action of retinoids is mediated in a manner similar to that of steroid hormones, we have analyzed mammary tissues during various physiological stages and have found both retinol- and retinoic acid-binding proteins to be present in normal mammary glands [41, 42] as well as in mammary tumors induced by both MNU and DMBA [41]. Furthermore, human breast cancers contain cytosolic retinoic acid-binding protein (CRABP) which sediments as a 2S component on sucrose density gradients and observes a strict specificity [43]. Unlabeled all-trans-retinoic acid at a 25-fold excess concentration competes effectively with the radioactive ligand for the binding sites. Certain retinoids which are effective against mammary carcinogenesis (HPR, retinyl acetate), however, fail to

Table II. Competition for [³H]-retinoic acid-binding sites by unlabeled retinoids[1]

Competitor	Concentration of competitor (x-fold excess)	Inhibition %
All-trans-retinoic acid	1	30
	10	49
	50	93
	100	100[2]
13-*cis*-retinoic acid	100	100
5,6-Epoxy retinoic acid	100	100
Retinyl acetate	100	8
N-(4-hydroxyphenyl)retinamide	100	0
Retinol	25	0
Retinyl methyl ether	100	0
Retinyl butyl ether	100	0
Axerophthene	100	0
Retinyl palmitate	25	0
17β-Estradiol	100	0

[1] Competition by unlabeled retinoid was determined using sucrose density gradient analysis.
[2] Inhibition in the presence of 100-fold excess unlabeled retinoic acid was considered as 100%.

compete for retinoic acid-binding sites (table II). This observation is supported by evidence showing that radioactive HPR does not bind with any protein of the tumor cytosol [41, 44]. These data suggest that HPR requires metabolism to an active component within the mammary cell which then allows it to effectively bind to the cytoplasmic retinoic acid-binding protein.

Our combination chemoprevention studies mentioned above indicate that ovarian hormone-independent tumors may be more responsive to retinoid treatment than ovarian hormone-dependent tumors. Thus, tumors appearing in intact animals (both ovarian hormone-dependent and independent tumors) as well as those arising in ovariectomized rats (ovarian hormone-independent tumors) were analyzed for their ability to specifically bind retinoic acid. As reported previously, mammary cancers arising in animals which were ovariectomized (hormone-independent) 1 week after MNU administration contained significantly greater concentrations of CRABP than did cancers appearing in intact animals [45].

Table III. Tumor response to ovariectomy and levels of CRABP in MNU-induced mammary carcinomas [from ref. 45, with permission]

Status of cancer after ovariectomy	Number of tumors	CRABP, pmol/mg protein mean ± SEM
Regressing	5	0.65 ± 0.16 (a)
Static	4	1.91 ± 0.35 (b)
Growing	6	4.02 ± 0.37 (c)

a vs b, p < 0.025; a vs c, p < 0.01; b vs c, p < 0.01.

Table IV. Levels of CRABP in tamoxifen-resistant MNU-induced mammary adenocarcinomas

Treatment	Number of tumors	CRABP, pmol/mg protein mean ± SEM
Vehicle	11	4.40 ± 0.57
Tamoxifen (10 µg/rat, 3 times/week)	11	4.53 ± 0.62

Table V. Comparison between steroid and retinoid receptors in human breast cancers [from ref. 43, with permission]

Steroid receptor status[1]	Number of tumors analyzed	CRABP[2], pmol/mg protein
ER+	17	5.3 ± 0.9
ER−	14	4.0 ± 1.1
PR+	16	5.4 ± 0.9
PR−	15	4.0 ± 1.1
ER+PR+	15	5.5 ± 0.9[3]
ER−PR−	13	4.3 ± 1.2[3]

[1] The levels of estradiol (E) and progesterone (P) receptors (R) were measured using sucrose density gradient analysis; less than 10 fmol/mg protein of ER and PR were considered negative.

[2] Mean CRABP ± standard error. Retinoic acid-binding proteins (CRABP) were measured using sucrose density gradient analysis. Area under the 2S region was calculated, specific binding was determined as a difference between the total and nonspecific binding in the 2S region.

[3] These values are not significantly different, p < 0.125.

Similar results were also obtained when animals bearing palpable tumors were ovariectomized; the tumors which regressed in size (dependent tumors) contained significantly lower levels of CRABP than the ovarian hormone-independent tumors which continued to grow (table III). Thus, an apparent correlation exists between the ability of retinoids to suppress mammary carcinogenesis and the level of CRABP in the cytoplasm of these mammary cancers. As mentioned earlier, tamoxifen did not exert any synergistic influence when the animals were treated with tamoxifen + HPR. The CRABP data also show that there was no observable difference between the tamoxifen-resistant tumors and control tumors with regard to their CRABP concentration (table IV).

Since we observed that the ovarian hormone-independent tumors contained increased levels of CRABP and that the occurrence of these tumors was selectively affected by the retinoid treatment, we compared the level of CRABP with the status of steroid receptor level in several human breast cancers. It would be of considerable importance if a significant difference in the level of CRABP could be demonstrated between steroid receptor-positive (estrogen receptor, ER^+ + progesterone receptor, PR^+) and steroid receptor-negative (ER^-PR^-) human breast cancers. However, as shown in table V, the data indicated that there was no significant correlation between the levels of steroid receptors and retinoid receptors in these tumors [43]. A possible reason for such a lack of correlation may be heterogeneity of the cell population of human breast cancers; the failure of approximately 40% of steroid receptor-positive human tumor patients to respond to endocrine therapy could result from such heterogeneity of cell populations.

A few investigators have studied the role of the retinoid-binding proteins on the interaction of the retinoid with the nucleus of target cells. Studies on the role of retinol-binding proteins in the interaction of retinoids with the nucleus, as well as the presence of retinoic acid-binding proteins in the nuclei of retinoblastoma cells, Lewis lung tumors and embryonal carcinoma cells, have been reported [46, 47]. Recent studies from our laboratory have indicated that formation of a retinoic acid-receptor complex in the mammary tumor cytoplasm is essential for the interaction of retinoic acid with the nucleus. Retinoic acid per se does not bind to nuclei or to nuclear components. The RABP which is isolated from purified nuclei of mammary cancers, following incubation of nuclei with cytoplasmic retinoic acid-receptor complex, sediments as a 2S component when subjected to sucrose density gradient analysis [48]. Furthermore, incubation of a constant amount of nuclei (constant DNA concentration, $\sim 100\ \mu g$) with an increas-

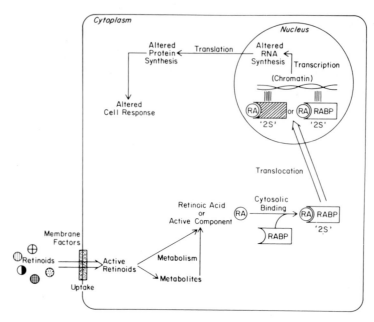

Fig. 3. Proposed steps in the mechanism of retinoid action [from ref. 44, with permission].

ing concentration of cytoplasmic retinoic acid-CRABP complex results in saturable nuclear binding. The data, when analyzed by a Scatchard plot, indicate that the nuclei bind retinoic acid with a high affinity (K_d = 1.7 × $10^{-9}\,M$) and that the number of nuclear binding sites approximates 4–5 pmol/100 μg DNA [48]. Although our results do not explain whether the retinoic acid-receptor complex enters the nucleus or simply delivers retinoic acid to the nucleus, they do provide evidence that the formation of cytoplasmic retinoic acid-receptor complex is essential for the interaction of retinoic acid with the nucleus of mammary cancer cells.

Based on the data presented above, a proposed interaction of retinoids at the cellular level is summarized in figure 3. The active retinoid may enter the target cell as an authentic retinoid or as a metabolite; some membrane factors may influence the entry of these compounds into the cell. Once in the cell, the retinoid may require further metabolism to an active component that binds to a 2S cytoplasmic binding protein which specifically binds retinoic acid. The retinoic acid-receptor complex then translocates to the nucleus; unlike steroid receptors, this step does not require temperature activation [48]. The retinoic acid or the retinoic acid-receptor complex in the nucleus may interact with the chromatin [49–51] and alter the synthesis of specific messenger RNA which, in turn, may influence translation of an enzyme or a protein responsible for the chemoprotective effect of the retinoid. The entire sequence of events is, however, poorly understood.

Acknowledgement

Studies cited in this presentation which were performed in our laboratory were supported by one or more of the following contracts or grants from the National Cancer Institute: N01-CP-23292, N01-CB-74207, N01-CP-75936, N01-CP-75939, N01-CP-05718, N01-CP-15742, CA-26030, CA-34664.

References

1   Hicks, R.M.: The scientific basis for regarding vitamin A and its analogues as anti-carcinogenic agents. Proc. Nutr. Soc. *42:* 83–93 (1983).

2   Rogers, A.E.; Herndon, B.J.; Newberne, P.M.: Induction by demethylhydrazine of intestinal carcinoma in normal rats fed high and low levels of vitamin A. Cancer Res. *33:* 1003–1009 (1973).

3   Cohen, S.M.; Wittenberg, J.F.; Bryn, G.T.: Effect of avitaminosis A and hypervitaminosis A on urinary bladder carcinogenicity of N-[4-(5-nitrozfuryl)-z-thiozolyl] formamide. Cancer Res. *36:* 2334–2339 (1976).

4   Sporn, M.B.; Dunlop, N.M.; Newton, D.L.; Smith, J.M.: Prevention of chemical carcinogenesis by vitamin A and its synthetic analogs (retinoids). Fed. Proc. *35:* 1335–1338 (1976).

5   Moon, R.C.; McCormick, D.L.; Mehta, R.G.: Inhibition of carcinogenesis by retinoids. Cancer Res. *43:* 2469s–2475s (1983).

6   Lotan, R.: Effects of vitamin A and its analogs (retinoids) on normal and neoplastic cells. Biochim. biophys. Acta *605:* 33–91 (1980).

7   Becci, P.J.; Thompson, H.J.; Grubbs, C.J.; Squire, R.A.; Brown, C.C.; Sporn, M.B.; Moon, R.C.: Inhibitory effect of 13-*cis*-retinoic acid in urinary bladder carcinogenesis induced in C57 BL/6 mice by N-butyl-*n*-4-hydroxy butyl)nitrosamine. Cancer Res. *38:* 4463–4466 (1978).

8   Moon, R.C.; McCormick, D.L.; Becci, P.J.; Shealy, Y.F.; Frickel, F.; Paust, J.; Sporn, M.B.: Influence of 15 retinoic acid amides on urinary bladder carcinogenesis in the mouse. Carcinogenesis *3:* 1469–1472 (1982).

9   Grubbs, C.J.; Becci, P.J.; Moon, R.C.: Characterization of 1-methyl-1-nitrosourea (MNU) induced tracheal carcinogenesis and the effect of feeding the retinoid N-(4-hydroxyphenyl)retinamide (4-HPR). Proc. Am. Ass. Cancer Res. *21:* 102 (1980).

10 Moon, R.C.; McCormick, D.L.: Inhibition of mammary carcinogenesis by retinoids. J. Am. Acad. Dermatol. *6:* 809–814 (1982).

11 Moon, R.C.; Grubbs, C.J.; Sporn, M.B.: Inhibition of 7,12-dimethylbenz[a]anthra-

cene-induced mammary carcinogenesis by retinyl acetate. Cancer Res. *36:* 2626–2630 (1976).

12   Grubbs, C.J.; Moon, R.C.; Spron, M.B.; Newton, D.L.: Inhibition by mammary cancer by retinyl methyl ether. Cancer Res. *37:* 599–602 (1977).

13   Moon, R.C.; Thompson, H.J.; Becci, P.J.; Grubbs, C.J.; Gander, R.J.; Newton, D.L.; Smith, J.M.; Phillips, S.R.; Henderson, W.R.; Mullen, L.T.; Brown, C.C.; Sporn, M.B.: *N*-(4 hydroxyphenyl)retinamide, a new retinoid for prevention of breast cancer in rats. Cancer Res. *39:* 1339–1346 (1979).

14   Thompson, H.J.; Becci, P.J.; Moon, R.C.; Sporn, M.B.; Newton, D.L.; Brown, C.C.; Nurrenbach, A.; Paust, J.: Inhibition of 1-methyl-1-nitrosourea-induced mammary carcinogenesis in the rat by the retinoid axerophthene. Drug Res. *30:* 1127–1129 (1980).

15   Welsch, C.W.; Goodrich-Smith, M.; Brown, C.K.; Crowe, N.: Enhancement by retinyl acetate of hormone-induced mammary tumorigenesis in female GR/A mice. J. natn. Cancer Inst. *67:* 635–638 (1981).

16   Welsch, C.W.; Dehoog, J.V.; Moon, R.C.: Inhibition of mammary tumorigenesis in nulliparous C3H mice by chronic feeding of the synthetic retinoid *N*-(4-hydroxyphenyl)retinamide. Carcinogenesis *14:* 1185–1187 (1983).

17   McCormick, D.L.; Burns, F.J.; Albert, R.E.: Inhibition of rat mammary carcinogenesis by short dietary exposure to retinyl acetate. Cancer Res. *40:* 1140–1143 (1980).

18   McCormick, D.L.; Moon, R.C.: Influence of delayed administration of retinyl acetate on mammary carcinogenesis. Cancer Res. *42:* 2639–2643 (1982).

19   Moon, R.C.: Influence of pregnancy and lactation on experimental carcinogenesis; in Pike, Sliteri, Welsch, Banbury report, vol. 8, pp. 353–364 (1981).

20   Huggins, C.: Two principles in endocrine therapy of cancers: hormone deprival and hormone interference. Cancer Res. *25:* 1163–1167 (1965).

21   Jordan, V.C.; Allen, K.E.; Dix, C.J.: Pharmacology of tamoxifen in laboratory animals. Cancer Treat. Rep. *64:* 745–759 (1980).

22   Welsch, C.W.; Goodrich-Smith, M.; Brown, C.K.; Mackie, D.; Johnson, D.: 2-Bromo-α-ergocryptine (CB 154 and tamoxifen C1C1 46474) induced suppression of the genesis of mammary carcinoma in female rats treated with 7-12-dimethylbenz[a]anthracene (DMBA): a comparison. Oncology *39:* 88–92 (1982).

23   McCormick, D.L.; Mehta, R.G.; Thompson, C.A.; Dinger, N.; Caldwell, J.; Moon, R.C.: Enhanced inhibition of mammary carcinogenesis by combination *N*-(4-hydroxyphenyl)retinamide and ovariectomy. Cancer Res. *42:* 508–512 (1982).

24   Mehta, R.G.; Moon, R.C.: Inhibition of DNA synthesis by retinyl acetate during chemically induced mammary carcinogenesis. Cancer Res. *40:* 1109–1111 (1980).

25   Kensler, T.W.; Muller, G.C.: Retinoic acid inhibition of the comitogenic action of mezerein and phorbol esters in bovine lymphocytes. Cancer Res. *38:* 771–775 (1978).

26   Yuspa, S.H.; Eigjo, K.; Morse, M.A.: Retinyl acetate modulation of cell growth kinetics and carcinogen-cellular interaction in mouse epidermal cell cultures. Chem.-Biol. Interact. *16:* 251–254 (1977).

27   Blalock, J.E.; Gifford, G.E.: Retinoic acid (vitamin A acid) induced transcriptional control of interferon production. Proc. natn. Acad. Sci. USA *74:* 5382–5386 (1977).

28 Brenckerhof, C.E.; Harris, E.D., Jr.: Modulation by retinoic acid and corticosteroids of collagenase production by rabbit fibroblasts treated with phorbol myristate acetate or poly(ethylene glycol). Biochim. biophys. Acta *677:* 424–432 (1981).

29 Deluca, L.M.: The direct involvement of vitamin A in glycol transfer reactions of mammalian membrane vitamins. Heron *35:* 1–57 (1977).

30 Wang, C.C.; Straight, S.; Hill, D.L.: Destabilization of mouse liver lysosomes by vitamin A compounds and analogs. Biochem. Pharmacol. *25:* 471–475 (1976).

31 Adamo, S.; Deluca, L.M.; Akalovsky, I.: Retinoid-induced adhesion in cultured transformed mouse fibroblasts. J. natn. Cancer Inst. *62:* 1473–1478 (1979).

32 Elias, P.M.; Grayson, S.; Caldwell, T.M.: Gap junction proliferation in retinoic acid-treated human basal cell carcinoma. Lab. Invest. *42:* 469–474 (1980).

33 Verma, A.K.; Boutwell, R.K.: Vitamin A (retinoic acid): a potent inhibitor of TPA-induced ornithine decarboxylase activity in mouse epidermis. Cancer Res. *37:* 2196–2201 (1977).

34 Strickland, S.; Smith, K.K.; Marotti, K.R.: Hormonal induction of differentiation in teratocarcinoma stem cells: generation of parietal ectoderm by retinoic acid and dibutyryl cAMP. Cell *21:* 347–355 (1980).

35 Sporn, M.B.; Roberts, A.B.: Role of retinoids in differentiation and carcinogenesis. Cancer Res. *43:* 3034–3040 (1983).

36 Chytil, F.; Ong, D.E.: Cellular retinol and retinoic acid-binding proteins in vitamin A action. Fed. Proc. *38:* 2510–2514 (1979).

37 Sani, B.P.; Corbett, T.H.: Retinoic acid-binding protein in normal tissues and experimental tumors. Cancer Res. *37:* 209–213 (1977).

38 Ong, D.E.; Chytil, F.: Retinoic acid-binding proteins in rat tissues. J. biol. Chem. *250:* 6113–6117 (1975).

39 Libby, P.R.; Bertram, J.S.: Lack of intercellular retinoid-binding protein in retinol-sensitive cell line. Carcinogenesis *3:* 481–484 (1982).

40 Lacroix, A.; L'Heureux, N.; Bhat, P.V.: Cellular retinoic acid-binding protein (CRABP) in retinoic acid-resistant human breast cancer. Sublines Am. Ass. Cancer Res. *24:* 17 (1983).

41 Mehta, R.G.; Cerny, W.L.; Moon, R.C.: Distribution of retinoic acid-binding protein in normal and neoplastic mammary tissues. Cancer Res. *40:* 47–49 (1980).

42 Mehta, R.G.; Moon, R.C.: Hormonal regulation of retinoic acid-binding proteins in the mammary gland. Biochem. J. *200:* 591–595 (1981).

43 Mehta, R.G.; Kute, T.E.; Hopkins, M.; Moon, R.C.: Retinoic acid-binding proteins and steroid receptor levels in human breast cancer. Eur. J. Cancer clin. Oncol. *18:* 221–226 (1982).

44 Moon, R.C.; Mehta, R.G.; McCormick, D.L.: Suppression of mammary carcinogenesis by retinoids; in Crispen, Cancer etiology and prevention, pp. 275–284 (Elsevier, Amsterdam 1983).

45 Mehta, R.G.; McCormick, D.L.; Cerny, W.L.; Moon, R.C.: Correlation between retinoid inhibition of *N*-methyl-*N*-nitrosourea-induced mammary carcinogenesis and levels of retinoic acid-binding proteins. Carcinogenesis *3:* 89–91 (1982).

46 Takase, S.; Ong, D.E.; Chytil, F.: Cellular retinol-binding protein allows specific interaction of retinol with the nucleus in vitro. Proc. natn. Acad. Sci. USA *76:* 2204–2208 (1979).

47 Wiggert, B.; Russell, P.; Lewis, M.; Chader, G.: Differential binding of soluble nuclear

receptors and effects in cell viability of retinol and retinoic acid in cultured retino-blastoma cells. Biochem. biophys. Res. Commun. *79:* 218–225 (1977).

48   Mehta, R.G.; Cerny, W.L.; Moon, R.C.: Nuclear interaction of retinoic acid binding protein in chemically induced mammary adenocarcinomas. Biochem. J. *208:* 731–736 (1982).

49   Tsai, C.H.; Chytil, F.: Effect of vitamin A deficiency on RNA synthesis in isolated rat liver nuclei. Life Sci. *23:* 1461–1472 (1978).

50   Liau, G.; Ong, D.E.; Chytil, F.: Interaction of the retinol/cellular retinol-binding protein complex with isolated nuclei and nuclear components. J. Cell Biol. *91:* 63–68 (1981).

51   Mehta, R.G.; Cerny, W.L.; Moon, R.C.: Alteration in DNA-dependent RNA poly-merase activity by retinoids. Proc. Am. Ass. Cancer Res. *23:* 21 (1982).

R.C. Moon, PhD, Laboratory of Pathophysiology, Life Sciences Division,
IIT Research Institute, Chicago, IL 60616 (USA)

Prasad (ed.), Vitamins, Nutrition, and Cancer, pp. 33–45 (Karger, Basel 1984)

Vitamin A (Retinol) and Epithelial Cancer in Man

T.K. Basu[a], *Una Chan*[a], *A. Fields*[b]

[a] Department of Foods and Nutrition, University of Alberta, Edmonton, Alberta;
[b] Cross Cancer Hospital, University of Alberta, Canada

Introduction

Vitamin A occurs physiologically as the alcohol (retinol), the aldehyde (retinaldehyde), the acid (retinoic acid) and the ester (retinyl ester). *Sporn* et al. [1] have coined the term 'retinoids' to describe all moieties of vitamin A molecules. The retinoids are well known for their importance in the general growth and differentiation and maintenance of epithelial tissues [2]. If vitamin A is deficient, differentiation switches in the pathway leading to keratinization of squamous cells which replace normal epithelium, a process known as squamous metaplasia (fig. 1). During the process of squamous metaplasia, mucous membranes change from a single layer of mucin-secreting and ciliated epithelium to multiple layers of epithelial cells, with overlying keratin resembling those of the skin [3, 4]. The mode of action of vitamin A in normal epithelial differentiation and maintenance of the mucous membranes is not well defined. It is believed that retinoic acid is the major biologically active form of vitamin A in somatic epithelial cells, where the vitamin influences cellular differentiation [5], while retinol is a labilizer of biological membranes [6].

Epithelial tissues that depend upon retinoids for normal cellular differentiation and growth account for over half of the total primary cancer in both men and women. Epithelial cancer includes squamous metaplasia and carcinoma of a wide variety of sites of the body (table I).

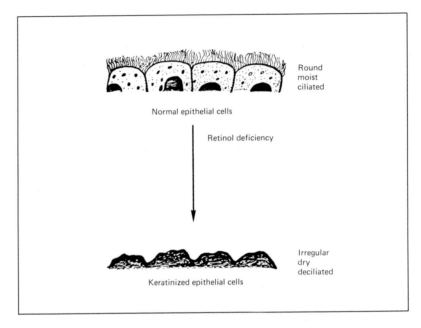

Fig. 1. Effect of retinol deficiency on the morphology of the epithelial cell.

Retinol and Carcinoma: Animal Studies

A connection between vitamin A and cancer was detected as early as 1926, when the development of carcinomas was found in rats fed a vitamin A-deficient diet [7]. However, only recently there have been intensive efforts to investigate the possible role of vitamin A in relation to epithelial cancer in man.

Experimental studies have revealed that vitamin A deficiency is related to cancer of the stomach, nasopharynx, lower respiratory tract and endocervix which are lined by glandular epithelium [8, 9]. Vitamin A deficiency may change the glandular epithelium to squamous and, whenever such 'squamous metaplasia' occurs, there are grounds for suspecting increased risk of cancer development.

Convincing evidence of the significance of vitamin A in protecting against cancer has come from experimental studies in which tissues in organ culture or in intact animals are exposed to carcinogenic polycyclic aromatic

Table I. Organs and tissue sites which are most susceptible to epithelial cancer

Contact epithelia	Excretory epithelia	Secretory epithelia
Skin	colon	pancreas
Buccal cavity and pharynx	rectum	breast
Esophagus	gallbladder	prostate
Larynx	kidney	testis
Trachea, bronchus and lung	bladder	uterus
Cervix uteri		ovary
		thyroid
		stomach
		small intestine

hydrocarbons (PAH) to develop squamous cancer. Furthermore, a number of studies have shown that systemic prophylactic administration of vitamin A in its ester, alcohol or acid form both before and after exposure to various chemical carcinogens (3-methylcholanthrene, 3-MCA; benzopyrene, BP; dimethylbenzanthracene, DMBA) inhibits the induction of metaplasia and carcinomas in various sites. Thus, vitamin A protected rats against the early development of squamous neoplasms in response to a carcinogen (3-MCA) given by endotracheal instillation [10]. Retinoids administration reduced the development of squamous metaplasia and carcinomas in rodents subjected to intratracheal administration of carcinogenic polycyclic hydrocarbons [8]. Supplemental vitamin A has been reported to prevent cancer of the forestomach and cervix in hamsters treated with polynuclear aromatic hydrocarbons [9]. Vitamin A also inhibits squamous metaplasia induced by BP on organ culture of hamster tracheas [11].

The prevention of epithelial cancer by retinoids was demonstrated by *Bollag* [12] using the classical two-stage skin carcinogenesis system. In this study, topical application of DMBA on mouse skin was followed by applications of the promoter, croton oil, inducing benign papillomas which progressed to carcinomas. Oral retinoic acid during the promotion phase delayed the appearance, retarded the growth, and led to regression of papillomas. The appearance of carcinomas was also delayed and their incidence reduced. More recently, several experimental studies have included the inhibition by oral 13-*cis*-retinoic acid (a synthetic retinoid analog) of lung tumors in hamsters given intratracheal BP [13] and the protection of rats against DMBA-induced breast cancer by oral retinyl methyl ether [21].

There is also evidence that the carcinogens are more potent in vitamin A-deficient animals. Various carcinogens bind more tightly to DNA in cultured tracheas from hamsters fed a vitamin A-deficient diet than from healthy animals [14]. In the absence of vitamin A intake, the susceptibility of rats to pulmonary carcinogens has increased even in the presence of substantial liver stores of vitamin A and in the absence of deficiency symptoms [15].

Squamous metaplasia appears to occur as an early phenotypic change following exposure to a carcinogen. The similarity in appearance of the histological change of retinol deficiency and a carcinogen-induced squamous metaplasia leads to speculations that the two conditions are similar in more fundamental ways, namely (a) that a retinol-deficient epithelium is more prone to malignant change either 'spontaneously' (i.e. without application of a specific carcinogenic agent) or in response to a carcinogen, and (b) that retinol may reverse the early metaplastic changes induced by carcinogens and so inhibit or delay the appearance of carcinoma.

Indeed, animal studies have demonstrated that retinol deficiency increases susceptibility to chemical carcinogenesis in the respiratory system [16], skin [17], bladder [18], and colon [19]. Small amounts of retinyl acetate or palmitate in the diet appear to abolish this enhanced susceptibility. Large doses of the natural retinoids have been reported to provide additional protection against carcinoma of the trachea and bronchus [8], esophagus, stomach and intestine [9], lung [10], and breast [20].

Vitamin A and Cancer in Man

Although evidence based on laboratory animal models has become increasingly voluminous, information relating to humans is sparse. Nonetheless, the evidence to support a link in man between vitamin A deficiency and cancer comes from three sources: biochemical studies involving comparison of serum vitamin A levels in cancer cases and controls, epidemiological studies of dietary intake and cancer incidence, and biochemical studies of vitamin A status in those who are destined to develop cancer.

Serum Vitamin A Levels in Cancer

In 1976, *Basu* et al. [22] studied 28 newly diagnosed patients with bronchial carcinoma. The serum vitamin A levels of these patients were compared with two age, sex and smoking habit-matched control groups – a group of nonmalignant lung diseases (such as bronchopneumonia, acute and chronic bronchitis), and a group of healthy subjects. This study revealed that the patients with either squamous or oat cell carcinoma had significantly lower serum vitamin A than those of the 2 control groups, and the patients with large undifferentiated bronchial carcinoma.

Ibrahim et al. [23] measured serum vitamin A and carotene levels in 203 cases of squamous cell carcinoma of the oral cavity and oropharynx in Pakistan and compared them with 112 controls. They found low vitamin A and carotene levels in 51% of patients according to WHO criteria. Subsequently, *Atukorala* et al. [24] measured serum carotene and vitamins A and E levels in 26 newly diagnosed lung cancer patients, 10 patients with non-malignant lung disease and 11 other hospital patients. This study showed that the lung cancer patients were associated with low serum vitamin A, but not carotene levels, when compared with the 2 control groups. It was of particular interest that vitamin E level in the cancer patients remained unaffected, indicating the effect on vitamin A being rather specific.

In recent years, attention has been paid to the relationship of zinc to vitamin A metabolism in an attempt to demonstrate that the trace element is vital in mobilizing vitamin A from the liver into the circulation [25, 26]. Although the exact mechanism by which zinc influences the mobilization of vitamin A is not at present clear, there have been reports indicating that zinc may be involved in the synthesis of vitamin A carrier protein, retinol-binding protein (RBP). It was of interest that *Atukorala* et al. [24] found that the newly diagnosed patients with lung cancer were associated with not only low serum vitamin A but also with low zinc and RBP levels. These results indicate that the depressed serum concentration of vitamin A in lung cancer patients may be caused, at least in part, by impaired mobilization of the vitamin from the liver. In order to determine whether the low serum levels of vitamin A and RBP were specific for epithelial cancer, *Basu* et al. [27] measured the concentration of the vitamin and its carrier protein in 28 patients with epithelial cancer (e.g. bronchus, lungs, bladder and endometrium) and 54 patients with cancer of the reticulo-endothelial system (e.g. myeloma). All patients had serum vitamin A below the normal range. However, the effect was found to be more marked in patients with epithelial cancer (30–55% of normal value) than with myeloma (70% of normal value), and that the serum concentrations of RBP fell in parallel with vitamin A in the former group, while the protein concentrations remained unaffected in the patients with myeloma, suggesting that the underlying cause for low vitamin A levels may be different in these 2 groups of patients. It is possible that the depressed serum concentration of vitamin A in epithelial cancer patients may be due to both reduced dietary intake and impaired mobilization of the vitamin from the liver.

Taken together, these biochemical studies present a consistent picture as to the associationship between vitamin A deficiency and cancer of epithelial cell origin in man. It must be, however, argued that the studies were carried out in those patients who had an established malignant disease; hence, the observations do not ascertain the cause-or-effect relationship.

A number of factors may account for the subnormal vitamin A status in patients with epithelial cancer. Thus, vitamin A deficiency may be precipitated either due to its low dietary intake or due to deficiencies of zinc and protein which are required for metabolic availability of vitamin A. The vitamin A deficiency may cause abnormalities in epithelial differentiation resulting in an increased susceptibility to the external insults, such as smoking and environmental chemicals. The resultant malignant condition, in turn, may be associated with a decreased food intake due to loss of appetite, and an increased requirement of nutrients, such as protein, zinc and vitamin A, exacerbating vitamin A status [28]. It is, therefore, of paramount importance that prospective studies are carried out in order to establish the cause-or-effect relationship between vitamin A status and an increased risk of epithelial cancer in various population groups.

Diet and Cancer Incidence

A number of studies (table II), in recent years, have associated a relative deficiency of vitamin A intake with an increased risk of lung cancer. In 1975, *Bjelke* [29] reported results of a 5-year follow-up study involving 8,278 men who had responded to a questionnaire on their smoking and dietary habits. An index of vitamin A intake, essentially based on reported consumption of carrots, eggs and milk, was negatively associated with lung cancer incidence; for a low vitamin A index were greatest in heavy smokers (relative risk, RR 2.86), less for light smokers (RR 2.27) and close to unity for non-smokers. The overall RR was 2.63 ($p < 0.01$). Higher risks were found when incidences of histologically confirmed carcinomas other than adenocarcinomas were compared.

More recently, *Hirayama* [31] reported results of a 10-year follow-up study involving 2,417,844 Japanese who had responded to questionnaires as to their diet and smoking habits. 807 deaths from lung cancer were

Table II. Questionnaire studies of cancer in relation to dietary intake of vitamin A

References	Relative risks (lower:higher intake)	Number and sites of cancer
29	2.6:1	36 lung
29	1.7:1	228 stomach
30	1.9:1	338 larynx
31	1.3:1	611 male lung
31	1.5:1	196 female lung
32	1.7:1	272 lung
33	2.1:1	569 bladder
34	2.2:1	233 lung

observed, the RR was found to be reduced by half in those who consumed green-yellow vegetables daily as compared to non-consumers. The consumers of green-yellow vegetables showed a lower risk of lung cancer in both smokers and non-smokers, and this was true for both males and females. A similar report was made by *MacLennan* et al. [34] who found in a case-control study that low consumption of green vegetables was related to lung cancer in both sexes. The estimated risk of low versus high vegetable intake was 2.23.

A research group in the Roswell Park Memorial Institute (RPMI) in the USA has conducted a number of studies concerning vitamin A intake and cancer. These studies have indicated that individuals with lower vitamin A intake are associated with higher incidence of cancer of the bladder [34], lung [32], and larynx [30]. One of the case-control studies they conducted was the association between vitamin A intake and the relative risk of lung cancer [32]. Retrospective dietary and smoking data were collected by interviewing 292 patients with lung cancer and 801 control patients who had neither cancer nor disease of the respiratory system during 1957–1965. The measure of vitamin A intake was obtained by interviewing patients as to their usual frequency of consumption of 21 different items which are considered to be rich in vitamin A, during the time 1 year prior to the onset of symptoms. The vitamin A content of the diet was determined by reference to the US Department of Agriculture tables of food values for a standard portion of each item. The Mantel-Haenszel age and smoking-adjusted RR for patients with lower vitamin A level was 1.7 times of their controls (p < 0.05). Increased risk of bladder cancer in association with a low value of an index of vitamin A intake has been reported by *Mettlin and Graham* [33]. Over 500 bladder cancer patients were compared with at least 1,000 age-matched controls, and a RR of 2.07 (p < 0.01) for low versus high vitamin A index was determined. Milk and carrot intakes were the major sources of ascertained vitamin A intake.

These studies present a consistent picture as to the associationship between low vitamin A intake and increased RR of cancers of epithelial cell origin. It may be argued that in most studies, specific interest in vitamin A arose after completion of an investigation undertaken for unrelated reasons so that only some of the sources of vitamin A could be assessed, and hence the index of vitamin A should be regarded as a crude measure. In most studies, the vitamin A index was primarily based on the intake of milk, carrots and green-yellow vegetables. Omissions of foods, such as liver, fortified margarine, and vitamin supplements may indeed have resulted in an underestimation of the relative risk of low vitamin A. Therefore, it is of paramount importance that the evidence of negative associationships between vitamin A intake and cancer is further substantiated by biochemical assessment of vitamin A status.

Serum Vitamin A and Cancer Incidence

A prospective study [35] was carried out where vitamin A levels were measured in the stored sera of 85 cancer cases and twice the number of matched controls from a community of over 3,000 individuals in Evans County, Georgia. The serum was obtained at least 1 year before overt manifestation of the cancer. This study indicated that those with low vitamin A values had a 6-fold increased risk of later developing cancer. This association was independent of age, smoking habits and serum cholesterol.

More recently, another prospective study was conducted by *Wald* et al. [36] involving 16,000 males aged between 35 and 64. These people attended the research center for a comprehensive health-screening examination between March 1975 to December, 1978. The sera were stored at −40 °C. By the end of 1976, 86 men had developed cancer. Controls were 172 males from the remainder study population who were alive and without cancer. Mean retinol for all cancer patients was significantly (p < 0.025) lower than for controls. The difference being greatest for gastrointestinal and lung cancer. The RR of cancer associated with retinol levels at the lowest quintile was 2.2 times that in the highest quintile. These authors suggested that serum retinol levels have a predictive value for subsequent cancer.

Table III. Serum retinol and RBP values in subjects destined to develop cancer, and in control subjects

Subjects	Retinol µg/dl	RBP mg/dl	Zinc mmol/dl
Controls (n = 81)	86.0	4.9	10.1
Subjects who subsequently developed lung cancer (n = 27)	56.8*	4.5	10.0

*p < 0.005.

In a case-control study by *Haines* et al. [37], plasma levels of vitamin A, RBP and zinc were measured in samples taken 2–7 years before the development of clinically manifest tumors. 27 participants later developed cancer of the lung after entry to the study. Each cancer was matched with 3 controls. Results indicated that there is no difference of RBP and zinc but vitamin A levels between cases and controls (table III).

Significance of Serum Vitamin A and RBP in Epithelial Cancer
The overall retrospective and prospective biochemical data indicate that vitamin A deficiency may be present long before one develops cancer of epithelial origin, and that serum RBP levels change only in the presence of the tumor. On the basis of these observations, it is not unreasonable to suggest that vitamin A deficiency may be one of the predisposing factors to the epithelial cancer, and that serum RBP level could be used as a tumor marker. The later aspect could be further substantiated by the observations made in a recent study [38] where serum vitamin A and RBP levels were measured in postoperative apparently disease-free colorectal cancer patients. According to the Dukes' classification, these patients were divided into two groups – 'B2' involving the full thickness of the bowel wall without node involvement, and 'C' with regional lymph node metastases. Both groups were found to be associated with subnormal serum vitamin A levels, while RBP levels appeared to be below normal only in patients with colorectal C (table IV). Furthermore, in follow-up studies to date, of the 103 disease-free colorectal cancer patients (B2 and C types), 12 subjects subsequently had recurrences of the disease who showed lower serum levels of vitamin A as well as RBP than those who remained disease-free (table V).

Table IV. Plasma vitamin A and retinol-binding protein in postoperative colorectal cancer patients

Groups	Average age years	Vitamin A µg/dl	Retinol-binding protein, mg/dl
Controls (n = 65)	46.5 ± 1.4	75.4 ± 2.5	5.7 ± 0.3
Colorectal B2 (n = 66)	62.4 ± 1.2	50.1 ± 2.9[1]	5.0 ± 0.3
Colorectal C (n = 37)	62.9 ± 1.6	49.6 ± 3.8[1]	3.8 ± 0.4[1, 2]

Each value is the mean ± SEM for the number of subjects shown in parentheses.
[1] Significantly different from the controls, $p < 0.001$.
[2] Significant difference between colorectal B2 and C patients, $p = 0.01$.

Table V. Plasma vitamin A and retinol-binding protein in patients with subsequent recurrence of cancer and in patients who remained disease-free

Groups	Vitamin A, µg/dl	Retinol-binding protein mg/dl
Disease-free (n = 91)	50.9 ± 1.8	4.6 ± 0.3
Recurrence (n = 12)	40.4 ± 6.7	3.7 ± 0.4
Significance	0.05	n.s.

Conclusions

A high proportion of human cancers is attributable to environmental factors [39]. Evidence to date obtained from studies with experimental animals and from human populations implicates vitamin A deficiency in the causation of epithelial cancer. Considering this evidence, the public at large should be advised to take a well-balanced diet containing vitamin A and zinc to meet the recommended dietary allowances. Such a measure must be taken from an early age before the onset of squamous metaplasia induced by environmental chemicals. As to the use of vitamin A (natural or analog) in chemoprevention of cancer, further studies are certainly warranted. The need for caution before recommending this form of prophylaxis is emphasized by the results of some animal experiments. Thus, the vitamin has been reported to enhance tumor growth in chickens [40] and promote metastasis in mice bearing spontaneous mammary tumors [41]. Furthermore, both cellular retinol-binding protein which binds retinol and cellular retinoic acid-binding protein which binds retinoic acid have been detected in human lung, breast and stomach carcinomas [42–45] but not in the adjacent normal tissue, indicating that there is an increased requirement or utilization of vitamin A in these target cells. Indeed, the decreased serum vitamin A levels in tumor-bearing subjects may be the reflection of an increased utilization of the vitamin by the tumor tissue.

Acknowledgements

Part of this project was funded by the Alberta Cancer Board, Research Project No. R-92. We wish to thank Dr. *T.A. McPherson,* Director of the Department of Medicine, Cross Cancer Institute for his helpful co-operation with this study.

References

1 Sporn, M.B.; Dunlop, N.S.; Newton, D.L.; Smith, J.M.: Prevention of chemical carcinogens by vitamin A and its synthetic analogs (retinoids). Fed. Proc. *25:* 1332–1338 (1976).

2 De Luca, L.; Maestri, N.; Bonanni, F.; Nelson, D.: Maintenance of epithelial cell differentiation. The mode of action of vitamin A. Cancer *30:* 1326 (1972).

3 Moore, T.: Effects of vitamin A deficiency in animals; in Sebrell, Harris, The vitamins, vol. 1, p. 245 (Academic Press, New York 1967).

4 Toyoshima, K.; Leighton, J.: Vitamin A inhibition of keratinization in rat urinary bladder cancer cell line Nara Bladder Tumor No. 2 in meniscus gradient culture. Cancer Res. *35:* 1873 (1975).

5 De Luca, L.; Anderson, H.; Wolf, G.: The in vivo and in vitro biosynthesis of lung tissue glycopeptides. Archs intern. Med. *127:* 853–857 (1971).

6 Roels, O.A.; Anderson, O.R.; Liu, N.S.T.; Shah, D.O.; Trout, M.E.: Vitamin A and membrane. Am. J. clin. Nutr. *22:* 1020–1032 (1969).

7 Fujamaki, Y.: Formation of carcinoma in albino rats fed on deficient diets. J. Cancer Res. *10:* 469–471 (1926).

8 Saffiotti, U.; Montesano, R.; Sellakumar, A.R.; Borg, S.A.: Experimental cancer of the lung. Inhibition by vitamin A of the induction of tracheobronchial squamous metaplasia and squamous cell tumors. Cancer *20:* 857–864 (1967).

9 Chu, E.W.; Malmgren, R.A.: An inhibitory effect of vitamin A on the induction of tumors of forestomach and cervix in the Syrian hamster by carcinogenic polycyclic hydrocarbons. Cancer Res. *25:* 884–885 (1965).

10 Cone, M.V.; Nettlesheim, P.: Effects of vitamin A on 3-methylcholanthrene-induced squamous metaplasia and early tumors in the respiratory tract of rats. J. natn. Cancer Inst. *50:* 1599–1606 (1973).

11   Crocker, T.T.; Sanders, L.L.: Influence of vitamin A and 3,7-dimethyl-2,6-octadienal (citral) on the effect of benzo[a]pyrene on hamster trachea in organ culture. Cancer Res. *30:* 1312–1316 (1970).

12   Bollag, W.: Therapy of epithelial tumors with an aromatic retinoic acid analog. Chemotherapy *21:* 236–247 (1975).

13   Port, C.D.; Sporn, M.B.; Kaufman, D.G.: Prevention of lung cancer in hamsters by 13-*cis*-retinoic acid. Proc. Am. Ass. Cancer Res. *16:* 21 (1975).

14   Genta, V.M.; Kaufman, D.G.; Harris, C.C.; Smith, J.M.; Sporn, M.D.; Saffiotti, U.: Vitamin A deficiency enhances binding of benzo[a]pyrene to tracheal epithelial DNA. Nature, Lond. *247:* 48–49 (1974).

15   Nettlesheim, P.; William, M.L.: The influence of vitamin A on the susceptibility of the rat lung to 3-methyl-cholanthrene. Int. J. Cancer *17:* 351–357 (1976).

16   Nettesheim, P.; Snyder, C.; Williams, M.L.; Cone, M.V.; Kim, J.C.: Effects of vitamin A on lung tumor induction in rats. Proc. Am. Ass. Cancer Res. *16:* 54 (1975).

17   Davies, R.E.: Effect of vitamin A on 7,12-dimethyl benz[a]anthracene-induced papillomas in rhino mouse skin. Cancer Res. *27:* 237–241 (1967).

18   Cohen, S.M.; Wittenberg, J.F.; Bryan, G.T.: Effect of hyper and avitaminosis A on urinary bladder and carcinogenicity of *N*-(-4(5-nitro-2-fury))-2-thiazolyl)formamide (FANFT). Cancer Res. *36:* 2334–2339 (1976).

19   Newberne, P.; Rogers, A.E.: Rat colon carcinomas associated with aflatoxin and marginal vitamin A. J. natn. Cancer Inst. *50:* 439–448 (1973).

20   Moon, R.C.; Grubbs, C.J.; Sporn, M.B.; Goodman, D.G.: Retinyl acetate inhibits mammary carcinogenesis induced by *N*-methyl-*N*-nitrosourea. Nature, Lond. *267:* 620–621 (1977).

21   Grubbs, C.J.; Moon, R.C.; Sporn, M.B.; Newton, D.L.: Inhibition of mammary cancer by retinyl methyl ether. Cancer Res. *37:* 599–602 (1977).

22   Basu, T.K.; Donaldson, D.; Jenner, H.; Williams, D.C.; Sakula, A.: Plasma vitamin A in patients with bronchial carcinoma. Br. J. Cancer *33:* 119–121 (1976).

23   Ibrahim, K.; Jafarey, N.A.; Zuberi, S.I.: Plasma vitamin A and carotene levels in squamous cell carcinoma of the oral cavity and oro-pharynx. Clin. Oncol. *3:* 203–207 (1977).

24   Atukorala, S.; Basu, T.K.; Dickerson, J.W.T.; Donaldson, D.; Sakula, A.: Vitamin A, zinc and lung cancer. Br. J. Cancer *40:* 927–931 (1979).

25   Smith, J.C.; McDaniel, E.G.; Fan, F.F.; Halstead, J.A.: Zinc: a trace element essential in vitamin A metabolism. Science, N.Y. *181:* 954–955 (1973).

26   Ette, S.I.; Basu, T.K.; Dickerson, J.W.T.: Short-term effect of zinc-sulphate on plasma and hepatic concentrations of vitamins A and E.in normal weanling rats. Nutr. Metab. *23:* 11–16 (1979).

27   Basu, T.K.; Rowlands, L.; Jones, L.; Kohn, J.: Vitamin A and retinol-binding protein in patients with myelomatosis and cancer of epithelial origin. Eur. J. Cancer clin. Oncol. *18:* 339–342 (1982).

28   Atukorala, T.M.S.: Vitamin A and lung cancer; PhD thesis, Surrey (1980).

29   Bjelke, E.: Dietary vitamin A and human lung cancer. Int. J. Cancer *15:* 561–565 (1975).

30   Graham, S.; Mettlin, C.; Marshall, J.; Priore, R.; Rzepka, T.; Shedd, D.: Dietary factors in the epidemiology of cancer of the larynx. Am. J. Epidem. *113:* 675–680 (1981).

31 Hirayama, T.: Diet and cancer. Nutr. Cancer *1:* 67–81 (1979).

32 Mettlin, C.; Graham, S.; Swanson, M.: Vitamin A and lung cancer. J. natn. Cancer Inst. *62:* 1435–1438 (1979).

33 Mettlin, C.; Graham, S.: Dietary risk factors in human bladder cancer. Am. J. Epidem. *110:* 235–238 (1979).

34 MacLennan, R.; Da Costa, J.; Day, N.E.; Law, C.H.; Ng, Y.K.; Shanmugaratnam, K.: Risk factors for lung cancer in Singapore Chinese, a population with high female incidence rates. Int. J. Cancer *20:* 854–860 (1977).

35 Kark, J.D.; Smith, A.H.; Switza, B.R.; Haines, C.G.: Serum vitamin A (retinol) and cancer incidence in Evans County, Georgia. J. natn. Cancer Inst. *66:* 7–16 (1981).

36 Wald, N.; Idle, M.; Boreham, J.; Bailey, A.: Low serum vitamin A and subsequent risk of cancer. Lancet *ii:* 813–815 (1980).

37 Haines, A.P.; Thompson, S.G.; Basu, T.K.; Hunt, R.: Cancer, retinol binding protein, zinc and copper. Lancet *i:* 52 (1982).

38 Chan, V.: Retinol (vitamin A) and post-operative colorectal cancer; MSc thesis, Edmonton (1983).

39 Doll, R.: Strategy for detection of cancer hazards to man. Nature, Lond. *265:* 589–596 (1977).

40 March, B.; Biely, J.: Increased incidence of ovarian leukosis in response to excess vitamin A. Nature, Lond. *214:* 287–288 (1967).

41 Weiss, L.; Holyoke, E.: Some effects of hypervitaminosis A on metastasis of spontaneous breast cancer in mice. Cancer Inst. *43:* 1045–1054 (1969).

42 Clamon, G.H.; Nugent, K.M.; Rossl, N.P.: Cellular retinoic acid-binding protein in human lung carcinomas. J. natn. Cancer Inst. *67:* 61–63 (1981).

43 Lotan, R.; Ong, D.E.; Chytil, F.: Comparison of the level of cellular retinoid-binding proteins and susceptibility to retinoid-induced growth inhibition of various neoplastic cell lines. J. natn. Cancer Inst. *64:* 1259–1262 (1980).

44 Ong, D.E.; Page, D.L.; Chytil, F.: Retinoic acid-binding protein: occurrence in human tumor. Science *190:* 60–61 (1975).

45 Ong, D.E.; Chytil, F.: Presence of cellular retinol and retinoic acid-binding proteins in experimental tumors. Cancer Lett. *2:* 2530 (1976).

Dr. T.K. Basu, Faculty of Home Economics, Department of Foods and Nutrition, University of Alberta, Edmonton, Alberta T6G 2M8 (Canada)

Prasad (ed.), Vitamins, Nutrition, and Cancer, pp. 46–67 (Karger, Basel 1984)

Influence of the Antioxidants Vitamins C and E and of Selenium on Cancer

Paul M. Newberne, Voranunt Suphakarn

Department of Nutrition and Food Science, Massachusetts Institute of Technology, Cambridge, Mass., USA

Introduction

There is a continuing interest in the effects of nutrients on susceptibility to cancer in man and animals. The public has developed an intense interest during the past few years primarily because several epidemiologic studies have clearly indicated dietary effects on cancer incidence in human populations; these pieces of evidence include: (1) geographic distribution of tumors in subsets of populations; (2) changing incidence in migrant populations, (3) and tumor distribution by socioeconomic groups. Moreover, data from experimental animals support those, for the most part, gathered from observations in humans. A most fruitful area for cancer research [1–3] is that of anticarcinogenesis, a concept presented by *Falk* [4] more than a decade ago. He pointed out that the idea was already 20 years old at that time and was first put forth in the recorded literature in 1947 by *Crabtree* [5].

In order to put the subject into perspective we must realize that food is a complex mixture and that it contains more than just nutrients. Table I illustrates effects of semisynthetic diets, compared to a natural unrefined ingredient diet, on the response of rats to a few carcinogens; many more examples are available. While the target organs and the chemical structures of the carcinogens vary in all but one instance (diethylstilbestrol, DES), generally, the natural products had a protective effect against the development of cancer at the target site, indicating the presence of anticarcinogenic materials in the unrefined materials used to make the diets. In the single instance where diet was not effective (DES) the total effect is much more complicated and probably related in some way to the complexity of the synthetic character of the hormone. These data clearly imply that there are

Table I. Chemical carcinogenesis in rats: variation in incidence associated with type of diet fed

Chemical	Target organ	% rats with tumors	
		semisynthetic diet	natural ingredient diet
Acetylaminofluorene (AAF)	mammary gland	91	33
	liver	67	29
	ear duct	57	46
Estradiol, ethinyl	liver	96	48
	ovary/uterus	63	11
Diethylstilbestrol (DES)	ovary/uterus	67	67
Dimethylhydrazine (DMH)	colon	67	42

factors in natural foods consumed by animals and man which offer some protection from the effects of carcinogens, whatever the origin.

Table II lists only a few contaminants which occur in commercially prepared rodent diets used in animal experimentation. These variations represent a true variation in the average human diet as well. The nutrient content of animal and human diets varies over a wide range of values, in terms of essential nutrients as well as in environmental toxicants; these variations complicate attempts to interpret effects of human and animal diets on the development of cancer. Aflatoxins, nitrosamines, cadmium and lead, among others should be of concern to the investigator using them to test other types of chemicals since they can modify the response of animals to other chemicals. In addition, these observations emphasize the potential role of diet in cancer investigations, where nutrients or contaminants can either enhance or inhibit tumor induction. Of special interest are the vitamins C and E and selenium which also serve as antioxidants.

Table III lists a few of the known promoters and co-carcinogens of suggested consequence to human cancer. Based on epidemiologic observations, some of which are supported by animal studies, it seems likely that many of the essential dietary nutrients can be involved in predisposing or protecting human and animal populations to cancer. It is significant that protein, fat, and total calories, can markedly affect tumor induction in animals [6–10] and have been associated with a higher incidence of certain types of tumors in human populations [11–17]. The role of vitamins and vitamin analogues in the development of certain types of tumors has raised

Table II. Contaminants found in natural product diets [abridged from ref. 99 with permission]

Toxin	Dietary content, various lots
Aflatoxin B_1, ppb	10; 200; 120; 4; 21; 80
Nitrosamines, ppb	
N-Dimethylnitrosamine	8; 32; 18; 5; 83; 12
N-Nitrosopyrrolidine	7; 16; 5; 2; 11; 22
Nitrates, ppm	23; 41; 180; 5; 90; 3
PCBs, ppm	9; 3; 28; 15; 23; 5
Arsenic, ppm	0.3; 0; 3; 1; 4; 2
Lead, ppm	0.8; 4.2; 3.2; 1.0; 0.2; 2
Cadmium, ppm	0.5; 1.2; 0.9; 2.0; 1.3; 0.4
Mercury, ppm	0.7; 1.2; 0.5; 0.3; 0.8; 1.0

Table III. Dietary nutrients and other factors which act as promoters and co-carcinogens of probable consequence to human cancer

Dietary constituents	Non-nutrient factors
Lipotropes	alcohol
Protein	tobacco
Fat	endogenous hormones
Total calories	chlorinated hydrocarbons
Vitamins	drugs
Fiber	viruses

Table IV. Nitrite, amines, ascorbate and mouse lung adenomas [from ref. 35]

Treatment	Adenoma yield (mean)	Inhibition %
Piperazine + $NaNO_2$	8.3 ± 0.6	$-$[1]
Piperazine + $NaNO_2$ + vitamin C, 5.75 g/kg	5.2 ± 0.5	37
Piperazine + $NaNO_2$ + vitamin C, 23 g/kg	0.7 ± 0.2	91
Morpholine + $NaNO_2$	9.9 ± 0.8	$-$[1]
Morpholine + $NaNO_2$ + vitamin C, 5.75 g/kg	2.8 ± 0.4	72
Morpholine + $NaNO_2$ + vitamin C, 23 g/kg	1.1 ± 0.2	89

[1] Tumor incidence without added vitamin C.

possibilities for intervention, particularly for epithelial tumors where vitamin A and the retinoids have a profound inhibiting effect on tumor induction under controlled conditions [18–21]. This will be discussed in more detail later. In regard to other factors (table III), alcohol and tobacco are unquestionably associated with increases in certain types of tumors, especially those of the head and neck, including nasopharyngeal and esophageal tumors [1–3]. Hormones which are produced in the tissues of individuals have been suspect for years as possible tumor promoters; but chlorinated hydrocarbons, widely used as pesticides, are also suspect without convincing solid evidence. Drugs are known to modify the occurrence of cancer in man and in animals and viruses are implicated in human liver cancer [22–24]. These must be considered as potential co-carcinogens or synergistic substances in other human cancers.

The highly significant work that is now being done in large-scale epidemiologic studies and in laboratory experiments relative to the interactions of viruses and chemical carcinogens in human liver cancer are clearly pointing the way to an elucidation of etiologic agents and mechanisms of action [25–27]. Now that carriers of hepatitis B virus can be identified in populations at high or low risk for liver cancer, along with capabilities for measuring environmental exposure to other chemicals, including aflatoxins, means are at hand for a better understanding of the complex nature of cancer in human populations. These observations also point the way toward promising methods for intervention [28].

Effects of dietary factors on cancer, primarily in the experimental systems, have produced results which indicate an inhibitory effect of natural products, some of which are listed in table IV. In addition to these inhibiting agents there are many other dietary or environmental factors which modify chemical carcinogenesis. These include other chemical carcinogens, radiation, factors which affect rate of DNA repair, age, sex, hormones, immunologic status, genetic constitution, metabolism of chemical carcinogens (either activation or detoxification) and diet, nutrition and life-style [11].

The investigator, from a scientific point of view, interested in identifying nutrients which may influence cancer, is confronted by interests concerned more with financial gain than sincere health interests. If one enters a food store selling 'natural' products, for example, there are implications or specific statements about many factors which are presumably of great importance to the health of individuals and, by analogy, they aid in preventing cancer. There are books on diets that propose to prevent rapid aging, miracle foods which serve as medicines, instructions on how to triumph over disease by following a number of patterns of a dietary nature and, invariably, miracle vitamins and minerals, designed to lengthen your life and to prevent cancer [29]. For this reason those who are sincerely interested in providing information relative to dietary habits that may be of some help are sometimes reluctant to release factual information. Nevertheless, it is important to provide the public with information which may be of value, even though there is the danger of alerting individuals, with less interest in promoting health than in economic gain.

Ascorbic Acid and Cancer

Much has been written in recent years about the value of ascorbic acid in disease prevention [30, 31]. A great deal of research has been done relative to the effects of ascorbate on cancer induction and on the prevention of infectious disease. The clinical reports have received the most attention [32]. *Linus Pauling* is probably best known for his writings and discussions on the nature, causes, prevention and treatment of cancer with special reference to the value of vitamin C. We do not infer that *Pauling* is wrong because there is emerging evidence now that ascorbic acid may indeed be effective in preventing some forms of cancer [32, 33]. Certainly one cannot doubt the real or potential value of dietary ascorbic acid to prevent the nitrosation of amines which are in themselves highly carcinogenic to animal species [34–36].

It was early in the 1960s when reports appeared in the literature noting that consuming foods rich in ascorbic acid was inversely related to the appearance of certain types of cancer [37–39]. These reports suggest that vitamin C protects against gastric cancer, perhaps by blocking the reaction of secondary amines with nitrite to form *N*-nitroso compounds, some of which are gastric carcinogens but also by other mechanisms as well.

Some of the epidemiologic studies conducted early in the 1970s were concerned with human populations along the Caspian littoral of Iran [34]. In these studies there was an inverse association between esophageal cancer and the consumption of fresh fruits which contain ascorbic acid [34]. More recently another report has appeared which indicates an inverse relationship between vitamin C consumption and uterine cervical dysplasia in women in New York [39]. On the other hand, *Jain* et al. [40] have failed to find an association between ascorbic acid consumption and colon cancer in a case-control study.

Table V. Reported untoward effects of ascorbic acid [abridged from ref. 36]

Acidosis	Renal stones
Oxaluria	Gastrointestinal disturbances
Fatigue	Destruction of other vitamins
Sterility	

There is additional evidence suggesting a role for ascorbic acid from human and animal studies [41–45]. It has been shown conclusively that ascorbic acid can prevent nitrosation of amines which in turn prevents the formation of nitrosamines, some of which are gastric carcinogens [41–45]. Table IV illustrates data taken from the work of *Mirvish* [35]. Vitamin C significantly inhibited the nitrosation of two important amines.

Despite the fact that there is some encouraging data relative to the anticarcinogenic effects of ascorbic acid there are also some reported untoward effects of vitamin C. Table V lists some of these that have been reported by a number of investigators. Other cases of adverse effects can be listed but these in table V serve to indicate that the use of higher than recommended levels of ascorbic acid can, under some conditions, result in unwanted side effects [37].

Some groups of American populations subsist on diets somewhat different from the major population groups; these include the Seventh-Day Adventists (SDA) [13] and the Mormons, as well as vegetarians with no religious persuasion. Table VI lists some of the differences in the dietary intake of SDA, a subset of our population known to have a remarkably diminished incidence of cancer of most sites compared to the non-SDA population of the USA. These data, listed in table VI, indicate a significant difference in the intake of animal fat, carbohydrates, vitamin A and, in particular, vitamin C. One cannot infer, however, that this is directly related to the differences but there is an association.

Additional data are available from both experimental studies and epidemiologic studies relative to an association of increased ascorbic acid and decreased cancer. One of the more interesting aspects is the association of salt-cured meats, pickled and smoked foods which correlate with an increased incidence of esophageal and stomach cancer [46]. There is a high stomach cancer rate in Japan which moderates when individuals migrate to either Hawaii or to California. Following migration those individuals generally assume the life-style and food habits of the local population and also

Table VI. Dietary intake of Seventh Day Adventists (SDA) compared to all USA White population [abridged from ref. 13]

Nutrient	Mean calories, %		All USA Whites
	California lacto-ovo vegetarians	White SDA use meat 4 times/week	
Total fat	36.1	40.7	42.6
Vegetable fat	24.7	17.6	18.3
Animal fat	8.6	19.5	24.3
Total protein	13.5	15.6	16.2
Vegetable protein	7.8	5.1	5.9
Animal protein	5.5	10.1	10.3
Starch	17.1	15.4	14.7
Vitamin A, IU/day	10,396	10,193	5,216
Vitamin C, mg/day	314	250	83

assume a similar cancer incidence. When Japanese move to the USA there is reduction in stomach cancer and an accompanying increase in colon tumors. Thus, the life-style and food habits may involve more than one target organ; cancer frequency in the migrants generally approaches that of the population native to the area to which they migrate.

Pickled, salt-cured, spicy foods are often associated with the formation of nitrosamines in foods; their consumption by populations that have had a high incidence of stomach cancer suggests that conditions that promote the formation of nitrosamines increase the risk of cancer of the stomach. While this has not been established in human populations it is clearly the case in experimental animal studies. Ascorbic acid inhibits the formation of nitrosamines; this appears to be a result of reacting with nitrite before it can react with amines in the diet to form the toxic and carcinogenic nitrosamines [35, 47]. This then is the likely means by which ascorbic acid prevents some forms of cancer in animals and perhaps in human populations. The evidence for such mechanisms in human populations, however, is yet to be produced.

It is of interest to cite at this point some other experimental data. Ascorbic acid prevented the nitrosation of a broad variety of amines, including drugs such as oxytetracycline, morpholine, piperazine, and other amines including *N*-methylamine, methylurea and dimethylamine [47].

Table VII. Results of a double-blind study on high-dose vitamin C in cancer patients [abridged from ref. 48]

| | Treatment | |
	placebo	vitamin C
Number of patients	63	60
Tumor sites		
Colorectal	26	24
Pancreas	12	12
Lung	6	6
Stomach	5	5
Other	16	12
Results		
Survival	no difference	
Symptoms	no difference	

There are numerous examples of drugs and chemicals, many of which are common in human environments. Thus, naturally occurring amines in our daily diets are nitrosatable to form nitrosamines [47].

Table VII lists a summary of the results of the double-blind study conducted by *Creagan* et al. [48] relative to high doses of ascorbic acid in cancer patients. The study reported in 1979 revealed no differences between those that were given ascorbic acid (60 patients) and those given a placebo (63 patients). There were no differences in survival time or in symptoms between the two subsets of cancer patients.

Table VIII lists additional experimental evidence for an association between cancer and ascorbic acid. From these data, provided by a number of investigators [41–44], it seems clear that the influence of ascorbic acid on different types of tumors is varied and has a mixed result. From the data shown in the foregoing tables, and from additional observations, it is evident from the results of animal studies that the data are conflicting, the epidemiologic studies in humans are weak, but it is established that vitamin C inhibits the formation of some carcinogens by interfering primarily with nitrosation of amines. Thus, the ingestion of vitamin C-containing foods appears to lower the risk of certain types of tumors. A few comments on the possible mechanisms which may account for these observations are in order.

Table VIII. Effects of ascorbic acid on a variety of tumors in animal studies [from ref. 41–44]

Carcinogen	Tumor type	Animal	Effect
Dimethylhydrazine	carcinoma	rat	decrease
Benzo[a]pyrene	sarcoma	rat	decrease
FANFT	carcinoma	rat	none
3-MCA	sarcoma	guinea pig	increased
3-MCA	sarcoma	guinea pig	none

Ascorbic acid affects the mixed function oxidase system in animals; this may be another mechanism by which it influences carcinogenesis. Most of the chemical carcinogens that have been studied require metabolic activation often by way of the MFO activity in the liver [49]. Furthermore, ascorbic acid has an inhibitory action both in vitro and in vivo on the nitrosation of secondary amines as pointed out earlier. It is likely that one of the most significant anticancer effects of ascorbic acid is through its blocking of nitrosation of amines by reacting with a large number of nitrosating agents [47]. However, an earlier report [50] indicated that vitamin C selectively destroyed malignant cells, an observation yet to be confirmed. *Edgar* [45] found that carcinogens, such as carbon tetrachloride, and some of the nitrosamines deplete the body stores of ascorbic acid, and *Banic* [51] reported that a high intake of ascorbic acid had an enhancing effect on the induction of sarcoma by 3-methylcholanthrene (3-MCA).

Vitamin E

Vitamin E is present in a wide variety of natural foods including vegetable oils, eggs, whole grains and many of the cereals. The primary form of vitamin E is α-tocopherol, a methyl substituted 6-hydroxycoumarin derivative with a 16 carbon side chain. The concentration of vitamin E in the various foods is usually proportional to the amount of linoleic acid present, which is particularly high in safflower oil. A minimum daily requirement is estimated to be about 30 IU or 15 mg, an amount that is likely to be present in almost every type of diet consumed by human populations [52]. Vitamin E appears to be nontoxic in moderate doses; the ingestion of 800 IU daily for 3 years caused no ill effects in man [53]. A major physiologic role of vitamin E is its ability to function as an antioxidant and as a free radical scavenger. It is especially active in inhibiting lipid peroxidation [54].

The biological effects of vitamin E deficiency have been well described in animals; they vary considerably from one species to another. A deficiency results in disorders of the reproductive, musculoskeletal, central nervous and vascular systems. A deficiency of vitamin E in human populations has not been clearly identified. There were no appreciable clinical disorders observed in human volunteers maintained on vitamin E deficiency diets for 6 years. However, the red blood cells of the volunteers became more sensitive to in vitro oxidative hemolysis [55]. In addition, a hemolytic anemia, which is vitamin E-responsive, has been described in premature infants, a condition caused apparently by insufficient development of free radical defense mechanisms. A wide variety of clinical signs and symptoms have been attributed to vitamin E deficiency but there is no substantial scientific evidence to support the claims.

To date there is no epidemiologic evidence that vitamin E has an influence on tumor induction in humans. The only remotely possible correlation has been through studies related to the consumption of certain foods that contain vitamin E. These, however, are still speculative and will not be covered in this report.

There are data in the literature indicating that vitamin E or α-tocopherol can have an influence on tumors induced in experimental animals [56–63]. There is some indication that vitamin E acts similarly to ascorbic acid in blocking the formation of nitrosamines. Since vitamin E is fat-soluble, its effect on the inhibition of nitrosation would likely take place in a lipid milieu; this is in contrast to vitamin C which inhibits nitrosation in an aqueous environment.

Several investigators have studied the effects of α-tocopherol on dimethylbenzanthracene (DMBA)-induced mammary tumors in animals [56, 57, 59]. It has been reported that the ingestion of high levels of α-tocopherol during the initiation stage of mammary tumors had no effect. However, other reports indicate that a large vitamin E supplement fed prior to DMBA exposure decreased tumor incidence by as much as 50%. *Lee and Chen* [64] reported that α-tocopherol at a reduced level in the diet resulted in an increased tumor incidence. There was no significant difference in the tumor incidence between mice fed the high or the low doses of vitamin E; however, the average number of tumors per animal was less if the mice were fed the high vitamin E diet.

Shamberger [65] reported an effect of vitamin E on skin tumors promoted by croton oil in mice. If vitamin E were applied topically a number of days after the carcinogen was applied there was a significant decrease in the number of tumors. Mice with benzo[a]pyrene-induced sarcomas survived longer if they were given vitamin E (α-tocopherol). *Haber and Wissler* [57] noted that there was a marked decrease in the carcinogenicity of methylcholanthrene in mice if the animals were given diets containing supplemental vitamin E. A number of other investigators have reported some effects of vitamin E on tumorigenesis. From these studies it is clear that the results of vitamin E and its effects on tumorigenesis is variable. The results appear to depend in part on the carcinogen that is used and in part on the animal species that is used as a model.

The well-known effect of vitamin E as a blocking agent in nitrosation confirms a role as a protective agent in the environment. Vitamin E competes for available nitrite and in this way, as with ascorbic acid, it blocks the nitrosation of amines and amides, reducing the amount of nitrosamines in foods and in the environment. Segregating effects of ascorbic acid from α-tocopherol on blocking nitrosation is yet to be done, but should prove to be informative; vitamin C is a hydrophilic and vitamin E is lipophilic.

Additional data of interest have been reported. *Shklar* [66] has observed an inhibition of oral carcinogenesis in hamsters by vitamin E. A most interesting review of effects of vitamin E, selenium and other antioxidants on cancer, through immunosurveillance, is provided by *Baumgartner* [67]. A large body of evidence now exists to clearly indicate that vitamin E has an important enhancing effect on the immune system, perhaps one mechanism for its influence on carcinogenesis.

Selenium

Selenium is an essential constituent of the diet of animals and probably is required for humans as well; in excess, however, it is toxic. The World Health Organization has reviewed selenium as to its role as a nutrient for animals and man but has made no recommendation about dietary intakes or tolerable levels for man [68]. The Food and Nutrition Board of the National Academy of Sciences, National Research Council [69] suggested a daily requirement of 60–120 µg of selenium for humans based on data from animal studies. It was pointed out that supplements considered for those living in low selenium areas might need to be in a range of 50–100 µg of selenium/person/day which from animal studies would appear to be safe.

An excellent review [70] brings the subject up to date from about 1974 and points out the more relevant information published in the interim. These authors have concluded that the role of selenium is still an open question. Early reports of cause and effect appear to be unfounded; selenium is not carcinogenic to the liver of experimental animals, as was recorded earlier. More recently evidence has been presented to support the contention that selenium may have anticarcinogenic properties in rats and mice. Table IX lists some of the data from a number of experimental studies.

There is an estimated daily intake of selenium of about 4–35 µg/person in infants and 60–250 µg in adults. Furthermore, it has been shown that animal feed supplementation can increase the meat content of selenium by as much as 30%. Studies to date have shown that most selenium is absorbed from the gastrointestinal tract and up to 50% is excreted in the urine. The remaining portion is retained primarily in the liver and the kidney, from which it is slowly released.

Selenium is increased in human tissues in some disease states. For example, it is increased in the synovia of patients with rheumatoid arthritis. It is increased in patients with leukemia or cancers of the reticuloendothelial system and it is increased in pregnancy, primarily as glutathione peroxidase (GSH-PX) in red blood cells. At the termination of pregnancy, however, it returns to a normal concentration. In normal healthy humans, the serum mean concentration of selenium is 0.118 µg/ml and in whole blood it varies from 0.10 to 0.34 µg/ml. In two conditions, however, where selenium deficiency has been suggested (kwashiorkor and sudden infant death

Table IX. Selenium inhibition of carcinogenesis

Tumor model		Target organ	Change in tumor incidence
species	carcinogen		
Mouse	DMBA	mammary gland	
Mouse	MMTV	mammary gland	
Rat	DMH	colon	
Rat	MAM	colon	
Rat	3'-MeDAB	liver	
Rat	AAF	liver	

in children), serum levels range from 0.08 to 0.11 μg/ml – well within normal ranges.

A biological role for selenium has been well established in animals. Selenium-dependent enzymes have been most studied; these include GSH-PX in red blood cells, in kidney, heart, and liver; other selenium-containing enzymes include formate dehydrogenase, glycine reductase, and nicotinic acid hydrolase [71]. The most important of these selenium dependent enzymes appears to be GSH-PX which is widely distributed in mammalian cells. Selenium as a selenoprotein is also found in heart muscle, in testes and in fetal calf serum. Furthermore, selenium-containing transfer RNAs have been identified which may play a regulatory role in nucleic acid metabolism.

Clayton and Bowman [72] first noted an effect of selenium on carcinogenesis in 1949. These investigators fed rats semisynthetic diets and gave them a 3′-Me-dimethylaminoazobenzene (3′-MeDAB) diet for 2 weeks; a diet free of the azo dye and supplemented with 5 ppm of selenium was then fed for 4 weeks. This was followed by an additional 4-week exposure to the dye. This regimen resulted in a 50% reduction in liver tumors in those animals given supplementary selenium during the intermediate period of exposure to the carcinogen. The early work of *Shamberger* [65] also showed that sodium selenite inhibited carcinogenesis. Many other studies have attested to a role for selenium in protecting against carcinogenesis in animal models [73–87].

Griffin [87] has shown in a series of studies that selenium, as sodium selenite in the drinking water, decreased the number of colon tumors in rats given injections of dimethylhydrazine. Furthermore, they have also shown that liver tumors in rats given 3′-MeDAB or 2-acetylaminofluorene (2-AAF) were also reduced in number in animals given supplementary sodium selenite. Table IX illustrates protective effects of selenium on experimentally induced cancer.

Wilt et al. [88] reported that selenium must be present during the initiation phase for inhibition of the formation of papillomas in mice exposed to DMBA, followed by a promoting agent. The recent report of *Soullier* et al. [89] is of significance. Rats fed a high fat diet and treated with azoxymethane to induce intestinal cancer exhibited a marked reduction in the number of tumors, particularly in the upper part of the colon, when they were given 8 ppm of selenium in the drinking water.

The long-standing interest and investigations of *Schrauzer* [90] have shown that the administration of selenium reduced the number of spontaneous tumors in mice. These observations have been confirmed by *Medina and Shepherd* [91]. *Thompson and Becci* [92] reported that sodium selenite inhibited mammary carcinogenesis in rats given methylnitrosourea. Furthermore, these investigators have shown that mammary tumors induced in rats by DMBA were inhibited by sodium selenite in the diet. The various studies referred to above clearly indicate that selenium in some as yet obscure manner does influence carcinogenesis in experimental animals.

The more recent work of *Ip* et al. [93–97] has shown that supplementation with selenium had an effect on mammary tumor induction, reducing the incidence and increasing lag time of the mammary tumors that were induced. In further studies comparing quality and quantity of dietary fat it was observed that while GSH-PX levels in the mammary tissue were affected by both the quality of fat and supplementation with selenium, these modifications in tumor incidence were not associated with tissue peroxidation.

Studies at the Massachusetts Institute of Technology have clearly indicated an effect of selenium on the induction of liver tumors. Tables X and XI list the effects of selenium on acute and chronic exposure to a carcinogen. Liver tumor induction by aflatoxin in animals given selenium was observed using selenium in amounts varying from a deficiency level (0.05 ppm) to an excess of 5 ppm [98–100]. The interesting aspect of these data is that while a low but adequate concentration of selenium did not seem to affect the induction of liver tumors, there was a pronounced protective effect at levels of 10-fold that considered to be adequate under normal conditions. Furthermore, as an excess was reached there was an enhancing effect of selenium on liver injury and tumor induction. This latter observation would appear to be related in some way to the liver injury as a result of excess selenium which was then more susceptible to the effects of cancer. This may in turn relate to the production of epigenetic events, aberrant methylation of DNA and the effects of peroxidation and tissue injury. This hypothesis is untested but seems reasonable and is under study in our laboratory. Based on preliminary observations, however, peroxidation does not appear to be a highly significant factor in tumor induction in some models, but this requires further study.

Studies which may have predicted some of the more recent observations clearly indicated a profound effect of selenium on prenatal and perinatal development of important organs and systems [89] and on the acute response to toxins [100]. Unpublished studies on-going in our laboratories showing that selenium appears to have a protective effect on the induction

Table X. Influence of selenium on body weight and mortality of rats exposed to aflatoxin B$_1$ [from ref. 98]

Se content of diet, ppm	Body weight, g[1]		
	initial	2 weeks	2-week mortality
0.03	100 ± 2	208 ± 4	28/29
0.10	104 ± 1	202 ± 3	20/30
1.00	101 ± 2	187 ± 5	7/28
5.00	103 ± 2	190 ± 6	27/29

[1] $\pm$ standard error.

Table XI. Effect of selenium on liver carcinogenesis

Group	Treatment, ppm		Liver injury	Nodular hyperplasia	Hepatocellular carcinoma
	aflatoxin B$_1$	selenium			
1	−	0.05	0	0	0/20
2	+	0.10	0	0	0/20
3	+	0.50	0	0	0/20
4	+	1.00	0	0	0/20
5	+	2.00	0	1/20	0/20
6	+	3.50	+	3/20	0/20
7	+	5.00	+	20/20	14/20

Aflatoxin B$_1$ was administered after 8 weeks on diet, 5 daily doses of 10 μg each. Rats were kept on respective diets 12 months.

of esophageal tumors induced by methylbenzylnitrosamine are of interest and will be reported in another communication on completion. Preliminary results equate in part with the report from *Sparnins* et al. [102] that there is an enhancement of glutathione *s*-transferase activity in the esophagus of animals treated with phenols, lactones and benzylisothioxyanide. While the relationship of glutathione *s*-transferase and glutathione peroxidase has not been completely elucidated, it is likely that this enhancement of glutathione *s*-transferase is similar to the enhancement of glutathione peroxidase and the protective effect by selenium may act through this mechanism to diminish the induction of tumors.

The situation in human populations relative to selenium deficiency or excess and its relation to carcinogenesis is still an open question. It is well known that selenium compounds possess a high degree of toxicity; either a deficiency or an excess may have severe consequences and result in a number of diseases in animals. A recent report from the mainland of China [103] regarding a cardiomyopathy which occurs in children living in some areas that are markedly deficient in selenium is of interest in regard to human needs for selenium. This syndrome, which occurs seasonally, responds to selenium administration. Cardiomyopathies have been reported from other parts of the world, including some regions of the USA and Finland, but the scientific basis for a relation between cardiomyopathies and selenium in the USA is not currently available.

Some recent studies from New Zealand, where the soil content of selenium is low and there is a known low level of selenium in the serum and tissues of natives, are of interest in the context of this presentation. *Robinson* et al. [104] have examined the situation in cancer patients and have looked at a number of parameters including the selenium levels of whole blood and GSH-PX activities. Table 17 of *Robinson* et al. [104] lists blood, selenium and GSH-PX levels in New Zealand cancer patients. The patients, with cancer of the stomach, colon, bladder, breast, liver and pancreas, as well as other sites, had selenium levels and enzyme activities equivalent to normal healthy individuals from the same geographic areas. It was concluded from these studies that even though there was some decrease in selenium status of cancer patients it was no lower than that of other elderly subjects and of patients without cancer. However, the levels were less than half that of US values. Despite these findings the investigators concluded that the low selenium status of cancer patients in New Zealand was most likely a consequence of illness or of age and not a cause of cancer.

References

1   Hiatt, H.H.; Watson, J.D.; Winsten, J.A. (eds): Origins of human cancer. Cold Spring Harbor Laboratory, vols. 1–3 (Cold Spring Harbor, New York 1977).
2   Cairns, J.: Cancer: science and society (Freeman, San Francisco 1978).
3   Doll, R.; Peto, R.: The causes of cancer: quantitative estimates of avoidable risks of cancer in the United States today. J. natn. Cancer Inst. *66:* 1191–1308 (1981).

4 Falk, H.L.: Anticarcinogenesis – an alternative. Prog. exp. Tumor Res., vol. 14, pp. 105–137 (Karger, Basel 1971).

5 Crabtree, H.G.: Anticarcinogenesis – an alternative. Br. med. Bull. *4:* 345–347 (1947).

6 Carroll, K.K.; Khor, H.T.: Dietary fats in relation to tumorigenesis. Prog. Biochem. Pharmacol. *10:* 308–353 (1975).

7 Rogers, A.E.; Wetsel, W.C.: Mammary carcinogenesis in rats fed different amounts and types of fat. Cancer Res. *41:* 3735–3737 (1981).

8 Silverstone, H.; Tannenbaum, A.: Proportion of dietary protein and the formation of spontaneous hepatomas in the mouse. Cancer Res. *11:* 442–446 (1951).

9 Wells, P.; Alftergood, L.; Alfin-Slater, R.B.: Effect of varying levels of dietary protein on tumor development and lipid metabolism in rats exposed to aflatoxin. J. Am. Oil Chem. Soc. *53:* 559–562 (1976).

10 Tannenbaum, A.: The dependence of tumor formation on the degree of caloric restriction. Cancer Res. *5:* 609–615 (1945).

11 Armstrong, B.; Doll, R.: Environmental factors and cancer incidence and mortality in different countries with special reference to dietary practices. Int. J. Cancer *15:* 617–631 (1975).

12 Kolonel, L.H.; Hankin, J.H.; Lee, J.; Chu, S.Y.; Nomura, A.M.Y.; Hunds, M.W.: Nutrient intakes in relation to cancer incidence in Hawaii. Br. J. Cancer *44:* 332–339 (1981).

13 Phillips, R.L.; Garfinkel, L.; Kuzma, J.W.; Beeson, W.L.; Lotz, T.; Brin, B.: Mortality among California Seventh-Day Adventists for selected cancer sites. J. natn. Cancer Inst. *65:* 1097–1107 (1980).

14 Blair, A.; Fraumeni, J.F., Jr.: Geographic patterns of prostate cancer in the United States. J. natn. Cancer Inst. *61:* 1379–1384 (1978).

15 Schuman, L.M.; Mandele, J.S.; Radke, A.; Seal, U.; Halberg, F.: Some selected features of the epidemiology of prostate cancer: Minneapolis-St. Paul, Minnesota, case-control study 1976–1979; in Magnus, Trends in cancer incidence: causes and practical implications, pp. 345–354 (Hemisphere Publishing, Washington 1982).

16 deWaard, F.; Cornelis, J.P.; Saki, K.; Yoshida, M.: Breast cancer incidence according to weight and height in two cities of the Netherlands and in Sichi Prefecture. Jap. Cancer *40:* 1269–1275 (1977).

17 Lew, E.A.; Garfinkel, L.: Variations in mortality by weight among 750,000 men and women. J. chron. Dis. *32:* 563–567 (1979).

18 Newberne, P.M.; Suphakarn, V.: Preventive role of vitamin A in colon cancer in rats. Cancer Res. *40:* 2553–2556 (1977).

19 Smith, D.M.; Rogers, A.E.; Herndon, B.J.; Newberne, P.M.: Vitamin A (retinyl acetate) and benzo[a]pyrene-induced respiratory tract carcinogenesis in hamsters fed a commercial diet. Cancer Res. *35:* 11–16 (1975).

20 Newberne, P.M.; Rogers, A.E.: Rat colon carcinomas associated with aflatoxin and marginal vitamin A. J. natn. Cancer Inst. *50:* 439–448 (1973).

21 Sporn, M.B.; Newton, D.L.: Chemoprevention of cancer with retinoids. Fed. Proc. *38:* 2528–2534 (1979).

22 Schottenfeld, D.: Cancer risks of medical treatment. Ca-A Cancer J. Clinicians *32:* 258–279 (1982).

23 O'Gara, R.W.; Adamson, R.H.; Kelly, M.G.: Neoplasms of the hemopoietic system

in non-human primates: report of one spontaneous tumor and two leukemias induced by procarbazine. J. natn. Cancer Inst. *46:* 1121–1130 (1971).

24 Kripke, M.L.; Boros, T.: Immunosuppression and carcinogenesis. Israel J. med. Scis *10:* 888–903 (1974).

25 Blumberg, B.S.; Larouze, B.; London, W.T.; et al.: The relation of infection with hepatitis B agent to hepatic carcinoma. Am. J. Path. *81:* 669–682 (1975).

26 Trichopoulos, D.; Tabor, E.; Gerety, R.J.; et al.: Hepatitis B and primary hepatocellular carcinoma in a European population. Lancet *ii:* 1217–1219 (1978).

27 O'Kuda, K.; Nakashima, T.; Sakamoto, K.; et al.: Hepatocellular carcinoma arising in noncirrhotic and highly cirrhotic livers. Cancer *49:* 450–455 (1982).

28 Beasley, R.P.; Hwang, L.Y.; Lin, C.C.; Chien, C.S.: Hepatocellular carcinoma and hepatitis B virus. A prospective study of 22,707 men in Taiwan. Lancet *ii:* 1129–1131 (1981).

29 Young, V.R.; Newberne, P.M.: Vitamins and cancer prevention. Issues and dilemmas. Cancer *47:* 1226–1240 (1981).

30 Johnson, F.C.: The antioxidant vitamins. CRC crit. Rev. Food Sci. Nutr. *11:* 217–310 (1979).

31 Cameron, E.; Pauling, L.; Leibowitz, B.: Ascorbic acid and cancer: a review. Cancer Res. *39:* 663–681 (1979).

32 Pauling, L.: Vitamin C therapy of advanced cancer. New Engl. J. Med. *302:* 694–698 (1980).

33 Graham, S.; Mettlin, C.; Marshall, J.; Priore, R.; Rzepka, T.; Shedd, D.: Dietary factors in the epidemiology of cancer of the larynx. Am. J. Epidem. *113:* 675–680 (1981).

34 Cook-Mozaffari, P.: The epidemiology of cancer of the esophagus. Nutr. Cancer *1:* 51–60 (1979).

35 Mirvish, S.S.: Inhibition of the formation of carcinogenic *N*-nitroso compounds by ascorbic acid and other compounds; in Burchenal, Oettgen, Cancer: achievements, challenges and prospects for the 1980s, vol. 1, pp. 557–587 (Grune & Stratton, New York 1981).

36 Mirvish, S.; Cardesa, A.; Wallcane, L.; Shubik, P.: Induction of mouse lung adenomas by amines or urea plus nitrite. J. natn. Cancer Inst. *55:* 633–636 (1975).

37 Ivankovic, S.; Preussmann, R.; Schmahl, D.; Zeller, J.W.: Prevention of ascorbic acid of in vivo formation of *N*-nitroso compounds; in Bogowski, Walker, *N*-nitroso compounds in the environment, IARC publ. No. 9, pp. 101–102 (IARC, Lyon 1975).

38 Graham, S.; Mettlin, C.; Marshall, J.; et al.: Dietary factors in the epidemiology of cancer of the larynx. Am. J. Epidem. *113:* 675–680 (1981).

39 Wassertheil-Smoller, S.; Romney, S.L.; Wylie-Rosett, J.; Slagle, G.; Miller, D.; Lucido, C.; Duttagupta, P.; Palan, R.: Dietary vitamin C and uterine cervical dysplasia. Am. J. Epidem. *114:* 714–724 (1981).

40 Jain, M.; Cook, G.M.; Davis, F.G.; Grace, G.; Howe, R.; Miller, A.B.: A case-control study of diet and colorectal cancer. Int. J. Cancer *26:* 757–768 (1980).

41 Logue, T.; Frommer, D.: The influence of oral vitamin C supplements on experimental colorectal tumor induction (Abstract). Aust. N.Z. J. Med. *10:* 588 (1980).

42 Kallistratos, G.; Fasske, E.: Inhibition of benzo[a]pyrene carcinogenesis in rats with vitamin C. J. Cancer Res. clin. Oncol. *97:* 91–96 (1980).

43 Soloway, M.S.; Cohen, S.M.; Dekernion, J.B.; Peroky, L.: Failure of ascorbic acid to inhibit FANFT-induced bladder cancer. J. Urol. *113:* 483–486 (1975).

44 Russell, W.O.; Ortega, L.R.; Wynne, E.S.: Studies on methylcholanthrene induction of tumors in scorbutic guinea pigs. Cancer Res. *12:* 216–218 (1952).

45 Edgar, J.A.: Ascorbic acid and biological alkylating agents. Nature, Lond. *248:* 136–137 (1974).

46 Wynder, W.L.; McCoy, G.D.; Reddy, B.S.; Cohen, L.; Hill, P.; Spingarn, N.E.; Weisburger, J.H.: Nutrition and metabolic epidemiology of cancers of the oral cavity, esophagus, colon, breast, prostate and stomach; in Newell, Ellison, Nutrition and cancer: etiology and treatment, pp. 11–48 (Raven Press, New York 1981).

47 National Academy of Sciences: The health effects of nitrate, nitrite and *N*-nitroso compounds (National Academy Press, Washington 1981).

48 Creagan, E.T.; Moertel, C.G.; O'Fallon, J.R.; et al.: Failure of high dose vitamin C (ascorbic acid) therapy to benefit patients with advanced cancer. New Engl. J. Med. *301:* 687–690 (1979).

49 Zannoni, V.G.; Flynn, E.J.; Lynch, M.: Ascorbic acid and drug metabolism. Biochem. Pharmacol. *21:* 1377–1392 (1972).

50 Benade, L.; Howard, T.; Burk, D.: Synergistic killing of Ehrlich ascites carcinoma cells by ascorbate +3-amino-1,2,4-thiazole. Oncology *23:* 33–43 (1969).

51 Banic, S.: Vitamin C acts as a co-carcinogen to methylcholanthrene in guinea pigs. Cancer Lett. *11:* 239–242 (1981).

52 Horwitt, M.: Vitamin E; in Goodhart, Shils, Modern nutrition in health and disease, pp. 181–191 (Febiger, Philadelphia 1980).

53 Farrell, P.; Bieri, J.: Megameanis supplementation in man. Am. J. clin. Nutr. *28:* 1381–1385 (1975).

54 Oski, F.: Metabolism and phyisologic role of vitamin E. Hosp. Pract. *12:* 79–85 (1977).

55 Horwitt, M.; Harvey, C.; Duncan, G.; Wilson, W.: Effect of limited tocopherol intake in man with relationship to erythrocyte hemolysis and lipid peroxidation. Am. J. clin. Nutr. *4:* 408–419 (1956).

56 Jaffe, W.G.: The influence of wheat germ oil on the production of tumors in rats by methylcholanthrene. Expl Med. Surg. *4:* 278–282 (1946).

57 Haber, S.L.; Wissler, R.W.: Effect of vitamin E on carcinogenicity of methylcholanthrene. Proc. Soc. exp. Biol. Med. *111:* 774–775 (1962).

58 Epstein, S.S.; Joshi, S.; Audrea, J.; Forsyth, J.; Mantel, N.: The null effect of antioxidants on the carcinogenicity of 3,4,9-10-dibenzpyrene of mice. Life Sci. *6:* 225–233 (1967).

59 Wattenberg, L.W.: Inhibition of carcinogenic and toxic effects of antioxidants and ethoxyquin. J. natn. Cancer Inst. *48:* 1425–1430 (1972).

60 Harman, D.: Dimethylbenzanthracene-induced cancer: inhibiting effect of dietary vitamin E. Clin. Res. *17:* 125–128 (1969).

61 Cook, M.G.; McNamara, P.: Effect of dietary vitamin E on dimethylhydrazine-induced colonic tumors in mice. Cancer Res. *40:* 1329–1331 (1980).

62 Kamm, J.J.; Dashman, T.; Newmark, H.; Mergens, W.J.: Inhibition of amine-nitrite hepatotoxicity by α-tocopherol. Toxicol. appl. Pharmacol. *41:* 575–583 (1977).

63 Mergens, W.J.; Kamm, J.J.; Newmark, H.L.; Fiddler, W.; Pensabene, J.: Alpha-

tocopherol: uses in preventing nitrosamine formation; in Walker, Castegnaro, Griciute, Lyle, Environmental aspects of *N*-nitroso compounds, No. 19, pp. 199–212 (IARC, Lyon 1978).

64 Lee, C.; Chen, C.: Enhancement of mammary tumorigenesis in rats by vitamin E deficiency (Abstract). Proc. Am. Ass. Cancer Res. *20:* 132 (1979).

65 Shamberger, R.J.: Relationship of selenium to cancer. I. Inhibitory effect of selenium on carcinogenesis. J. natn. Cancer Inst. *44:* 931–936 (1970).

66 Shklar, G.: Oral mucosal carcinogenesis inhibition by vitamin E. J. natn. Cancer Inst. *68:* 791–797 (1982).

67 Baumgartner, W.A.: Antioxidants, cancer and the immune response; in Kharasch, Trace metals in health and disease, pp. 287–305 (Raven Press, New York 1979).

68 WHO: Trace elements in human nutrition. Tech. Rep. Ser. Wld Hlth Org. *532* (1973).

69 National Academy of Sciences, National Research Council. Food and Nutrition Board: Are selenium supplements needed by the general public? J. Am. Dietetic Ass. *70:* 249–250 (1977).

70 Lo, M.T.; Sandi, E.: Selenium: Occurrence in foods and its toxicological significance. A review. J. envir. Path. Toxicol. *4:* 193–218 (1980).

71 Stadtman, P.C.: Selenium dependent enzymes. A. Rev. Biochem. *49:* 93–110 (1980).

72 Clayton, C.C.; Bowman, C.A.: Diet and azotumors: effect of dietary period when the diet is not fed. Cancer Res. *9:* 575–582 (1949).

73 National Academy of Sciences: Selenium in nutrition. A Report of the Subcommittee on Selenium, Committee on Animal Nutrition (National Academy of Sciences, Washington 1971).

74 Shamberger, R.J.; Frost, D.V.: Letter to the editor: possible protective effect of selenium against human cancer. Can. med. Ass. J. *100:* 682 (1969).

75 Shamberger, R.J.; Willis, C.E.: Selenium distribution and human cancer mortality. CRC crit. Rev. clin. Lab. Sci. *2:* 211 (1971).

76 Shamberger, R.J.; Tytko, S.A.; Willis, C.E.: Antioxidants and cancer. VI. Selenium and age-adjusted human cancer mortality. Archs envir. Hlth *31:* 231 (1976).

77 Shamberger, R.J.; Rukovena, E.; Longfield, A.K.; Tytko, S.A.; Deodhar, S.; Willis, C.E.: Antioxidants and cancer. I. Selenium in the blood of normals and cancer patients. J. natn. Cancer Inst. *50:* 863 (1973).

78 Schrauzer, G.N.: Selenium and cancer: a review. Bioinorg. Chem. *5:* 275 (1976).

79 Schrauzer, G.N.; White, D.A.; Schneider, C.J.: Cancer mortality correlation studies. III. Statistical associations with dietary selenium intakes. Bioinorg. Chem. *7:* 23 (1977).

80 Schrauzer, G.N.; White, D.A.; Schneider, C.J.: Cancer mortality correlation studies. IV. Associations with dietary intakes and blood levels of certain trace elements, notably Se-antagonists. Bioinorg. Chem. *7:* 35 (1977).

81 Nelson, A.A.; Fitzhugh, O.G.; Calvery, H.O.: Liver tumors following cirrhosis caused by selenium in rats. Cancer Res. *3:* 230 (1943).

82 Volgarev, M.N.; Tscherkes, L.A.: Further studies in tissue changes associated with sodium selenate; in Symp. Selenium in Biomedicine. 1st Int. Symp., p. 179 (AVI Publishing, Westport 1967).

83 Schrauzer, G.N.; White, D.A.; Schneider, C.J.: Selenium and cancer: effects of sele-

nium and of the diet on the genesis of spontaneous mammary tumors in virgin inbred female C$_3$H/St mice. Bioinorg. Chem. *8:* 387 (1978).

84 Harr, J.R.; Exon, J.H.; Whanger, P.D.; Weswig, P.H.: Effect of dietary selenium on *N*-2-fluorenyl-acetamide (FAA)-induced cancer in vitamin E-supplemented, selenium-depleted rats. Clin. Toxicol. *5:* 187 (1972).

85 Ip, C.; Sinha, D.K.: Enhancement of mammary tumorigenesis by dietary selenium deficiency in rats with a high polyunsaturated fat intake. Cancer Res. *41:* 31 (1981).

86 Clayton, C.C.; Baumann, C.A.: Diet and azo dye tumors: effect of diet during a period when the dye is not fed. Cancer Res. *9:* 575 (1949).

87 Griffin, A.C.: The chemopreventive role of selenium in carcinogenesis; in Arnott, van Eys, Wang, Molecular interrelations of nutrition and cancer, pp. 401–408 (Raven Press, New York 1982).

88 Wilt, S.; Pereira, M.; Couri, D.: Selenium effect on initiation and promotion of tumors by benzo[a]pyrene and 12-*O*-tetradecanoylphorbol (Abstract). Proc. Am. Ass. Cancer Res. *20:* 21 (1979).

89 Soullier, B.K.; Wilson, P.S.; Nigro, N.D.: Effect of selenium on azoxymethane-induced intestinal cancer in rats fed high fat diet. Cancer Lett. *12:* 343–348 (1981).

90 Schrauzer, G.N.: Selenium and cancer: a review. Bioinorg. Chem. *5:* 275–281 (1976).

91 Medina, D.; Shepherd, F.: Selenium-mediated inhibition of mouse mammary tumorigenesis. Cancer Lett. *8:* 241–245 (1980).

92 Thompson, H.J.; Becci, P.J.: Selenium inhibition of *N*-methyl-*N*-nitrosourea-induced mammary carcinogenesis in the rat. J. natn. Cancer Inst. *65:* 1299–1301 (1980).

93 Ip, C.; Sinha, K.: Enhancement of mammary tumorigenesis by dietary selenium deficiency in rats with a high polyunsaturated fat intake. Cancer Res. *41:* 31–34 (1981).

94 Ip, C.: Factors influencing the anticarcinogenic efficacy of selenium in DMBA-induced mammary tumorigenesis in rats. Cancer Res. *41:* 1683–1686 (1981).

95 Ip, C.; Ip, M.M.: Chemoprevention of mammary tumorigenesis by a combined regimen of selenium and vitamin A. Carcinogenesis *2:* 915–918 (1981).

96 Ip, C.: Prophylaxis of mammary neoplasia by selenium supplementation in the initiation and promotion phases of chemical carcinogenesis. Cancer Res. *41:* 4386–4390 (1981).

97 Ip, C.; Sinha, D.: Anticarcinogenic effect of selenium in rats treated with dimethyl-benz[a]anthracene and fed different levels and types of fat. Carcinogenesis *2:* 435–438 (1981).

98 Newberne, P.M.; Conner, M.W.: Effect of selenium on acute response to aflatoxin B$_1$; in Hemphill, Trace substances in environmental health, vol. VIII, pp. 323–328 (University of Missouri Press, Columbia 1974).

99 Newberne, P.M.; McConnell, R.G.: Nutrient deficiencies in cancer causation. J. envir. Path. Toxicol. *3:* 323–356 (1980).

100 Sprinker, L.H.; Harr, J.; Newberne, P.M.; Whanger, P.D.; Weswig, P.: Selenium deficiency lesions in rats fed vitamin E-supplemented rations. Nutr. Rep. int. *4:* 335–340 (1971).

101 Grant, K.E.; Conner, M.W.; Newberne, P.M.: Effect of dietary sodium selenite on

lesions induced by repeated small doses of aflatoxin B_1 (Abstract). Toxicol. appl. Pharmacol. *41:* 166 (1977).

102 Sparnins, V.L.; Chuan, J.; Wattenberg, L.W.: Enhancement of glutathione *S*-transferase activity on the esophagus by phenols, lactone and benzyl isothiocyanate. Cancer Res. *42:* 1205–1207 (1982).

103 Chen, X.; Yang, G.; Chan, J.; Wen, Z.; Ge, K.: Relation of selenium deficiency to the occurrence of Keshan disease; in Selenium in biology and medicine; 2nd Int. Symp., Lubbock (AVI Press, Westport 1980).

104 Robinson, M.F.; Godfrey, P.J.; Thomson, C.D.; Rea, H.M.; Van Rij, A.M.: Blood, selenium and glutathione peroxidase activity in normal subjects and in surgical patients with and without cancer. Am. J. clin. Nutr. *32:* 1477–1485 (1979).

Dr. Paul M. Newberne, Massachusetts Institute of Technology,
50 Ames Street, E18-611, Cambridge, MA 02139 (USA)

Prasad (ed.), Vitamins, Nutrition, and Cancer, pp. 68–75 (Karger, Basel 1984)

Role of Vitamins C and E in the Etiology of Human Cancer

E. Bright-See

Ludwig Institute for Cancer Research, Toronto Branch for Human Cancer Prevention, Toronto, Ont., Canada

Vitamins C and E are among the nutrients being considered as potentially protective against cancer. The basis for such a suggestion arises from many studies in animal models and cell culture systems. The majority of the animal work has centered on the fact that vitamins C and E can block the formation of nitrosamines both in vitro [27] and in vivo [19, 20, 26]. As nitrosamines and other N-nitroso compounds induce a wide variety of tumors in many species of animals [24], it has been suggested that these compounds may also be contributing factors in a number of types of human cancers, including those of the esophagus [1, 22], urinary bladder [15], lung [5] and stomach [37]. If nitrosamines are indeed responsible for human cancers, blocking agents such as vitamins C and E would prove useful in cancer prevention.

Humans are exposed to nitrosamines. The estimated average daily exposure is 1.1 µg from the diet and 17 µg from each pack of American filter cigarettes smoked [8]. Since blocking agents such as vitamins C and E are not effective against the preformed nitroso-compounds, attempts have been made to use these vitamins to block nitrosation in foods [28].

Humans are also exposed to a variety of nitrosating agents in food and water [38, 39], cigarette smoke [5] and polluted air [27]. It has been suggested that endogenous formation of N-nitrosamines from these precursors account for the largest proportion of nitrosamines found that in human biological fluids [9, 35]. *Ohshima and Bartsch* [29] found that subjects given 500 mg proline and 250 ml beet juice (containing 375 mg nitrate) excreted an average of 14.9 μg of the noncarcinogenic nitrosoproline (NPRO) in urine over 24 h. Thus, somewhere in the human body, probably the stomach, an environment exists in which nitrates can be connected to nitrite, which then can nitrosate exogenous and, presumably, endogenous amines. This system provides a means of measuring endogenous nitrosamine formation and also of studying factors that may promote or block nitrosation.

Ohshima and Bartsch [29] found that consumption of 1 g of vitamin C with the proline and beet juice completely blocked NPRO excretion and therefore presumably its formation. Consumption of 500 mg of α-tocopherol (equivalent to a little less than one fifth of the vitamin C on a molar basis) decreased NPRO excretion by one half.

In a further study with rats [30], the effect of several phenols was tested. Both resorcinol and catechin promoted nitrosation while chlorogenic acid reduced the NPRO excretion to below control values.

Human Studies

The proposed relationship of nitrosamines and of blocking agents to cancer has not been extensively tested in human studies. One of the simplest forms of human studies is a comparison of food or nutrient availability and cancer death rates. We have recently compared per capita vitamin C availability [10] and age-adjusted death rates of several types of cancer [33]. The correlations were essentially zero (stomach, $R = -0.001$; breast, $R = -0.09$; prostate $R = -0.06$; uterine, other than cervix, $r = -0.07$) with the exception of cancer of the uterine cervix which showed a negative correlation of $R = -0.53$ with vitamin C availability. This finding for cervical cancer is interesting in light of the report of *Wassertheil-Smoller* et al. [36] that a group of women with cervical dysplasia had lower vitamin C intakes than a group of controls (calculated from 24-hour intake recalls or 3-day food records).

The death rate of cervical cancer also correlated with a number of other foods and food components. Adjustments were made for each of these individually (table I). The cervical cancer-vitamin C association was still highly significant after the adjustments were made for each of the factors, except total calories where the association approaches significance at the 5% level.

Multiple regression analysis identified total energy and fruit availability (either as percent of energy or fruit fibre) as two factors, other than

Table I. Examination of the relationship between the 1974 age-adjusted death rate from cervical cancer and the per capita availability of vitamin C and other foods or nutrients

	R	p
Vitamin C	−0.53	0.001
Adjusted for:		
Total energy	−0.32	0.056
Fat energy, %	−0.50	0.0015
Pulse energy, %	−0.51	0.0012
Fruit fibre	−0.39	0.018
Fruit energy, %	−0.48	0.0025
Vegetable energy, %	−0.52	0.0010
Retinol	−0.58	0.0002
Retinol equivalents	−0.43	0.0086
Carotene	−0.47	0.0036
Alcohol energy, %	−0.43	0.0087
Total energy + fruit energy, %	−0.22	0.21
Percent of energy from fruit, adjusted for:		
Total energy + vitamin C	−0.15	0.37

vitamin C, making major contributions to the variations in cervical cancer rates. When both total energy and energy from fruit were taken into account, the cervical cancer-vitamin C association was no longer significant (table I). On the other hand, controlling for both vitamin C and total calories eliminated the significant association between fruit availability and cervical cancer. Thus, at this point, one cannot say whether the important factor associated with cervical cancer is vitamin C availability or some other food or food factor associated or correlated with fruit intake.

Butterworth and Norris [7] have suggested that folic acid rather than vitamin C may be the critical nutrient in cervical dysplasia; the relationship of mild folate deficiency to cervical dysplasia has been documented [6, 23]. In the study of *Wassertheil-Smoller* et al. [36], vitamin C intake correlated with the intake of folic acid (R = 0.35). There are no data on the international availability of folate, but vitamin C availability is associated with the availability of vegetables (R = 0.69), cruciferous vegetables (R = 0.55) and fruit (R = 0.41) – all known sources of dietary folate.

Table II. Studies of 'vitamin C' and human cancer

Cancer	Reference	Type of measurement
Stomach	*Meinsma,* 1964 [25]	food use
	Higginson, 1967 [16]	food use
	Graham et al., 1967 [11]	food use
	Graham et al., 1972 [12]	food use
	Haenszel et al., 1972 [14]	food use
	Kolonel et al., 1981 [40]	calculated intake
Esophagus	*Aoki* et al., 1982 [2]	food use
Larynx	*Graham* et al., 1981 [13]	food use index
Lung	*Hirayama,* 1977 [17]	food use
	Bjelke et al., 1982 [4]	vitamin C index
	Kvale et al., 1982 [21]	vitamin C index

A second type of human study used to investigate diet-cancer relationships is the case-control study. Several of these have been used to implicate vitamin C in the prevention of cancer. (No similar studies have been made of vitamin E, because this nutrient is widely distributed in foods and no adequate food tables exist for it.) Some of the studies often cited in support of the 'vitamin C hypotheses' are listed in table II. With one exception, these studies have not attempted to assess vitamin C intakes, either by calculations or by biochemical markers, but have simply dealt with frequency of use of different foods and food groups.

In the case of stomach cancer, individuals with cancer were found to have lower intakes of fruits [25], lettuce [11], total raw vegetables [12], Western vegetables [14] or fresh fruits and vegetables [16] than did control subjects. *Hirayama* [17] reported that Japanese who ate yellow and green vegetables daily had a lower risk of lung cancer; this was true for both smokers and nonsmokers. Fruit and vegetable intake was also negatively associated with risk of lung cancer in Norway [4]. Cases with esophageal cancer had low intakes of a series of 'Western' fruits and vegetables [2] and low total vegetable consumption was as strongly associated with laryngeal cancer as was the 'vitamin C index' [13].

Current data from human studies offer little if any support for the view that vitamin C intake is associated with several types of human cancer. In case-control studies this may be due to the fact that the 'measures' of vitamin C were not sensitive enough. Further studies of this nature will contribute little unless more precise markers of vitamin C intakes are used.

Vitamin C intakes can be calculated from food records. However, due to the daily variability in intake, up to 21-day records may be necessary to estimate 'usual' intake for an individual [18]. Shorter records may be adequate to estimate differences between groups. Assuming that accurate records of adequate length can be obtained, several problems remain.

Vitamin C is one of the most labile nutrients. Values from food tables may not represent the amounts in the foods actually consumed. Biochemical markers could be used to avoid this problem. For example, *Shier* et al. [34] reported that 24-hour urinary vitamin C was proportional to calculated vitamin C intake up to about 400 mg/day. This observation needs to be expanded to evaluate output against analyzed intake and to cover the range of some of the doses now being consumed as supplements (up to 5,000 mg/day). Urinary vitamin C might then prove useful as the sole measure of intake or as a periodic check on the adequacy of intake records.

Both intake records and urinary output illustrate one of the continuing problems with dietary studies: they represent only current intake. In the case of vitamin C this may be particularly important as massive use of vitamin C supplements has only occurred recently.

White blood cell (WBC) vitamin C shows less day-to-day variation than either serum or urinary levels and therefore may reflect 'usual' intake [32]. However, the measure is technically difficult [3] and the value again does not represent vitamin C status a long time prior to the study. Data compiled by *Sauberlich* et al. [31] show that there is a close association between dietary, serum and WBC vitamin C (dietary vs serum R = 0.94; diet vs WBC, R = 0.91; serum vs WBC, R = 0.96). The dietary intakes, however, were only up to 133 mg/day, a value much below that consumed by many people today. At the higher level, WBC may become saturated [31] and therefore no longer serve as a good marker of intake.

From a practical standpoint, the best approach for studying vitamin C seems to be use of food records (4 days or more) and urinary vitamin C. Information must be collected on current and past use of vitamin C supplements. In addition, comprehensive data on total food intake, including biochemical markers where available, must be obtained, in order to ensure that any association that may be found between a type of human cancer and vitamin C intake cannot be explained by other dietary factors.

References

1 Ackerman, L.V.; Weinstein, I.B.; Kaplan, H.S.: Cancer of the esophagus; in Kaplan, Tsuchitaui, Cancer in China, pp. 111–136 (Liss, New York 1978).

2 Aoki, K.; Okada, H.; Takeda, S.; Sigi, M.; Ohno, Y.; Sasaki, R.; Tominaga, S.: Case control study on esophageal cancer in Japan. Proc. 13th Int. Cancer Congr., Seattle 1982, abstr. 986.

3 Attwood, E.C.; Robey, E.D.; Ross, J.; Bradley, F.; Kramer, J.J.: Determination of platelet and leucocyte vitamin C and the levels found in normal subjects. Clin. chim. Acta 54: 95–105 (1974).

4 Bjelke, E.; Schuman, L.M.; Gart, J.J.; Houch, I.: Dietary factors and lung cancer mortality. The Luthern Brotherhood study 1966–1977. Proc. 13th Int. Cancer Congr., Seattle 1982, abstr. 985.

5 Bokhoven, C.; Niessen, H.J.: Amounts of oxides of nitrogen and carbon monoxide in cigarette smoke, with and without inhalation. Nature, Lond. 192: 458 (1961).

6 Butterworth, C.E.; Hatch, K.D.; Gore, H.; Mueller, H.; Krumdieck, C.L.: Improvement in cervical dysplasia associated with folic acid therapy in users of oral contraceptives. Am. J. clin. Nutr. 35: 73–82 (1982).

7 Butterworth, C.E.; Norris, D.: Folic acid and vitamin C in cervical dysplasia. Am. J. clin. Nutr. 37: 332–333 (1983).

8 Committee on Nitrite and Alternative Curing Agents in Foods, National Academy of Science-National Research Council: The health effects of nitrate, nitrite and N-nitroso compounds (National Academy Press, Washington 1981).

9 Fine, D.H.; Ross, R.; Rounbehler, D.P.; Silvergleid, A.; Song, I.: Formation in vivo of volatile N-nitrosamines in man after ingestion of cooked bacon and spinach. Nature, Lond. 265: 753–755 (1977).

10 Food and Agricultural Organization, United Nations Provisional Food Balance Sheets, 1972–74 Average, Rome 1977.

11 Graham, S.; Lilienfeld, A.M.; Tidings, J.E.: Dietary and purgation factors in the epidemiology of gastric cancer. Cancer 20: 2224–2234 (1967).

12 Graham, S.; Schotz, W.; Martino, P.: Alimentary factors in the epidemiology of gastric cancer. Cancer 30: 927–938 (1972).

13 Graham, S.; Mettlin, C.; Marshall, J.; Priore, R.; Rzopka, T.; Shedd, D.: Dietary factors in the epidemiology of cancer of the larynx. Am. J. Epidem. 113: 675–680 (1981).

14 Haenszel, W.; Kurihara, M.; Segi, M.; Lee, R.K.C.: Stomach cancer among Japanese in Hawaii. J. natn. Cancer Inst. 49: 969–988 (1972).

15 Hicks, R.M.; Gough, T.A.; Walters, C.L.: Demonstration of the presence of nitrosamines in human urine: preliminary observations of the possible etiology for the bladder cancer in association with chronic urinary tract infection; in Walker, Environmental aspects of N-nitroso compounds, pp. 465–475 (International Agency for Research on Cancer, Lyon 1978).

16 Higginson, J.: Etiology of gastrointestinal cancer in man. Natn. Cancer Inst. Monogr. 25: 191–198 (1967).

17 Hirayama, T.: Epidemiological evaluation of the role of naturally occurring carcinogens and modulators of carcinogenesis; in Miller, Naturally occurring carcinogens –

mutagenic and modulators of carcinogenesis, pp. 359–380 (University Press, Baltimore 1977).

18   James, W.P.T.; Bingham, S.A.; Cole, T.J.: Epidemiological assessment of dietary intake. Nutr. Cancer 2: 203–212 (1981).

19   Kamm, J.J.; Dashman, T.; Conney, A.H.; Burns, J.J.: Effect of ascorbic acid on amine-nitrite toxicity. Ann. N.Y. Acad. Sci. 258: 169–174 (1975).

20   Kamm, J.J.; Dashman, T.; Newmark, H.; Mergens, W.J.: Inhibition of amine-nitrite hepatotoxicity by α-tocopherol. Toxicol. appl. Pharmacol. 41: 578–583 (1977).

21   Kvale, G.; Bjelke, E.; Gart, J.J.: Dietary habits and lung cancer risk. Proc. 13th Int. Cancer Congr., Seattle 1982, abstr. 984.

22   Li, M.; Lu, S.; Ji, C.; Wang, M.; Chung, S.; Jin, S.: Formation of carcinogenic N-nitroso compounds in corn-bread inoculated with fungus. Scientia Sinica 22: 471–477 (1979).

23   Lindenbaum, J.; Whitehead, N.; Reyner, F.: Oral contraceptive hormones, folate metabolism and the cervical epithelium. Am. J. clin. Nutr. 28: 346–353 (1975).

24   Lijinsky, W.: Structure-activity relationships among N-nitroso compounds; in Scalan, Tannenbaum, N-nitroso compounds, pp. 89–99 (Am. Chemical Society, Washington 1981).

25   Meinsma, L.: Voeding en Kanker. Voeding 25: 357–365 (1964).

26   Mirvish, S.S.; Cardisa, A.; Wallcove, L.; Sherbik, P.: Induction of lung adenomas by amines or ureas plus nitrite and by N-nitroso compounds: effect of ascorbic acid, gallic acid, thiocyanate and caffeine. J. natn. Cancer Inst. 55: 633–636 (1975).

27   Newmark, H.L.; Mergens, W.J.: α-Tocopherol (vitamin E) and its relationship to tumor induction and development; in Zodeck, Lipkin, Inhibition of tumor induction and development, pp. 127–168 (Plenum Publishing, New York 1981).

28   Newmark, H.L.; Mergens, W.J.: Application of ascorbic acid and tocopherols as inhibitors of nitrosamine formation and oxidation in foods; in Solms, Hall, Criteria of food acceptance, pp. 379–390 (Forster Publishing, Zürich 1981).

29   Ohshima, H.; Bartsch, H.: Quantitative estimation of endogenous nitrosation in humans by monitoring N-nitrosoproline excreted in the urine. Cancer Res. 41: 3658–3662 (1981).

30   Pignatelli, B.; Bereziat, J.C.; O'Neill, I.K.; Bartsch, H.: Catalytic role of some phenolic substances in endogenous formation of N-nitroso compounds. IARC scient. Publ. 41: 413–426 (1982).

31   Sauberlich, H.E.; Dowdy, R.P.; Skale, J.H.: Laboratory tests for the assessment of nutritional status; in King, Faulkner, CRC crit. Rev. Clin. Lab. Sci. 4: 227–236 (1973).

32   Sauberlich, H.E.: Vitamin C status: methods and findings. Ann. N.Y. Acad. Sci. 258: 438–449 (1975).

33   Segi, M.: Age-adjusted death rates for cancer for selected sites (A-classification) in 46 countries in 1975 (Segi Institute of Cancer Epidemiology, Nagoya 1980).

34   Shier, M.W.; Heinrichs, T.F.; Hart, W.: Effects of diet on urinary 1-ascorbic acid in the human. J. Food Sci. 47: 334–337 (1981).

35   Walker, E.A.; Castegnaro, M.; Pigatelli, B.; Munoz, N.; Crespi, M.: N-Nitrosamines in gastric juice and atrophic gastritis: a pilot study; in Walker, N-Nitroso compounds: analysis, formation and occurrence. IARC scient. Publ. 31: 633–641 (1980).

36   Wassertheil-Smoller, S.; Romney, S.L.; Wylie-Rosett, J.; Slagle, S.; Miller, G.; Luci-

do, D.; Duttagupta, C.; Palan, P.R.: Dietary vitamin C and cervical dysplasia. Am. J. Epidem. *114:* 714–724 (1981).

37 Weisberger, J.H.; Raineri, R.: Dietary factors and the etiology of gastric cancer. Cancer Res. *35:* 3469–3474 (1975).

38 White, J.W., Jr.: Relative significance of dietary sources of nitrate and nitrite. J. agric. Fd Chem. *23:* 886–891 (1975).

39 White, J.W., Jr.: Correction: relative significance of dietary sources of nitrate and nitrite. J. agric. Fd Chem. *24:* 202 (1976).

40 Kolonel, L.N.; Nomura, A.M.Y.; Hirohata, T.; Hankin, J.N.; Hinds, M.W.: Association of diet and place of birth with stomach cancer incidence in Hawaii, Japanese and Caucasians. Am. J. clin. Nutr. *34:* 2478–2485 (1981).

E. Bright-See, PhD, Ludwig Institute for Cancer Research, Toronto Branch for Human Cancer Prevention, 9 Earl Street, Toronto, Ontario M4Y 1M4 (Canada)

Prasad (ed.), Vitamins, Nutrition, and Cancer, pp. 76–104 (Karger, Basel 1984)

Modification of the Effect of Pharmacological Agents, Ionizing Radiation and Hyperthermia on Tumor Cells by Vitamin E

K.N. Prasad, B.N. Rama

Center for Vitamins and Cancer Research, Department of Radiology, School of Medicine, University of Colorado Health Sciences Center, Denver, Colo., USA

Introduction

The transformation from normal cells to cancer cells due to the effect of ionizing radiation, chemical carcinogen, viruses or any combination of these probably frequently occur in the body; however, these transformed cells do not always establish themselves in the host as a clinical cancer. This suggests that the host exerts considerable selection pressure against the first or first few transformed cells. This selection pressure is exerted by the host's immune system and by certain endogenous substances. The transformed cells probably escape the selection pressure of the host by undergoing additional mutations. Since the transformed cells escape the selection pressure exerted by certain endogenous substances at physiological concentrations, these substances at pharmacological concentrations should exhibit antitumor activity either by inducing normal phenotype and/or by causing cell death. Indeed, recent studies suggest that vitamin A, vitamin C and vitamin E may be the endogenous substances which exert the selection pressure against the transformed cells. We discuss here the biological basis for using vitamin E in the treatment of tumors.

In vitro Studies: Introduction of Normal Phenotype

D-α-Tocopheryl (vitamin E) acid succinate induces morphological changes in mouse melanoma cells (B-16) in culture [1]. These morphological changes include enlargement of soma, enlongation of bipolar cytoplas-

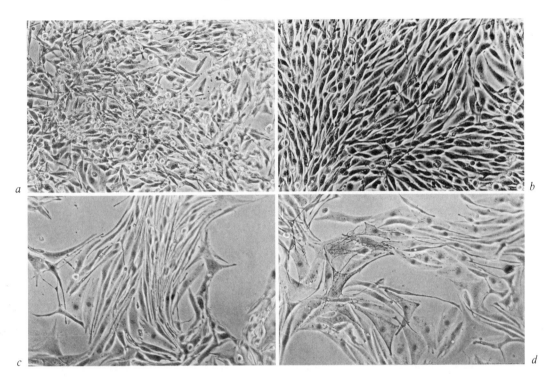

Fig. 1. Melanoma cells (10^5) were plated in Lux tissue culture dishes (60 mm), and *D*-α-tocopheryl (vitamin E) acid succinate (soluble in ethanol) and sodium succinate plus ethanol were added to separate cultures 24 h after plating. Drugs and medium were changed at 2 and 3 days after treatment. Photomicrographs were taken 4 days after treatment. Control culture contains fibroblastic cells as well as round cells in clumps (*a*). Cultures treated with ethanol (1 %) and sodium succinate (5–6 μg/ml) also exhibited fibroblastic morphology with fewer round cells (*b*). Vitamin E acid succinate-treated cultures (5 μg/ml, *c*; 6 μg/ml, *d*) showed a dramatic change in morphology. × 300 [1].

mic processes, and tendency of cells to arrange themselves in parallel to each other. The above changes resemble those observed in cultures of normal melanocytes. The untreated melanoma cells form clumps during growth and exhibit mostly round cell morphology (fig. 1a). It is interesting to note that the effective concentration range of vitamin E acid succinate is very narrow. A concentration of 6 μg/ml produces a more marked change (fig. 1d) in comparison to that produced by a concentration of 5 μg/ml (fig. 1c). A concentration of 10 µg/ml was lethal. Sodium succinate at similar concentrations with or without an equivalent volume of ethanol was ineffective (fig. 1b). Other forms of vitamin E, such as aquasol *DL-α*-tocopheryl acetate (up to 10 µg/ml), *DL-α*-tocopheryl nicotinate (up to 200 µg/ml), and *DL-α*-tocopherol free alcohol (up to 10 µg/ml), were also ineffective. Higher concentrations of vitamin E acetate and vitamin E free alcohol could not be used because of the toxicity of specialized solvents in which aquasol vitamin E acetate and vitamin E free alcohol are solubilized. These studies suggest that vitamin E acid succinate is the most potent form of vitamin E for inducing morphological differentiation and growth inhibition in mouse melanoma cells in culture.

Vitamin E acid succinate-induced morphological changes are primarily irreversible [1]. This is shown by the fact that when the drug is removed after 4 days of treatment, the differentiated phenotype is maintained. However, vitamin E acid succinate-resistant cells exist in culture. They exhibit morphology which is similar to that observed in untreated cultured cells.

Results show that vitamin E acid succinate-induced morphological changes in hormone-supplemented serum-free medium (SFM) were similar to those observed in serum-supplemented medium [1]; however, the concentration needed to produce the effect was about 5 times less (table I). This suggests that the effect of vitamin E acid succinate on melanoma cells is not mediated by serum factors. The serum factors only modify the effect of vitamin E in the quantitative sense.

To study the generality of the effect of vitamin E acid succinate on mammalian cells in culture, we investigated the effect of vitamin E acid succinate on mouse fibroblasts (L cells), rat glioma (C-6) and mouse neuroblastoma (NBP$_2$) cells in culture. Results show that vitamin E acid succinate at a concentration of 5 µg/ml did not affect the morphology or growth of mouse fibroblasts in culture; however, it inhibited the growth of mouse neuroblastoma (NB) cells and rat glioma cells in culture. These results are similar to those described previously with aquasol vitamin E acetate [5, 6]. Vitamin E succinate also inhibits the growth of human NB cells in culture and in nude mice [2] and human prostate cells in culture [*Weber and Prasad,* unpublished observation]. *D-* and *DL-* forms of α-tocopheryl succinate were equally effective on NB and melanoma cells in culture [3]. A recent study [4] has shown that *DL-α*-tocopherol induces morphological differentiation in mouse myeloid leukemia cells in culture without affecting the growth rate. These studies show that vitamin E inhibits the growth and causes morphological changes in several tumor cells in culture.

In vitro Studies: Induction of Growth Inhibition

The effect of vitamin E acid succinate on the growth of melanoma cells was investigated using three different methods: number of viable cells per dish, protein content per dish, and colony formation. The concentrations of vitamin E acid succinate needed to inhibit the growth of melanoma cells by 50% were similar irrespective of the methodologies (table I). Vitamin E acid succinate inhibited the growth of mouse melanoma cells in culture in a dose-dependent fashion (fig. 2). However, aquasol vitamin E acetate, vitamin E-free alcohol at similar concentrations were ineffective. It was important to note that the solvents of vitamin E acetate and vitamin E-free alcohol at higher concentrations by themselves markedly inhibited the growth of melanoma cells, and the presence of the vitamin E in the solvents

Table I. Effect of *D-α*-tocopheryl acid succinate on growth of melanoma (B-16) and fibroblast (L) cells in culture using different assay methods

Technique of assay	Concentration (μg/ml) needed to inhibit growth by 50%
Protein content/dish (B-16)	6
Protein content/dish (L cells)	10
Number of viable cells/dish (B-16; cells grown in serum)	5.5
Number of viable cells/dish (B-16; cells grown in SFM[1])	1.2
Colony formation (B-16; cells grown in serum)	5.7

Cells (melanoma, 10^5; L cells, 1×10^5) were plated in Lux tissue culture dishes (60 mm), and *D-α*-tocopheryl acid succinate at various concentrations was added to culture 24 h after plating. Drug and medium were changed 2 days after treatment. To study the effect of vitamin E acid succinate on melanoma cells growing in the absence of serum, cells were plated in serum-supplemented medium as described. After 24 h of plating, cells were washed twice with SFM, and then cells were incubated in the presence of SFM for 15 min before the addition of vitamin E acid succinate. Drug and medium were changed 2 days after treatment. The growth inhibition was determined 3 days after treatment. The growth inhibition (percentage of untreated controls) as function of concentration of vitamin E acid succinate was plotted on linear paper. Each point on the curve represents an average of 6 samples. From this curve, the concentration of vitamin E acid succinate needed to inhibit the growth by 50% was determined [1].
[1] Serum-free medium.

reduced the solvent-induced growth inhibition (fig. 2). These data suggest that vitamin E acetate and vitamin E-free alcohol solubilized in these solvents are not suitable for in vitro studies.

The growth inhibitory effect of vitamin E acid succinate on mouse melanoma cells in culture is primarily irreversible [1]. This is shown by the observation that when vitamin E acid succinate is removed after 4 days of treatment, the growth does not begin for a period of 24 h. However, a slight increase in growth is observed at 2 days after removal of vitamin E (fig. 3). This may be due to the existence of vitamin E acid succinate-resistant melanoma cells as well as only partially affected cells which eventually grow to confluency. The reasons for the resistance of melanoma cells to vitamin E succinate are unknown.

Our results show that vitamin E acid succinate is the most potent form of vitamin E in causing morphological changes and growth inhibition in melanoma cells in culture. The exact reasons for this are unknown: however, the following possibilities can be suggested: (a) vitamin E acid succi-

---

Fig. 2. Effect of various forms of tocopherol (vitamin E) on the growth of mouse melanoma (B-16) cells in culture. Cells (10^5) were plated in Lux tissue culture dishes (60 mm). 24 h after plating, D-α-tocopheryl acid succinate (Sigma; soluble in ethanol), DL-α-tocopherol free alcohol (Hoffmann-La Roche; soluble in specialized solvent), and Aquasol DL-α-tocopheryl acetate (USV Laboratories; soluble in specialized solvent) at various concentrations were added individually to separate dishes. Growth medium and drug were changed at 2 days after treatment, and the growth inhibition, based on the amount of protein per dish, in the treated culture was determined at 3 days after treatment. The average value of the untreated controls was considered 100%, and the growth inhibition of treated cultures was expressed as percentage of untreated controls. The amount of protein per dish in the untreated cultures was 850 ± 67 µg. Each point on the curve represents an average of 9 samples. Bars = SD [1].

Fig. 3. Effect of D-α-tocopheryl acid succinate on the growth of melanoma cells in culture. Cells (10^5) were plated in Lux tissue culture dishes (60 mm). 24 h after plating, D-α-tocopheryl acid succinate (6 µg/ml) or sodium succinate (6 µg/ml) with an equivalent volume of ethanol (0.6%) was added to separate dishes. Growth medium and drug were changed 2 days after treatment and then every day thereafter. In one set of cultures the drugs were removed 4 days after treatment. In one set of cultures the drugs were removed 4 days after treatment. The protein content per dish was determined every day. Each point on the curve represents an average of 9 samples. Bars = SD. When bars are not shown SDs are equal to the sizes of the symbols [1].

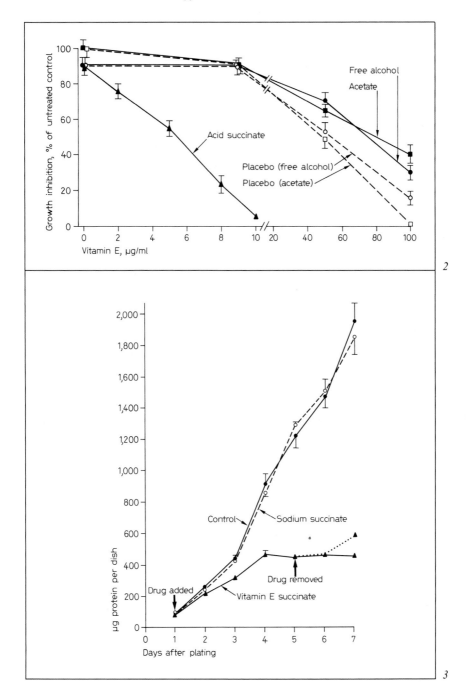

2

3

nate may be relatively more soluble and stable in growth medium or in solution; (b) it may easily cross the cell membrane, and (c) it may be converted to α-tocopherol more slowly, so that the intracellular level of α-tocopherol remains high for a longer period of time.

Modification of the Effect of Pharmacological Agents by Vitamin E

The concept that vitamins E and C can modify the effect of pharmacological agents on tumor cells in culture is novel [5–10]. The extent of modification depends upon the types of tumor cells, the types of vitamin, and the types of pharmacological agents. This concept is primarily based on in vitro systems. However, if this concept is applicable to in vivo conditions, the effectiveness of pharmacological agents can be greatly enhanced by manipulating the body levels of these vitamins.

Effects of Vitamin E in Combination with Vitamins A and C. Tumor cells resistant to vitamins A, C and E are present in tumors. The mechanisms of the effects of these vitamins on tumor cells appear in part to be different for each. Therefore, a combination of more than one vitamin may be more effective than the individual vitamins. Our preliminary data show that the combination of vitamin E and vitamin A is more effective on melanoma cells in culture on the criterion of growth inhibition; the combination of vitamin C and vitamin E is more effective on mouse NB cells than the individual vitamins [*Prasad,* unpublished observation]. Extensive studies are needed to develop a rational strategy for using multiple vitamins in high doses in the treatment of human tumors.

Modification of the Effects of Tumor Therapeutic Agents by Vitamin E. We believe that combinations of more than one vitamin may be more effective than the individual agent in the treatment of advanced metastatic tumor. Thus, any agent which enhances the effect of currently used therapeutic agents on tumor cells would be very useful in the management of advanced tumor. We have reported [5, 6, 11, 12] that vitamin E enhances the effect of tumor therapeutic agents on tumor cells in culture. Tumor therapeutic agents can be grouped into four categories: (a) ionizing radiation; (b) synthetic cytotoxic agents; (c) naturally occurring nontoxic agents; and (d) hyperthermia. The effects of vitamin E in modifying the effects of these agents will be discussed separately.

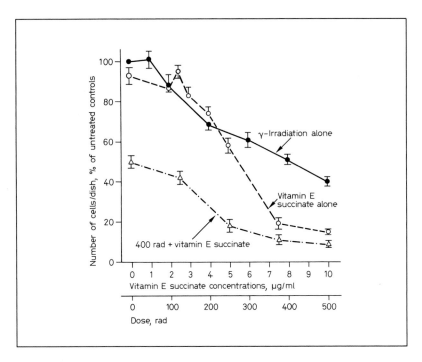

Fig. 4. Neuroblastoma cells (NBP₂) were plated-in Lux culture dishes (60 mm), and the cells were γ-irradiated 24 h after plating. Vitamin E succinate or the solvent (ethanol 0.25% and sodium succinate 5 μg/ml) was added immediately before irradiation. The drugs and medium were changed 2 days after treatment. The number of cells per dish was determined 3 days after treatment. Each experiment was repeated at least twice involving 3 samples per treatment. The average value ($172 \pm 7 \times 10^4$) of untreated control NB cells was considered 100%, and the growth in treated cultures was expressed as a percentage of untreated controls. The bar at each point is standard error of the mean [12].

Modification of Radiation Effects by Vitamin E

Several studies have shown that α-tocopherol protects normal tissue in vitro and in vivo against radiation damage [13–20], whereas others have reported that vitamin E is ineffective in protecting normal or tumor tissue [21–24]. A few studies have shown that vitamin E enhances the effect of radiation on tumor cells in vivo [25, 26] and in vitro [12, 61]. Another study has shown that *DL*-α-tocopheryl succinate enhances the effect of γ-irradiation on mouse neuroblastoma (NBP₂) cells in culture (fig. 4); how-

Table II. Modification of the radiation response of mouse neuroblastoma (NBP$_2$) by *DL*-α-tocopheryl succinate

Treatments	Number of cells/dish % of untreated controls	Trypan blue-stained cells % of attached cells
400 rad	51 ± 2.7[1]	< 1
Vitamin E succinate (5 μg/ml)	58 ± 3.5	< 1
400 rad plus vitamin E succinate	18 ± 3.0	< 2
No radiation, sodium succinate (5 μg/ml) and ethanol (0.25 %, final concentration)	94 ± 6	< 1
400 rad plus sodium succinate and ethanol	59 ± 2.1	< 1
Butylated hydroxyanisole (2 μg/ml)	56 ± 2.5	< 1
400 rad plus butylated hydroxyanisole	31 ± 1.8	< 1

Neuroblastoma cells (50,000 cells) were plated in Lux culture dishes (60 mm), and the cells were irradiated 24 h after plating. Vitamin E succinate or the solvent was added immediately before irradiation. The drugs and medium were changed 2 days after treatment. The number of cells per dish was determined 3 days after treatment. Each experiment was repeated at least twice involving 3 samples per treatment. The average value (172 ± 7 × 10^4) of untreated control NB cells was considered 100 %, and the growth in treated cultures was expressed as a percentage of untreated controls.
[1] Standard error of the mean.

ever, it does not enhance the effect of irradiation on fibroblasts (L cells) [12]. The exact mechanisms of the vitamin E-induced enhancement of radiation effects are unknown, but we have observed that butylated hydroxyanisole (BHA), a lipid-soluble antioxidant, also enhances the effect of γ-irradiation on NB cells in culture (table II). In addition, vitamin C, a water-soluble antioxidant, increases the effect of radiation on NB cells in culture [7]. These studies suggest that vitamin E-induced enhancement of the effect of radiation may in part be mediated by antioxidant mechanisms. *DL*-α-Tocopheryl acetate also enhances the effect of irradiation on glioma cells in culture [6].

These studies suggest that vitamin E may increase growth inhibition of tumor cells by ionizing radiation, whereas it may or may not protect normal tissue against radiation damage. If vitamin E produces similar results during radiation therapy of human tumors, it may markedly improve treatment effectiveness. Since vitamin E taken orally may not accumulate

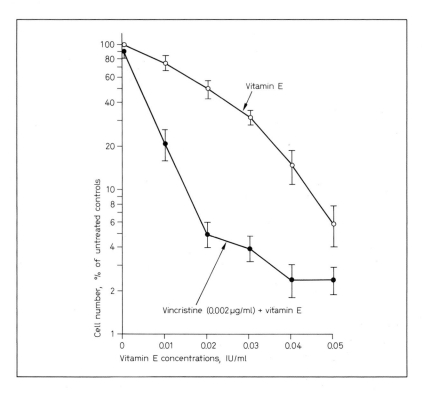

Fig. 5. Neuroblastoma cells (50,000) were plated in Lux culture dishes (60 mm), and vincristine and vitamin E were added 24 h later. Drugs and medium were changed 2 days after treatment. The cell number and the number of trypan blue-stained cells were determined 3 days after treatment. The number of stained cells was subtracted from the total naumber of cells to obtain viable cells per dish. The average value of control cultures was considered 100%. Each value represents an average of at least 6 samples. The bar of each point is standard deviation [6].

quickly in tumor tissue because of relatively poor absorption from the intestinal tract, it is important that vitamin E be given intravenously before irradiation and throughout the radiation therapy period.

Modification of the Effects of Synthetic Antitumor Agents by Vitamin E. Most of the currently used chemotherapeutic agents are immunosuppressive, toxic, and not naturally present in the body. These agents kill normal cells as well as tumor cells. It has been reported [6] that *DL*-α-tocopheryl acetate in combination with vincristine (fig. 5), 5-fluorouracil, adriamycin

Table III. Vitamin E effects on NB and glioma cells. Effect of vitamin E in combination with pharmacological agents on NB (P_2) and glioma (C-6) cells in culture

Treatments	Cell number, % of untreated control[1]	
	glioma	NB
Vitamin E	50 ± 6^2 (0.05 IU/ml)	53 ± 5 (0.02 IU/ml)
Bleomycin	77 ± 5 (0.004 U/ml)	54 ± 4 (0.002 U/ml)
Bleomycin + vitamin E	42 ± 3^3	29 ± 3^3
5-FU	71 ± 7 (0.1 µg/ml)	63 ± 4 (0.03 µg/ml)
5-FU + vitamin E	32 ± 3^3	15 ± 3^4
Adriamycin	36 ± 4 (0.004 µg/ml)	42 ± 3 (0.001 µg/ml)
Adriamycin + vitamin E	22 ± 2^3	12 ± 1.5^4
CCNU	43 ± 3 (20 µg/ml)	55 ± 6 (10 µg/ml)
CCNU + vitamin E	11 ± 2^4	38 ± 3^3
DTIC	57 ± 4 (20 µg/ml)	60 ± 5 (4 µg/ml)
DTIC + vitamin E	35 ± 5^3	31 ± 4^3
Sodium butyrate (NaB)	78 ± 4 (0.5 mM)	87 ± 6 (0.25 mM)
NaB + vitamin E	45 ± 6^5	36 ± 6^4
R020-1724	73 ± 6 (100 µg/ml)	45 ± 4 (100 µg/ml)
R020-1724 + vitamin E	16 ± 3^4	10 ± 1.8^4
Prostaglandin E_1 (PGE$_1$)	78 ± 7 (5 µg/ml)	40 ± 5 (10 µg/ml)
PGE$_1$ + vitamin E	46 ± 5^5	9 ± 1.3^4
Papaverine (µg/ml)	63 ± 5 (10 µg/ml)	41 ± 4 (5 µg/ml)
Papaverine + vitamin E	25 ± 4^3	18 ± 3^3
Mutamycin	46 ± 4 (0.01 µg/ml)	48 ± 4 (0.01 µg/ml)
Mutamycin + vitamin E	23 ± 3^3	24 ± 4^3
Chlorozotocin	84 ± 7 (1 µg/ml)	82 ± 4 (2 µg/ml)
Chlorozotocin + vitamin E	52 ± 5^5	36 ± 3^4
cis-Platinum	54 ± 4 (0.2 µg/ml)	43 ± 5 (0.2 µg/ml)
cis-Platinum + vitamin E	29 ± 5^3	18 ± 5^3

[1] Cells (5×10^4, NB; 10^5, glioma) were plated in Lux tissue culture dishes (60 mm), and drugs were added 24 h after plating. Fresh media and drugs were added 2 days after treatment. The number of viable cells were determined 3 days after treatment. The values in treated groups were expressed as a percentage of untreated controls. The number of cells per dish in untreated control, NB and glioma cells were 81×10^4 and 68×10^4, respectively. Each value represents an average of at least 6 samples.

[2] Standard deviation. To test whether the drug had any effect at all in combination with vitamin E in enhancing the growth inhibition of cells, the mean percentage of untreated control cultures for the drug + vitamin E-treated cultures with that of vitamin E-treated cultures was compared by use of 2 independent sample t tests at $p = 0.01$. If no significant effect of the drug was found, no further analysis was done. If there was a significant effect of the drug in conjunction with vitamin E, then an additional test was performed to establish whether the combination of vitamin E and a drug produced an additive or a synergistic effect [6].

[3] Additive effect.

[4] Synergistic effect.

[5] No effect.

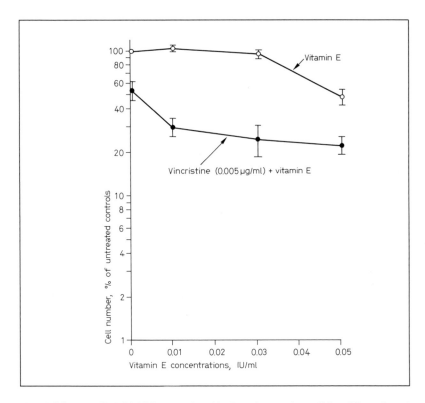

Fig. 6. Glioma cells (100,000) were plated in Lux tissue culture dishes (60 mm), and vincristine and vitamin E were added 24 h later. Drugs and medium were changed 2 days after treatment. The cell number and the number of trypan blue-stained cells were determined 3 days after treatment. The number of stained cells was subtracted from the total number of cells to obtain viable cells per dish. The average value of control cultures was considered 100%. Each value represents an average of at least 6 samples. The bar of each point is standard deviation [6].

or chlorozotocin produced a synergistic effect, whereas vitamin E in combination with bleomycin, 1-(2-chloroethyl)-3-cyclohexyl-1-nitrosourea (CCNU), 5-(3,3-dimethyl-1-triazeno)-imidazole-4-carboxamide (DTIC), mutamycin or *cis*-diamine dichloro-platinum II produced an additive effect on the criterion of growth inhibition of NB cells (table III). In glioma cell cultures, vitamin E acetate in combination with vincristine (fig. 6) or CCNU produced a synergistic effect, whereas vitamin E in combination with bleomycin, 5-fluorouracil, adriamycin, DTIC, mutamycin and *cis*-

platinum produced an additive effect on the criterion of growth inhibition (table III). Another form of vitamin E, *DL*-α-tocopheryl succinate, also enhances the effect of chemotherapeutic agents on NB and melanoma cells in culture [27]. These studies suggest that modification of the effect of chemotherapeutic agents on tumor cells depends upon tumor form and type of chemotherapeutic agent. Our in vitro observations cannot readily be extrapolated to in vivo conditions. However, if they can be, the addition of vitamin E to currently used treatment protocols involving chemotherapeutic agents may markedly increase their effectiveness in the management of tumors. It is also possible that the doses of chemotherapeutic agents required for effective treatment may be markedly reduced in the presence of vitamin E. Extensive studies are needed to test the above concepts on animal tumors before applying them to human tumors.

Modification of the Effects of Naturally Occurring Substances by Vitamin E. The use of cytotoxic drugs in the management of human tumors continues to be emphasized, but it cannot be accepted as the best way of treating human tumors. Recent experimental studies suggest that it may be possible to treat human tumors by using naturally occurring substances. These substances at higher concentrations induce differentiated phenotypes in tumor cells and/or inhibit their growth. Some of these include vitamin A [28, 29], vitamin C [10, 30, 31], adenosine 3′:5′-cyclic phosphate (cAMP) [32–35] and butyric acid [36, 37].

Our studies show that *DL*-α-tocopheryl acetate markedly enhances the antitumor effect of naturally occurring substances on NB, glioma and melanoma cells in culture. For example, vitamin E acetate enhances the effect of cAMP-stimulating agents (PGE$_1$, a stimulator of adenylate cyclase, and R020-1724, an inhibitor of cyclic nucleotide phosphodiesterase) [6], sodium butyrate (a four-carbon fatty acid) [6], vitamin A and vitamin C [*Prasad and Rama,* unpublished observation] on tumor cells in culture. The extent of vitamin E enhancement depends upon the form of tumor cell and the type of naturally occurring substance. For example, vitamin E in combination with PGE$_1$, R020-1724, or sodium butyrate produced a synergistic effect on NB cells (table III), whereas in glioma cell cultures, vitamin E in combination with R020-1724 produced a synergistic effect on the criterion of growth inhibition (table III). Vitamin E failed to enhance the effect of PGE$_1$ and sodium butyrate on glioma cells (table III). A combination of *DL*-α-tocopheryl acetate or *DL*-α-tocopheryl succinate with vitamin C is more effective on NB cells than the individual vitamin; however, vitamin E in the presence of vitamin C failed to be more effective on melanoma cells in culture [unpublished observation]. We have recently observed that the combination of vitamin A and vitamin E is more effective in inhibiting the growth of melanoma cells than the individual vitamins. Additional studies are needed on this subject using tissue culture and animal tumor models.

Modification of the Effects of Hyperthermia by Vitamin E. During the last 10 years, extensive experimental and clinical studies of the effect of hyperthermia alone or in combinaiton with X-rays and certain chemicals have been published [38–52]. However, the results of clinical trials have been disappointing because the temperature required to kill cells are 42–43 °C and are fatal when used systemically. Even in the management of local lesions, success has been very limited. Therefore, the use of hyperthermia in the management of tumors will continue to be restricted until the cell killing effects of hyperthermia can be achieved at temperatures around 40 °C, which can be reached systemically without toxicity. Since vitamin E enhances the effects of ionizing radiation and chemotherapeutic agents on tumor cells in culture [5, 12], the question has arisen whether vitamin E would enhance the growth inhibitory effect of hyperthermia on tumor cells in culture. Indeed, *DL-α*-tocopheryl succinate markedly enhanced the effect of hyperthermia at both 43 and 41 °C (table IV). The presence of vitamin E before heat treatment and during the entire period of observation was necessary for the above effect. BHA a lipid-soluble antioxidant, also enhanced the effect of heat, but to a lesser degree than that produced by vitamin E succinate. This suggests that the effect of vitamin E in enhancing the effect of heat on NB cells may be mediated, in part, by antioxidant mechanisms [11]. In a more recent study we have found that vitamin E succinate enhances the effect of heat even at 40 °C, which can be achieved systemically. If similar results are obtained in vivo, the addition of vitamin E to hyperthermia protocols may greatly improve their effectiveness in the management of tumors.

Vitamin E and Prostaglandins. The formation of prostaglandins involves oxygenation and cyclization of polyunsaturated fatty acids [53]. The cyclooxygenation of arachidonic acid leads to the formation of the PGE_2 series, prostacyclin and thromboxane, whereas the lipoxygenation of arachidonic acid leads to the formation of leukotrienes. Therefore, vitamin E as an antioxidant plays a regulatory role in prostaglandin biosynthesis by controlling the formation of key lipid hydroperoxides and cyclic endoperox-

Table IV. Modification of the effect of hyperthermia on neuroblastoma cells in culture by *DL*-α-tocopheryl succinate

Treatments	Number of cells/dish % of untreated controls	Trypan blue-stained cells % of attached cells
Sodium succinate (5 µg/ml) and ethanol (0.25 %)	102 ± 3[1]	< 1
Vitamin E succinate (5 µg/ml)	50 ± 3	5
Butylated hydroxyanisole (2 µg/ml)	51 ± 3	4
43 °C (20 min)	40 ± 1	4
Vitamin E succinate plus 43 °C[2]	9 ± 1	27
43 °C plus vitamin E succinate[3]	30 ± 2	6
Sodium succinate and ethanol plus 43 °C[2]	43 ± 4	5
Butylated hydroxyanisole plus 43 °C[2]	20 ± 3	10
41 °C (45 min)	56 ± 3	1
Vitamin E succinate plus 41 °C[2]	21 ± 2	12
41 °C plus vitamin E succinate[3]	32 ± 2	6
Sodium succinate and ethanol plus 41 °C[2]	62 ± 2	1
Butylated hydroxyanisole plus 41 °C[2]	20 ± 1	5

[1] Standard error of the mean.
[2] Agents were added before heating and remained in the culture during the entire period of observation.
[3] Vitamin E was added after heating and remained in the culture for the entire period of observation [11].

ides. Although it has been shown [54, 55] that vitamin E and/or selenium deficiency may severely impair hydroperoxide metabolism and, thereby, alter the biosynthesis of prostaglandins, the effects of excess concentrations of vitamin E on the biosynthesis of prostaglandins have not been adequately studied. α-Tocopherol may prevent the peroxidation of polyunsaturated fatty acids, components of cellular membranes, including arachidonic acid. It has been reported [56] that normal plasma concentrations of α-tocopherol enhance lipooxygenation of arachidonic acid, whereas higher concentrations suppress it in human neutrophils. Although the physiological concentration of vitamin E is necessary for an optimal cyclooxygenation of arachidonic acid in rabbit tissue [55], higher concentrations of vitamin E may inhibit the synthesis of prostaglandins [57]. Vitamin E deficiency causes an increase in cyclooxygenase activity and thereby enhances levels of

PGE_2 in the plasma [55, 58]; however, vitamin E at certain concentrations inhibits cyclooxygenase activity [54, 59–61]. A higher plasma concentration of the PGE series (especially PGE_2) has been implicated in suppressing the host's immune system in patients with cancer and in experimental tumor-bearing animals [62–66]. Thus, higher doses of vitamin E may reduce the level of PGE_2 in plasma by inhibiting cyclooxygenase activity and thereby spare the host's immune system from the adverse effects of PGE_2.

Reduction of Side Effects of Currently Used Tumor Therapeutic Agents by Vitamin E. Several animal studies have shown that vitamin E may reduce adriamycin-induced cardiac toxicity [67–70]; but one study [71] has failed to confirm this in the rabbit. The reasons for this discrepancy are unknown. Vitamin E has also been shown to protect against bleomycin-induced lung fibrosis [72]; however, it failed to reduce drug-induced bone marrow toxicity in animals [70]. A recent study [73] has shown that vitamin E acetate and vitamin E succinate reduced adriamycin-induced skin lesions. Vitamin E succinate was found to be more effective than vitamin E acetate [73]. This observation is similar to our previous study [1] in which vitamin E succinate was found to be more effective than vitamin E acetate on the criterion of growth inhibition of melanoma cells in culture.

Again these animal studies cannot be readily extrapolated to in vivo conditions in human beings; however, if they can be, the addition of vitamin E may reduce the side effects of certain chemotherapeutic agents which become severe during treatment. Frequently, severe side effects become the limiting factor for the continuation of therapy. In addition, doses of chemotherapeutic agents required for effective treatment may be reduced in the presence of vitamin E.

Stimulation of Immunity by Vitamin E. The host's immune system constitutes an important component of the host's selection pressure against the newly transformed cells. It is believed that impairment of the host's immune surveillance mechanisms may allow the transformed cells to escape the selection pressure and thereby allow development of clinically detectable cancer. Conversely, the presence of a responsive host immune system may kill the first or first few transformed cells. Thus, any agent which would stimulate the host's immune system should be of great value in reducing the incidence of cancer.

A responsive host's immune system may also be important during therapy of tumor. Vitamin E has been shown to stimulate humoral immunity [74–77] and cellular immunity [78–80], both in vitro and in animal systems. A recent study [81] has shown that DL-α-tocopherol free alcohol at high doses stimulates the immune system in humans.

Clinical Trials of Vitamin E. From studies of mouse and human tumor cells in culture [1, 5, 6], and of human NB cells in nude mice [2], it is likely that vitamin E at high doses may exhibit antitumor activity on human NB cells in vivo. Because of poor absorption of orally ingested vitamin E ester or free alcohol, it was felt that an oral intake of vitamin E may not increase the plasma vitamin E level enough to allow the accumulation of vitamin E in tumor cells in quantities known to be sufficient to kill or inhibit the growth of tumor cells in culture. Therefore, it was decided that intravenous infusion of vitamin E would be most suitable for treatment of human tumors. *Helson* [this volume] has initiated a phase I trial of vitamin E-free alcohol in the treatment of metastatic NB.

DL-α-Tocopherol free alcohol is being used in a phase I trial (after patients have become unresponsive to all known therapeutic modalities) for the treatment of metastatic human neuroblastomas, primitive neuroecto-dermal tumor, and retinoblastoma. Vitamin E was given intravenously over 3–6 h twice weekly, in dosages of 450–2,300 mg/m^2 or daily 24-hour infusions for 9 days. Some antitumor and analgesic effects were observed. If one considers that the biology of tumor cells in phase I patients is very complex as a result of extensive therapy, and that these cells have become unresponsive to all therapeutic agents, even a partial response by the infusion of vitamin E alone can be considered encouraging. The major untoward side effect of high doses of vitamin E was an increased bleeding tendency which was effectively counteracted with vitamin K infusions. It should be pointed out that DL-α-tocopherol free alcohol which is being used in the treatment of human tumor is much less potent than DL-α-tocopheryl succinate [1]; however, the latter cannot be used in the treatment until the pharmacology and toxicology of this form of vitamin E have been defined.

One clinical study [82] has shown that the administration of vitamin E produces a beneficial effect in patients with chronic cystic mastitis, the most common benign lesion of the female breast. In this study it was not apparent whether vitamin E produced a regression in the lesion.

In summary, vitamin E may influence the management of tumors through several modes of action. For example, it can directly inhibit growth by causing cell death and inhibiting cell division and can induce certain differentiated functions in tumor cells. Vitamin E can also inhibit growth by stimulating the host's immune system. It can increase the effectiveness of currently used tumor therapeutic agents by directly enhancing their lethal effects on tumor cells and reducing their adverse effects on normal cells.

Mechanisms of Vitamin E Effects on Tumor Cells

The exact mechanisms of the antitumor effects of vitamin E are unknown. A well-known characteristic of vitamin E in vitro and in vivo is its antioxidation property [83–88]. Consequently, the question has arisen as to whether the effects of vitamin E on tumor cells in culture are mediated, at least in part, by antioxidant mechanisms. To answer this question in an indirect manner, we have compared the effect of vitamin E succinate on the growth and morphology of NB, melanoma and glioma cells in culture with those of the lipid-soluble antioxidants, BHA and butylated hydroxytoluene (BHT).

We have found [3] inhibition of growth of melanoma cells after treatment with BHT and BHA to be less than that produced by vitamin E acid succinate (table V). Morphological changes produced by a concentration of 10 µg/ml of BHA were similar to those observed with 6 µg/ml of vitamin E succinate. Treated melanoma cells became very elongated and arranged in parallel in comparison to solvent-treated and untreated controls. The number of trypan blue-stained cells in treated cultures was less than 4%. BHT and BHA also inhibited the growth of NB (table VI) and glioma (table VII) cells in culture. The number of trypan blue-stained cells in treated cultures was not more than 2–4%. The fact that vitamin E succinate and other lipid-soluble antioxidants produce similar effects on cultured tumor cells suggests that the effects of vitamin E are mediated, at least in part, by antioxidation mechanisms [3].

Administration of additional DL-α-tocopherol to normal chicks causes significant reticulocytosis [89]. This has been interpreted to mean that maturation of reticulocytes to erythrocytes involves reduction in the amount of total lipid. If peroxidation is involved in the reduction of lipids, then antioxidants should retard differentiation and promote reticulocytosis. By altering the level of peroxidation, vitamin E may change the membrane structure in a way which would alter receptor sites, receptor sensitivity, transport functions and membrane-bound enzyme activities. These mem-

Table V. Effect of *D-* and *DL*-forms of vitamin E succinate and other lipid-soluble antioxidants on the growth inhibition of mouse melanoma (B-16) cells in culture

Treatments	Growth inhibition % of untreated controls	
	cell number	colony
Sodium succinate (5 μg/ml) + ethanol (0.5%)	109 ± 7[1]	96 ± 6[1]
DL-Vitamin E succinate (5 μg/ml)	59 ± 6	42 ± 4
D-Vitamin E succinate (5 μg/ml)	55 ± 5	36 ± 5
Butylated hydroxytoluene (5 μg/ml)	85 ± 5	66 ± 5
Butylated hydroxyanisole (5 μg/ml)	73 ± 4	76 ± 5
Trolox C (5 μg/ml)	83 ± 6	66 ± 6

Melanoma cells (10^5 cells for counting cell number; 100 cells for colony formation) were plated in Lux culture dishes (60 mm). The growth inhibition was determined on the basis of number of cells per dish and number of colonies per dish. The values of untreated control cultures ($62 \pm 6 \times 10^4$; plating efficiency 55%) were considered to be 100%. The growth inhibition was determined as a percentage of untreated controls. Each value represents an average of 9 samples [3].
[1] Mean ± SD.

Table VI. Effect of *D-* and *DL*-forms of vitamin E succinate and other lipid-soluble antioxidants on growth inhibition of NB cells (NBP$_2$) in culture

Treatments	Growth inhibition % of untreated controls
Sodium succinate (5 μg/ml) plus ethanol (0.5%)	86 ± 6[1]
DL-Vitamin E succinate (5 μg/ml)	54 ± 7
D-Vitamin E succinate (5 μg/ml)	52 ± 6
Butylated hydroxytoluene (5 μg/ml)	37 ± 4
Butylated hydroxyanisole (5 μg/ml)	31 ± 4
Trolox C (5 μg/ml)	65 ± 5

Cells (50,000) were plated in Lux culture dishes (60 mm), and the drugs were added separately 24 h later. The drugs and medium were changed 2 days after treatment. The number of cells per dish was determined 3 days after treatment. Each experiment was repeated 3 times involving 3 samples per treatment. The average value of untreated controls ($162 \pm 13 \times 10^4$) was considered 100%, and the growth inhibition in treated culture was expressed as a percentage of untreated controls. Each value represents an average of 9 samples [3].
[1] Mean ± SD.

brane changes could then alter the translation and transcriptional activities of the genome.

The fact that vitamin E and other lipid-soluble antioxidants (BHA and BHT) reduce growth and cause morphological changes in cultured tumor cells suggests that the maintenance of malignant phenotype and growth rate requires a high rate of lipid peroxidation in order to maintain reduced levels of lipids in the membrane [3]. If this is true, increased amounts of lipids in the membrane may favor differentiation and reduction in the growth of tumor cells. This possibility is supported by our studies in which vitamin E and other lipid-soluble antioxidants (BHA and BHT) induced cell differentiation associated with growth inhibition in mouse melanoma cells in culture [3].

Vitamin E obviously inhibits DNA synthesis in tumor cells, because it inhibits cell division, but the mechanism of its effect is unknown. Previous studies have shown that three distinct vitamin E-binding proteins exist in mammalian liver cells in vivo. Two of them are extranuclear components present in the cytosol of rat liver, while the third is associated with the nuclear fraction [90–94]. We have also demonstrated the presence of vitamin E-binding proteins in tumor cells in culture [95].

Table VII. Effects of *D-* and *DL-*α-tocopheryl succinate and other lipid-soluble antioxidants on growth inhibition of rat glioma cells (C-6) in culture

Treatment	Growth inhibition % of untreated controls
Sodium succinate (5 µg/ml) + ethanol (0.5%)	97 ± 6[1]
Ethanol (0.5%) or sodium succinate (5 µg/ml)	103 ± 4
*D-*α-Tocopheryl succinate (5 µg/ml)	29 ± 4
*DL-*α-Tocopheryl succinate (5 µg/ml)	66 ± 6
Butylated hydroxytoluene (5 µg/ml)	92 ± 5
Butylated hydroxyanisole (5 µg/ml)	63 ± 4
Trolox C (5 µg/ml)	73 ± 7

Cells (10^5) were plated in Lux tissue culture dishes (60 mm), and the drugs were added separately 24 h later. Drugs and medium were changed 2 days after treatment. The number of cells per dish was determined 4 days after treatment. Each experiment was repeated 3 times with 3 samples per treatment. The average value of untreated controls ($60 \pm 6.0 \times 10^4$) is considered to be 100%, and growth inhibition in treated cultures is expressed as a percentage of untreated controls. Each value represents an average of 9 samples [3].
[1] Mean $\pm$ standard deviation.

Although a single peak of vitamin E-binding protein occurred in the nuclear and pellet fractions of mouse neuroblastoma (NBP$_2$), mouse melanoma (B-16), and rat glioma (C-6) cells in culture, there were multiple vitamin E-binding proteins in their cytosol. The number depended upon the type of tumor cells; for example, there were five vitamin E-binding proteins in NB cells, two in glioma cells and only one in melanoma cells. The relationship of vitamin E-binding proteins to the mechanisms of action of vitamin E is unknown. The fact that a significant amount of radioactive vitamin E was associated with the purified chromatin suggests that vitamin E may modulate genetic expression in mammalian cells [95]. It has been shown [96] that when physiological doses of α-tocopherol were injected into vitamin E-deficient animals, a dramatic but transient increase in hepatic nuclear RNA synthesis was observed.

In addition to inhibiting the growth of tumor cells in culture, vitamin E appears to affect other cellular functions. These include stabilization of the membrane by physicochemical interaction between its phytyl side chain and the fatty acyl chains of polyunsaturated phospholipids [87, 88, 97–99], prevention of platelet aggregation [100–102] and release [103].

Toxicity of Vitamin E

Since vitamin E is being used clinically in the prevention and treatment of human cancer, it is important to discuss its possible toxicity. Assessment of available data in the literature suggests that the likelihood of serious side effects from consuming 100–1,000 IU/day appears to be very low [104, 105]. A review of another series of human data shows no toxic side effects of vitamin E after prolonged ingestion of 100–800 IU/day [106–109]. An unpublished review of trials in over 9,000 cases by *Salkeld* [1983] has shown that doses of vitamin E of 3,000 IU/day for up to 11 years and 53,000 IU for a few months in a few subjects had no serious effects on a variety of clinical and biochemical parameters. Only 8% of these patients complained, mostly about gastrointestinal problems. However, several reports [110–114] suggest that high doses of vitamin E could produce some toxicity. Unfortunately, as none of these studies was controlled and they were of a primarily anecdotal nature, the data cannot be considered convincing. Animal data appear similarly contradictory. For example, a high dose of *DL*-α-tocopheryl acetate (500 mg/kg of body weight) was not toxic in mice [115], whereas in another study [80], a dose of 400 mg/kg of body weight of *DL*-α-tocopheryl acetate was lethal to mice. The latter study reports that vitamin E at lower doses (5–20 IU/kg body weight daily) stimulates the immune system; however, higher doses (80 IU/kg body weight daily) inhibit phytohemagglutinin (PHA)-induced proliferation of lymphocytes. A chronic intake of supplemental vitamin E with food causes an increased deposit of fat in the rat liver [116]. Although there appears to be no adverse effects of high doses of vitamin E in human beings, possible toxicity must be monitored closely whenever ingestion of high doses (1,000 mg/day or more) of vitamin E over a long period of time is recommended.

Conclusions

α-Tocopherol (vitamin E) may be important in the prevention and treatment of cancer. There are sufficient experimental data to suggest that the presence of high levels of vitamin E may reduce the incidence of cancer. However, the role of vitamin E in the prevention of human cancer has not been demonstrated as yet. Vitamin E may inhibit the incidence of tumors through several mechanisms. For example, vitamin E can prevent the formation of mutagenic and carcinogenic substances in the lumen of the gut. Vitamin E blocks the action of certain tumor-promoting agents. It can also kill newly transformed cells directly or indirectly by stimulating the host's immune system and can reverse the malignant phenotype to a normal phenotype in certain tumors.

Vitamin E may also be useful in the treatment of human tumors by several mechanisms. For example, vitamin E inhibits growth and/or induces differentiated phenotypes in several types of tumors. However, vitamin E-resistant tumor cells exist in culture and in vivo. Vitamins A and E in combination are more effective than the vitamins individually. Vitamin E also enhances the growth inhibitory effect of several currently used tumor therapeutic agents. It enhances the effects of ionizing radiation on tumor cells in culture without affecting the radiation response of normal tissues. Vitamin E also enhances the effects of hyperthermia on tumor cells in culture and inhibits the production of prostaglandin E series which are known to suppress the host's immune system. Finally, vitamin E reduces the toxic effects of some chemotherapeutic agents. These studies suggest that vitamin E may be one of the important anticancer agents which could play a very significant role in the prevention and treatment of cancer.

Acknowledgment

This work was supported by Hoffmann-La Roche and The Hill Foundation. We thank Dr. *Hemmy Bhagavan* for a generous supply of *DL*-α-tocopheryl acetate and *DL*-α-tocopherol free alcohol. We also thank E.M. Laboratories, Elmsford, New York, for supplying *DL*-α-tocopheryl succinate.

References

1   Prasad, K.N.; Edwards-Prasad, J.: Effects of tocopherol (vitamin E) acid succinate on morphological alteration and growth inhibition in melanoma cells in culture. Cancer Res. *42:* 550–555 (1982).

2   Helson, L.; Verma, M.; Helson, C.: Vitamin E and human neuroblastoma; in Meyskens, Prasad, Modulation and mediation of cancer cells by vitamins, pp. 258–265 (Karger, Basel 1983).

3   Rama, B.N.; Prasad, K.N.: Study on the specificity of alpha-tocopheryl (vitamin E) acid succinate effects on melanoma, glioma and neuroblastoma cells in culture. Proc. Soc. exp. Biol. Med. *174:* 302–307 (1983).

4   Sakagami, H.; Asaka, K.; Abe, E.; Miyaura, C.; Suda, T.; Konno, K.: Effect of *DL*-alpha-tocopherol (vitamin E) on the differentiation of mouse myeloid leukemia cells. J. Nutr. Sci. Vitaminol. *27:* 291–300 (1981).

5   Prasad, K.N.; Ramanujam, S.; Gaudreau, D.: Vitamin E induces morphological differentiation and increases the effect of ionizing radiation on neuroblastoma cells in culture. Proc. Soc. exp. Biol. Med. *16:* 570–573 (1979).

6   Prasad, K.N.; Edwards-Prasad, J.; Ramanujam, S.; Sakamoto, A.: Vitamin E increases the growth inhibitory and differentiation effects of tumor therapeutic agents in neuroblastoma and glioma cells in culture. Proc. Soc. exp. Biol. Med. *164:* 158–163 (1980).

7   Prasad, K.N.; Sinha, P.K.; Ramanujam, M.; Sakamoto, A.: Sodium ascorbate potentiates the growth inhibitory effects of certain agents on neuroblastoma cells in culture. Proc. natn. Acad. Sci. USA *76:* 829–832 (1979).

8   Prasad, K.N.: Modulation of the effect of tumor therapeutic agents by vitamin C. Life Sci. *27:* 275–280 (1980).

9   Josephy, P.D.; Paleic, B.; Skarsgard, L.D.: Ascorbate-enhanced cytotoxicity of misonidazole. Nature, Lond. *271:* 370–372 (1978).

10 O'Connor, M.K.; Malone, J.F.; Moriarty, M.; Mulgrew, S.: A radioprotective effect of vitamin C observed in Chinese hamster ovary cells. Br. J. Radiol. *50:* 587–591 (1977).

11 Rama, B.N.; Prasad, K.N.: Modifications of the effect of hyperthermia on neuroblastoma cells in culture by *DL*-alpha-tocopheryl succinate. J. Nutr. Growth Cancer (in press).

12 Sarria, A.; Prasad, K.N.: *DL*-Alpha-tocopheryl succinate enhances the effect of γ-irradiation on neuroblastoma cells in culture. Proc. Soc. exp. Biol. Med. *175:* 88–92 (1984).

13 Srinivasan, V.; Jacobs, A.L.; Simpson, S.A.; Weiss, J.F.: Radioprotection by vitamin

E. Effect on hepatic enzymes, delayed type hypersensitivity and post-irradiation survival of mice; in Meyskens, Prasad, Modulation and mediation of cancer cells by vitamins, pp. 119–131 (Karger, Basel 1983).

14   Bacq, Z.M.; Herve, A.: Protection of mic,e against a lethal dose of X-rays by cyanide, azide and malononitrile. Br. J. Radiol. 24: 617–621 (1951).

15   Huber, R.; Schroeder, R.: Antioxydantien und Überlebensrate ganz körperbestrahlter Mäuse. Strahlentherapie 119: 308–315 (1962).

16   Sakamoto, K.; Sakka, M.: Reduced effect of irradiation on normal and malignant cells irradiated in vivo in mice pretreated with vitamin E. Br. J. Radiol. 46: 538–540 (1973).

17   Malick, M.A.; Roy, R.M.; Sternberg, J.: Effect of vitamin E on post-irradiation death in mice. Experientia 34: 1216–1217 (1978).

18   Londer, H.M.; Myers, C.E.: Radioprotective effect of vitamin E. Am. J. clin. Nutr. 31: 705 (1978).

19   Prince, E.W.; Lieele, J.B.: The effects of dietary fatty acids and tocopherol on the radiosensitivity of mammalian erythrocytes. Radiat. Res. 53: 49–64 (1973).

20   Hoffer, A.; Roy, R.M.: Vitamin E decreases erythrocyte fragility after whole body irradiation. Radiat. Res. 61: 439–443 (1975).

21   Furth, F.W.; Coulter, M.P.; Howland, J.W.: Failure of alpha-tocopherol to protect against radiation injury in the rat. University of Rochester Atomic Energy Report UR 152, p. 34 (1951).

22   Haley, T.K.; McCulloh, E.F.; McCormick, W.G.: Influence of water-soluble vitamin E on survival time in irradiated mice. Science 119: 126–127 (1954).

23   Ershoff, B.H.; Steers, C.W., Jr.: Antioxidants and survival time of mice exposed to multiple sublethal doses of X-irradiation. Proc. Soc. exp. Biol. Med. 104: 274–276 (1960).

24   Rostock, R.A.; Stryker, J.A.; Abt, A.B.: Evaluation of high-dose vitamin E as a radioprotective agent. Radiology 126: 763–765 (1980).

25   Kagerud, A.; Holm, G.; Larsson, H.; Peterson, H.I.: Tocopherol and local X-ray irradiation of two transplantable rat tumors. Cancer Lett. 5: 123–129 (1978).

26   Kagerud, A.; Peterson, H.I.: Tocopherol in irradiation of experimental neoplasms: influence of dose and administration. Acta radiol. oncol. 20: 97 (1981).

27   Prasad, K.N.; Rama, B.N.: Modification of the effect of pharmacological agents on tumor cells in culture by vitamin C and vitamin E; in Meyskens, Prasad, Modulation and mediation of cancer cells by vitamins, pp. 244–257 (Karger, Basel 1983).

28   Lotan, R.: Effect of vitamin A and its analogs (retinoids) on normal and neoplastic cells. Biochim. biophys. Acta 605: 33–91 (1980).

29   Meyskens, F.L., Jr.: Modulation of abnormal growth by retinoids: a clinical perspective of the biological phenomenon. Life Sci. 28: 2323–2327 (1981).

30   Cameron, E.; Pauling, L.; Leibovitz, F.: Ascorbic acid and cancer. A review. Cancer Res. 39: 663–681 (1979).

31   Benade, L.; Howard, T.; Burk, D.: Synergistic killing of Ehrlich ascites carcinoma cells by ascorbate and 3-amino-1,2,4-triazolo. Oncology 23: 33–43 (1969).

32   Prasad, K.N.: Differentiation of neuroblastoma cells in culture. Biol. Rev. 50: 129–165 (1975).

33   Prasad, K.N.: Maturation of neuroblastoma; in Stoll, Prolong arrest of cancer, pp. 281–308 (Wiley & Sons, New York 1982).

34   Pastan, I.; Johnson, G.S.; Anderson, W.: Role of cyclic nucleotide in growth control.
      A. Rev. Biochem. *44:* 491–522 (1975).

35   Puck, T.: Cyclic AMP, the microtubule-microfilament systems, and cancer. Proc.
      natn. Acad. Sci. USA *74:* 4491–4495 (1977).

36   Prasad, K.N.: Effect of sodium butyrate on mammalian cells in culture. In vitro *12:*
      125–132 (1975).

37   Prasad, K.N.: Butyric acid: a small fatty acid with diverse biological functions. Life
      Sci. *27:* 1351–1358 (1980).

38   Coley, W.B.: The treatment of malignant tumors by repeated inoculation of erysip-
      elas: with a report of ten original cases. Am. J. med. Sci. *105:* 487–511 (1893).

39   Cavaliere, R.; Cicatto, E.C.; Giovanella, B.C.; Heidelberger, C.; Johnson, R.O.; Mar-
      gottin, I.M.; Mondovi, B.; Morvicca, G.; Rossi-Fanelli, A.: Selective heat sensitivity
      of cancer cells. Cancer *20:* 1351–1381 (1967).

40   Overgaard, K.; Overgaard, J.: Investigation on the possibility of a thermic tumor
      therapy. I. Short-wave treatment of a transplanted isologous mouse mammary carci-
      noma. Eur. J. Cancer *8:* 65–78 (1972).

41   Kim, S.H.; Kim, J.H.; Hahn, E.W.: The radiosensitization of hypoxic tumor cells by
      hyperthermia. Radiology *114:* 727–728 (1975).

42   Dewey, W.C.; Hopwood, L.E.; Separeto, S.A.; Gerweck, L.E.: Cellular responses to
      combinations of hyperthermia and radiation. Radiology *123:* 463–474 (1977).

43   Harkedar, I.; Bleehen, N.M.: Experimental and clinical aspects of hyperthermia
      applied to the treatment of cancer with special reference to the role of ultrasonic and
      microwave heating. Adv. Radiat. Biol. *6:* 229–266 (1976).

44   Luk, K.H.; Purser, P.R.; Castro, J.R.; Meyer, T.S.; Phillips, T.L.: Clinical experiences
      with local microwave hyperthermia. Int. J. Radiat. Oncol. Biol. Phys. *2:* suppl. 5,
      pp. 215–216 (1979).

45   Larkins, J.M.; Edwards, W.S.; Smith, D.E.: Total body hyperthermia and preliminary
      results in human neoplasms. Surg. Forum *27:* 121–123 (1976).

46   Suit, H.D.; Shwayder, M.: Hyperthermia potential as an antitumor agent. Cancer *34:*
      122–129 (1974).

47   Overgaard, J.: Fractionated radiation and hyperthermia. Cancer *48:* 1116–1123
      (1981).

48   Urano, M.; Rice, L.; Epstein, R.; Suit, H.D.; Chu, A.M.: Effect of whole body hyper-
      thermia on cell survival, metastasis, frequency, and host immunity in moderately and
      weakly immunogenic murine tumors. Cancer Res. *43:* 1039–1043 (1983).

49   Song, C.W.; Kang, M.S.; Rhee, J.G.; Levitt, S.H.: Effect of hyperthermia on vascu-
      lar function in normal and neoplastic tissues. Ann. N.Y. Acad. Sci. *335:* 35–47
      (1980).

50   Manning, M.R.; Cetas, T.; Boone, M.L.M.; Miller, R.C.: Clinical hyperthermic
      results of the phase I clinical trial combining localized hyperthermia with or without
      radiation (high dose rate and low dose rate). Int. J. Radiat. Oncol. Biol. Phys. *2:*
      suppl., p. 173 (1979).

51   Hill, S.A.; Denekamp, J.: The response of six mouse tumors to combined heat and
      X-rays. Implication for therapy. Br. J. Radiat. *52:* 209–218 (1979).

52   Goldfeder, A.; Brown, D.M.: Radiosensitization of tumors by combined treatment
      with microwave hyperthermia and misonidazole; in Brady, Radiation sensitizers,
      pp. 509–511 (Masson, New York 1980).

53 Samuelson, B.: Prostaglandins, thromboxane, and leukotrienes: biochemical pathways; in Powles, Buckman, Honn, Ramwell, Prostaglandins and cancer, pp. 1–19 (Liss, New York 1982).

54 Hope, W.L.; Dalton, C.; Machlin, L.J.; Filipski, R.J.; Vane, F.M.: Influence of dietary vitamin E on prostaglandin biosynthesis in rat blood. Prostaglandins 10: 557–571 (1975).

55 Chan, A.C.; Allen, C.R.; Hegarty, R.V.J.: The effect of vitamin E depletion and repletion on prostaglandin synthesis in semitendinosus muscle of young rabbit. J. Nutr. 110: 66–73 (1980).

56 Goetzel, J.: Vitamin E modulates the lipoxygenation of arachidonic acid in leukocytes. Nature, Lond. 288: 183–185 (1980).

57 Machelin, L.: Vitamin E and prostaglandins; in deDuve, Hayashi, Tocopherol, oxygen, biomembrane, pp. 179–189 (Elsevier/North-Holland Biomedical Press, New York 1978).

58 Hwang, D.H.; Donovan, J.: In vitro and in vivo effects of vitamin E on arachidonic acid metabolism in rat platelets. J. Nutr. 112: 1233–1237 (1982).

59 Vanderhoek, J.Y.; Lands, W.E.M.: The inhibition of fatty acid oxygenase of sheep vascular glands by antioxidants. Biochim. biophys. Acta 296: 382–385 (1973).

60 Zenser, T.V.; Davis, B.B.: Antioxidant inhibition of prostaglandin production by rat renal medulla. Metabolism 27: 227–233 (1978).

61 Panganamala, R.V.; Miller, J.S.; Gweby, E.; Sharma, T.; Cornwell, D.G.: Differential inhibitory effects of vitamin E and other antioxidants on prostaglandin synthetase, platelet aggregation and lipoxygenase. Prostaglandins 14: 261–271 (1978).

62 Vane, J.R.; Weissman, G.; Zurieri, R.B.: Pain and prostaglandins. New clinical perspectives (Burroughs, Wellcome Research, Triangle Park 1977).

63 Metzger, Z.; Hoffeld, J.T.; Oppenheim, J.J.: Macrophage-mediated suppression. I. Evidence for participation of both hydrogen peroxide and prostaglandins in suppression of murine lymphocyte proliferation. J. Immun. 129: 983–988 (1980).

64 Plescia, O.T.: Does prostaglandin synthesis affect in vivo tumor growth by altering tumor/host balance? in Powles, Bockman, Henn, Ramwell, Prostaglandins and cancer, pp. 619–631 (Liss, New York 1982).

65 Tildon, A.B.; Dougherty, P.A.; Balch, C.M.: Differential effects of indomethacin and PGE$_2$ on the depressed responses of cancer patients; in Powles, Bockman, Honn, Ramwell, Prostaglandins and cancer, pp. 597–607 (Liss, New York 1982).

66 Parker, C.W.: Arachidonate metabolites and immunity; in Powles, Bockman, Honn, Ramwell, Prostaglandins and cancer, pp. 597–607 (Liss, New York 1982).

67 Myers, C.E.; McGuire, W.; Young, R.: Adriamycin: amelioration of toxicity by alpha-tocopherol. Cancer Treat. Rep. 60: 961–962 (1976).

68 Sonnevald, P.: Effect of alpha-tocopherol on cardiotoxicity of adriamycin in the rat. Cancer Treat. Rep. 62: 1033–1036 (1978).

69 Van Vleet, J.F.; Greenwood, L.; Ferrans, V.J.; Rebar, A.H.: Effect of selenium-vitamin E on adriamycin-induced cardiomyopathy in rabbits. Am. J. Vitam. Res. 39: 997–1010 (1978).

70 Wang, Y.M.; Madanat, F.F.; Kimball, J.C.; Gieiser, C.A.; Ali, M.K.; Kaufman, M.W.; Van Eys, J.: Effect of vitamin E against adriamycin-induced toxicity in rabbits. Cancer Res. 40: 1022–1027 (1980).

71 Breed, J.G.C.; Zimmerman, A.N.E.; Dormans, J.A.; Pinedo, H.M.: Failure of the

antioxidant vitamin E to protect against adriamycin-induced cardiotoxicity in the rabbit. Cancer Res. *40:* 2033–2038 (1980).

72 Yamanaka, N.; Fukushima, M.; Koizumi, K.; Nishida, K.; Kato, T.; Ota, K.: Enhancement of DNA chain breakage by bleomycin and biological free radical producing system; in deDuve, Hayaishi, Tocopherol, oxygen, and biomembranes, pp. 59–69 (Elsevier/North-Holland Biomedical Press, New York 1978).

73 Svingen, B.A.; Powis, G.; Appel, P.L.; Scott, M.: Protection against adriamycin-induced skin necrosis in the rat by dimethylsulfoxide and alpha-tocopherol. Cancer Res. *41:* 3395–3399 (1981).

74 Tengerdy, R.P.; Brown, J.C.: Effect of vitamins E and A on humoral immunity and phagocytosis in *E. coli*-infected chickens. Poultry Sci. *56:* 975–983 (1977).

75 Tengerdy, R.P.; Heinzerling, R.H.; Nockels, C.F.: Effect of vitamin E on immune response of hypoxic and normal chickens. Infect. Immunology *5:* 987–989 (1972).

76 Campbell, P.A.; Cooper, H.R.; Tengerdy, R.P.: Vitamin E enhances in vitro immune response by normal and non-adherent spleen cells. Proc. Soc. exp. Biol. Med. *146:* 465–469 (1974).

77 Nockels, C.F.: Protective effect of supplemental vitamin E against infection. Fed. Proc. *38:* 2139–2143 (1979).

78 Tanaka, J.; Fujiwara, H.J.; Toriso, M.: Vitamin E and immune response enhancement of helper T cells' activity by dietary supplementation of vitamin E in mice. Immunology *38:* 727–734 (1979).

79 Sheffy, B.E.; Schultz, R.D.: Influence of vitamin E and selenium on immune response mechanism. Fed. Proc. *38:* 2139–2143 (1979).

80 Yasumaga, T.; Kato, H.; Ohgaki, K., Inamoto, T.; Hgikasa, Y.: Effect of vitamin E as an immuno-potentiation agent for mice at optimal dosage and its toxicity at high dosage. J. Nutr. *112:* 1075–1084 (1982).

81 Black, M.M.; Zachrau, R.E.; Dion, A.S.; Katz, M.: Stimulation of prognostically favorable cell-mediated immunity of breast cancer patients by high dose vitamin A and vitamin E; in Prasad, Vitamins, nutrition, and cancer, pp. 134–146 (Karger, Basel 1984).

82 Abrams, A.A.: Use of vitamin E in chronic cystic mastites. New Engl. J. Med. *272:* 1080–1081 (1965).

83 Dam, H.; Granados, H.: Peroxidation of body fat in vitamin E efficiency. Acta physiol. scand. *10:* 162–171 (1945).

84 McCay, P.B.; King, M.M.: Vitamin E: its role as a biological free radical scavanger and its relationship to the microsomal mixed-function oxidase system; in Machlin, Vitamin E, pp. 289–317 (Dekker, New York 1980).

85 Tappel, A.L.: Vitamin E and free radical peroxidation of lipids. Ann. N.Y. Acad. Sci. *203:* 12–27 (1972).

86 Olcott, H.S.; Matill, H.A.: Constituents of fats and oils affecting the development of rancidity. Chem. Res. *29:* 257–268 (1941).

87 Lucy, J.A.: Structural interactions between vitamin E and polyunsaturated phospholipids; in deDuve, Hayaishi, Tocopherol, oxygen, and biomembranes, pp. 109–120 (Elsevier/North-Holland Biomedical Press, New York 1978).

88 Diplock, A.T.; Lucy, J.A.: The biochemical modes of action of vitamin E and selenium: a hypothesis. FEBS Lett. *29:* 205–210 (1973).

89 March, B.E.; Coates, V.; Biely, J.: Reticulocytosis in response to dietary antioxidants. Science *164*: 1398–1400 (1969).

90 Nair, P.P.; Patnaik, R.N.; Hauswirth, J.W.: Cellular transport and binding of *D*-alpha-tocopherol; in deDuve, Hayaishi, Tocopherol, oxygen and biomembranes, pp. 121–130 (Elsevier/North-Holland Biomedical Press, New York 1978).

91 Catignani, G.L.: An alpha-tocopherol-binding protein in rat liver cytoplasm. Biochem. biophys. Res. Commun. *67*: 66–72 (1975).

92 Patnaik, R.N.; Nair, P.P.: Studies on the binding of *D*-alpha-tocopherol to rat liver nuclei. Archs Biochem. Biophys. *178*: 333–341 (1977).

93 Rajaram, O.V.; Fatlerpaker, P.; Screenivasan, A.: Involvement of binding lipoproteins in the absorption and transport of alpha-tocopherol in the rat. Biochem. J. *140*: 509–516 (1974).

94 Patnaik, R.; Kessie, G.; Nair, P.; Biswal, N.: Vitamin E-binding proteins in mammalian cells; in Prasad, Vitamins, nutrition, and cancer, pp. 105–117 (Karger, Basel 1984).

95 Prasad, K.N.; Gandreau, D.; Brown, J.: Binding of vitamin E in mammalian tumor cells in culture. Proc. Soc. exp. biol. Med. *166*: 167–174 (1981).

96 Catignani, G.L.: An α-tocopherol binding protein in rat liver cytoplasm. Biochem. biophys. Res. Commun. *67*: 66–72 (1975).

97 Molenaar, I.; Vos, J.; Hommes, F.A.: Effect of vitamin E deficiency on cellular membranes. Vitams Horm. *30*: 45–82 (1972).

98 Huang, C.: Configurations of fatty acyl chains in EGG phosphatidylcholine-cholesterol mixed bilayers. Chem. Phys. Lipids *191*: 150–158 (1977).

99 Marusich, W.: Vitamin E as an in vivo lipid stabilizer and its effect on flavor and storage properties of milk and meat; in Machlin, Vitamin E, pp. 445–466 (Dekker, New York 1980).

100 Steiner, M.: Inhibition of platelet aggregation by alpha-tocopherol; in deDuve, Hayaishi, Tocopherol, oxygen, and biomembranes, pp. 143–163 (Elsevier/North-Holland Biomedical Press, New York 1978).

101 Machlin, J.J.; Flipski, R.; Willis, A.L.; Kuhn, D.C.; Brin, M.: Influence of vitamin E on platelet aggregation and thrombocythemia in the rat. Proc. Soc. exp. Biol. Med. *149*: 275–277 (1975).

102 Fang, J.S.C.: Alpha-tocopherol: its inhibition on human platelet aggregation. Experientia *32*: 6–9, 41 (1976).

103 Steiner, M.: Inhibition of platelet aggregation by alpha-tocopherol; in deDuve, Hayaishi, Tocopherol, oxygen and biomembranes, pp. 143–163 (Elsevier/North-Holland Biomedical Press, New York 1978).

104 Bieri, J.G.: Vitamin E. Nutr. Rev. *33*: 161–167 (1975).

105 Horwitt, M.K.; Mason, K.E.: Tocopherol. XIII. Pharmacology and toxicology; in Sebrill, Harris, The vitamins, pp. 309–312 (Academic Press, New York 1972).

106 Farrel, P.M.; Bieri, J.G.: Mega vitamin E supplementation in man. Am. J. Nutr. *28*: 1381–1386 (1975).

107 Farrel, M.P.M.: Deficiency status, pharmacological effects, nutritional requirements; in Machilin, Vitamin E, pp. 520–620 (Dekker, New York 1980).

108 Bieri, J.G.; Corash, L.; Hubbard, V.S.: Medical uses of vitamin E. New Engl. J. Med. *308*: 1063–1071 (1983).

109 Salkeld, R.M.: Safety and tolerance of high-dose vitamin E administration in man. A

review of the literature. Draft of unpublished data included in OTC vol 150121 (1982).

110 Robert, H.J.: Perspective on vitamin E as therapy. J. Am. med. Ass. *246:* 129–131 (1981).

111 Herbert, F.: Toxicity of vitamin E. Nutr. Rev. *35:* 158 (1977).

112 Corrigan, J.J., Jr.; Marcus, F.I.: Coagulopathy associated with vitamin ingestion. J. Am. med. Ass. *230:* 1300–1301 (1974).

113 Briggs, M.H.: Vitamin E in clinical medicine. Lancet *i:* 220 (1947).

114 Prasad, J.S.: Effect of vitamin E supplementation on leukocyte function. Am. J. clin. Nutr. *33:* 606–608 (1980).

115 Yamanaka, N.; Kato, T.; Nishida, K.; Fuzikawa, T.; Fukushima, M.; Ota, K.: Elevation of serum level lipid peroxide level associated with doorubicin toxicity and its amelioration by *DL*-alpha-tocopherol acetate or Co-enzyme Q10 in mouse. Cancer Chemother. Pharmacol. *3:* 223–227 (1979).

116 LeVander, O.A.; Morris, V.C.; Higgs, D.J.; Verma, R.N.: Nutritional interrelationship among vitamin E, selenium, antioxidants and ethyl alcohol in the rat. J. Nutr. *103:* 536–542 (1973).

K.N. Prasad, PhD, Center for Vitamins and Cancer Research,
Department of Radiology, School of Medicine,
University of Colorado Health Sciences Center, Denver, CO 80262 (USA)

Prasad (ed.), Vitamins, Nutrition, and Cancer, pp. 105–117 (Karger, Basel 1984)

Vitamin E-Binding Proteins in Mammalian Cells

Rabi Patnaik[a], *George Kessie*[a], *P.P. Nair*[a], *Nilamber Biswal*[b, 1]

[a] Department of Research Medicine, Sinai Hospital of Baltimore, Baltimore, Md.; Department of Biochemistry, The Johns Hopkins University School of Hygiene and Public Health, Baltimore, Md.; [b] Division of Molecular Biology, University of Maryland Cancer Center, University of Maryland School of Medicine, Baltimore, Md., USA

Introduction

In recent years studies have been initiated to examine the effects of vitamin E (D-α-tocopherol) alone and in combination with other nutritional factors such as vitamin C on metabolic, preneoplastic (high risk for neoplasia) and neoplastic diseases in human population as well as in experimental animals [1–3]. Although the preliminary findings are very encouraging, the mechanism of action of these factors is not known at the present time. One of the postulated hypotheses is that, in order to be effective at cellular level to bring about 'corrective/protective modification' in cell metabolism these factors are expected to enter into the cell by moving across its membrane. Once inside the cell, these may be transported to various intracellular sites and get 'associated' or 'bound' to specific cellular molecules to bring about changes at cellular and/or molecular level by specific mechanism.

Such binding species for various nutritional factors have been identified in many mammalian tissue. Occurrence of such species for vitamin E has been sporadically reported in the past few years. Vitamin E-binding proteins are shown to be present in rat liver [4], rabbit heart muscle [5], mouse neuroblastoma and glioma cells [6], human erythrocytes [7] and in human serum [8]. In rat liver vitamin E is associated with a cytosolic binding protein [4], a carrier lipoprotein [9] and nuclear binding protein [10]. This paper examines and describes some of the characteristics and site of association of intranuclear binding species in hepatic tissue. Further-

---

[1] We thank *Stephen Keoseian* for taking the photomicrographs of the rat liver nuclei.

more, it also examines the uptake, intracellular distribution and binding characteristics of vitamin E in human transformed cells such as human epithelial cells (HEp-2) and neuroblastoma cells (MNB-8) in culture.

Experimental Procedures

Experimental Animals. Male weanling rats of Sprague-Dawley strain maintained on vitamin E-deficient diet [11] were intravenously injected with ^{3}H-D-α-tocopherol (100 µCi/rat; 60 Ci/mmol) in a compatible solvent system containing dimethylsulfoxide and Tween 80. After 10–12 h the animals were sacrificed and perfused livers were used for subsequent analyses.

Cell Lines. Human epithelial cells (HEp-2) derived from laryngeal squamous carcinoma and human neuroblastoma cells (MNB) were grown in monolayers in minimum essential medium (MEM) with 10% calf serum. The cells were incubated with ^{3}H-D-α-tocopherol (10 µCi/ml) in MEM for 12 h and were washed 3 times in phosphate-buffered saline (PBS) and used for further studies.

Preparation of Rat Liver Nuclei and Chromatin. The liver was homogenized in 0.32 M sucrose with 3 mM MgCl$_2$ and the homogenate was centrifuged (800 g) to obtain crude nuclei which were recentrifuged (64,000 g) in 2.2 M sucrose to obtain purified nuclei. The nuclei were washed with 0.2% Triton X-100 in 0.32 M sucrose, 3 mM MgCl$_2$ to eliminate cytoplasmic contamination. Subsequently these nuclei were homogenized and washed several times with decreasing concentrations of Tris-HCl, pH 8.0, to obtain chromatin as per the method of *Huang and Huang* [12]. The average composition of chromatin was protein:DNA:RNA 1.96:1.0:0.043.

Extraction of Chromatin by Various Reagents. Chromatin-bound with labeled vitamin E was treated with various reagents known to solubilize or extract its specific components. The end point followed was the removal of radioactivity from chromatin.

Gel Filtration of Chromatin on Sepharose 4B Column. Chromatin solubilized in sodium chloride (0.6–1.0 M) in 0.01 M Tris·HCl, pH 7.4, was fractionated on Sepharose 4B column. Each fraction was assayed for radioactivity, protein and DNA content. In other experiments the high salt extract of chromatin was salted out and the supernatant fraction was fractionated as described above.

Reconstitution and Fractionation of Reconstituted Chromatin. Labeled vitamin E-bound chromatin was partially dissociated by high salt treatment and reconstituted by salting out as per the method of *Alberga* et al. [13]. By this method the proteins having high affinity for DNA precipitated as DNA-protein complex and those having lower affinity remained in solution. The reconstituted DNA-protein complex was fractionated by the method of *Teng* et al. [14] to obtain basic proteins, DNA and phenol-soluble nonhistone chromosomal proteins.

Heterogeneous Nuclear RNA (hnRNA) Synthesis. Vitamin E-deficient and control rats were intravenously injected with ^{3}H-orotic acid (100 µCi/rat). After various time intervals rats were sacrificed, hnRNA was extracted and prepared from purified nuclei by conventional phenol extraction procedure. Purified hnRNA samples were fractionated by 5–40% sucrose gradient ultracentrifugation. Fractions were assayed for radioactivity.

Intracellular Distribution of ^{3}H-D-α-Tocopherol in HEp-2 and MNB-8 Cells. The cells were incubated with ^{3}H-*D*-α-tocopherol (50 µCi/dish) for 12 h. The cells were washed extensively in PBS and homogenized. Various intracellular components were fractionated by conventional differential centrifugation method.

Intranuclear Localization of ^{3}H-D-α-Tocopherol in HEp-2 and MNB-8 Cells. The cells were homogenized in isotonic solution and nuclei were purified as described above. The nuclei were treated with 0.2% Triton X-100 and high concentrations of NaCl. Each fraction was assayed for radioactivity.

Gel Filtration of Cytosolic Fractions from Vitamin E-Labeled HEp-2 and MNB-8 Cells. The cells were homogenized in Hepes buffer [6] and the 105,000 *g* supernatant was fractionated on a Sephadex G-25 column. Each fraction was monitored for radioactivity and protein content. In some cases the cytosolic samples were fractionated on Sepharose 6B column. In each case fractionation was undertaken in Hepes buffer.

Sucrose Gradient Ultracentrifugation of Cytosolic Fractions from Vitamin E-Labeled HEp-2 and MNB-8 Cells. The cytosolic fractions were fractionated by 5–20% sucrose gradient ultracentrifugation at 40,000 rpm in SW 50.1 rotor for 16 h. Each fraction was assayed for radioactivity.

Electron Microscopy. Purified rat liver nuclei were prefixed in glutaraldehyde and fixed in 2% osmium tetraoxide. The encapsulated fixed nuclei were cut into sections, stained with Richardson's stain and examined under light microscope. Thin sections from specific thick samples were cut and stained with uranyl acetate and lead citrate, carbon-coated and observed under Hitachi electron microscope.

Analytical Methods. The purity of commercial labeled *D*-α-tocopherol and that bound to various hepatic and cellular fractions was established by thin-layer chromatography as described by *Bieri* [15]. Radioactivity was assayed by liquid scintillation counting using either the dioxane-based Bray's solution or the toluene-based liquifluor after solubilizing the samples in NCS solubilizer. Protein was assayed by the method of *Lowry* et al. [16], DNA by the method of *Burton* [17] and RNA by orcinol method [18].

Results

In order to obtain a precise knowledge about the magnitude and site of binding of vitamin E in the intranuclear domain, it is essential to prepare intact nuclei free from cytoplasmic contamination. Several reports have dealt with this problem by incorporating nonionic detergent Triton X-100 ranging from 0.1 to 0.5% in the isolation medium. However, we observed variable results in terms of vitamin E binding by using different concentrations of this detergent. This created suspicion of possible nuclear damage by this detergent. The purified hepatic nuclei looked intact with clearly visible single or multiple nucleoli under light microscope (fig. 1). However, electron micrographs showed a different picture (fig. 2a–d). Without any detergent the nuclei were contaminated with cytoplasmic debris and the outer

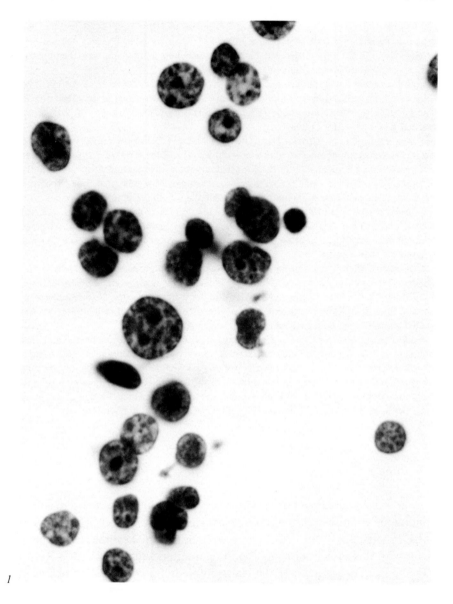

1

Fig. 1. Light microscopic appearance of purified rat liver nuclei. HE. × 980.

Fig. 2. Electron micrographs of purified nuclei treated with various concentrations of Triton X-100. *a* Untreated nuclei; *b* 0.1% Triton X-100; *c* 0.2% Triton X-100; *d* 0.5% Triton X-100. × 9,100–22,000.

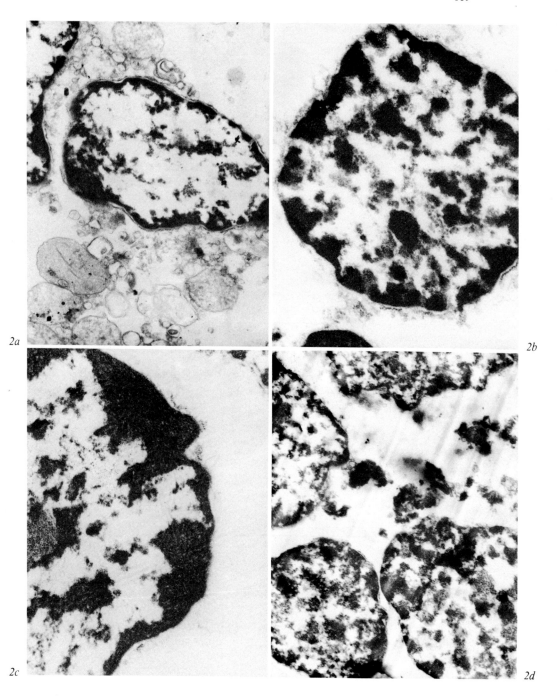

2a

2b

2c

2d

Table I. Solubility of intranuclear binding sites by reagents

Reagents	Radioactivity solubilized, dpm	Percent solubilized
0.32 M sucrose with 3 mM MgCl$_2$	781	8.9
0.2% Triton X-100 in 0.32 M sucrose, 3 mM MgCl$_2$	3,924	44.7
0.1 M Tris-HCl, pH 7.5	184	2.1
0.01 M Tris-HCl, pH 7.5 with 1.0 M NaCl	4,284	48.8
10% trichloroacetic acid	2,036	23.2

[3]H-D-α-Tocopherol-bound nuclei were divided into various fractions having 8,780 dpm radioactivity. Each fraction was extracted with different reagents and centrifuged to obtain soluble fraction.

Table II. Effect of various treatments on the release of ^{3}H-D-α-tocopherol from chromatin

Treatments	Radioactivity released, % total
10% trichloroacetic acid	44.9
0.15 M H$_2$SO$_4$	2.7
0.03 M sodium citrate, pH 4.0	2.8
0.01 M Tris-HCl, pH 7.0	7.4
0.02 M sodium phosphate, pH 7.6 with 1.0 M NaCl	56.3
0.02 M sodium phosphate, pH 12.0	47.5
Enzymes	
Control	7.7
RNase A	7.8
DNase I	11.6
Trypsin	22.0
Pronase	34.1
Lipase	8.4
Steapsin	6.9

and inner membranes were intact (fig. 2a). Use of 0.1% Triton X-100 did not solubilize the outer membrane completely (fig. 2b). This was successfully accomplished by raising the concentration to 0.2% (fig. 2c). However, at still higher concentrations (0.5%), both outer and inner membranes seemed to be solubilized releasing the nuclear content (fig. 2d). Consequently, 0.2% appeared to be the optimum concentration of the detergent which

Table III. Distribution of radioactivity among fractions obtained by partial dissociation and reconstitution of ^{3}H-*D*-α-tocopherol-bound chromatin

Fraction	Radioactivity, dpm
Residual pellet	3,073
Tris-EDTA-glycerol-soluble fraction	1,267
Tris-EDTA-glycerol-insoluble DNA-protein complex	7,321
0.25 *N* HCl	169
Phenol-insoluble aqueous phase	540
2-Mercaptoethanol phase	105
Phenol-soluble protein phase	6,437

EDTA = Ethylenediaminetetraacetic acid.

could be used for purifying the intact nuclei without damaging the inner membrane or loosing the nuclear content. Thus, this concentration was routinely used in all purification procedures.

The specific properties of vitamin E-associated binding sites is presented in table I. Major portion of nuclear associated vitamin E was associated with nucleoprotein complex (chromatin, 50%) and can be extracted by high concentration of salt. The vitamin E-associated sites were precipitable by trichloroacetic acid (TCA), an indication of being associated with macromolecules. Acidic conditions did not solubilize the binding species. On the other hand, raising pH to alkaline range progressively enhanced solubility, more particularly in the presence of salt in the medium. RNase, lipase, or steapsin did not release the vitamin whereas trypsin and pronase showed pronounced effect, pronase being more effective than trypsin. DNase I had limited effect. This suggested that the binding sites are proteins and possibly nonhistone in nature (table II).

In order to examine the site of association of vitamin E in the intrachromatin domain, chromatin-vitamin E complex was partially dissociated and subsequently reassociated by salting out procedure (table III). A major portion of vitamin E was associated with reassociated DNA-protein complex, showing that the vitamin E-associated sites have very high affinity for DNA. The reassociated DNA-protein complex was subfractionated into its components, such as acid extract, containing histones, phenol extracted aqueous phase containing nucleic acids and phenol-soluble fraction containing nonhistone proteins, possibly phosphoproteins. It is the phenol-soluble fraction which carried most of the vitamin E.

Table IV. Distribution of vitamin E among fractions obtained by Sepharose 4B chromatography

Fraction	^{3}H-D-α-tocopherol, dpm	
	before reconstitution 1.0 M NaCl extract	after reconstitution
Peak I (high molec. wt)	11,675	287[1]
Peak II (lower molec. wt)	9,500	734

[1] Most of DNA and significant amounts of protein were precipitated out as DNA-protein complex as a result of desalting. Major portion of radioactivity was recovered in the complex.

The affinity of vitamin-associated sites for DNA was further examined by Sepharose 4B fractionation of high salt extract of chromatin. In this experiment labeled vitamin E was associated with two peaks, peak I (high molecular weight, comprising of DNA and small amount of protein) and peak II (predominantly large amounts of protein). The chromatin extract was salted out and subsequently centrifuged to obtain DNA-protein complex and soluble fractions. When this fraction was fractionated on Sepharose 4B column there was dramatic decrease in radioactivity under both peak I and peak II, showing that most of the vitamin E-bound sites were associated with pelleted DNA-protein complex as a result of salting out (table IV).

In order to examine the effect of vitamin E on the synthesis of RNA, specifically hnRNA in liver, ^{3}H-orotic acid, a precursor of RNA synthesis, was intravenously injected to vitamin E-deficient and control (sufficient) rats. At various time periods postadministration, hepatic hnRNA was purified and was examined by sucrose gradient ultracentrifugation (fig. 3). The data under each fraction was first calculated as percentage of total activity in the sample to eliminate the differences in nucleotide pool in the different samples. Subsequently the data was plotted as net incorporation (vitamin E-sufficient-deficient) under each fraction. At an early period there appeared to be a general stimulation in hnRNA synthesis, except that of lower sedimentation values. But during the later period specific classes of hnRNA (4–7S, 11–19S and 27–35S) seemed to have been stimulated by the presence of vitamin E.

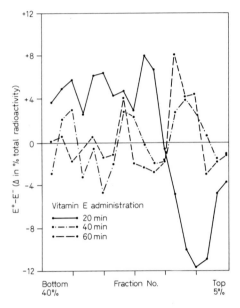

Fig. 3. 5–40% linear sucrose gradient ultracentrifugation of rapidly labeled heteroge-neous nuclear RNA (hnRNA) species from vitamin E-deficient and control rat liver.

The distribution of vitamin E among various subcellular components of HEp-2 cells and MNB-8 cells is presented in table V. Significant amounts of vitamin E were localized in the nuclear fraction in both cell lines. Higher amounts of vitamin E (50%) were observed to be present in the cytosolic fraction in HEp-2 cells as compared to that in MNB cells. On the other hand, crude nuclei in MNB cells carried more vitamin E (21%) as compared to those in HEp-2 cells (13%).

The cytosolic fractions from both cell lines were prepared and were examined by sucrose gradient ultracentrifugation (5–20%). Labeled vitamin E was more polydispersed in HEp-2 cells as compared to that in MNB cells. Most of the radioactivity sedimented between 2.7S and 4.2S. Thus, there is perhaps more than one class of vitamin E-binding species in these cell lines (fig. 4).

The cytosol from both cell lines was fractionated on Sephadex G-75 column. In both the cases a single peak of radioactivity was eluted with protein (fig. 5). However, when the cytosolic fraction from MNB-8 cells was fractionated on Sepharose 6B column, at least 3 radioactivity peaks were

Table V. Intracellular distribution of ^{3}H-*D*-α-tocopherol in mammalian cells in culture

Fraction	Total radioactivity, %	Specific activity cpm $\times$ 10^{-4}/mg protein
HEp-2		
Total	100	0.4227
Cytosol	50.9	0.2717
Cytoplasmic particulate	35.3	0.3606
Crude nuclei	13.7	0.3360
MNB-8		
Total	100	0.4705
Cytosol	13.28	0.0652
Cytoplasmic particulate	64.79	14.6345
Crude nuclei	21.19	4.7596

Table VI. Intranuclear distribution of ^{3}H-*D*-α-tocopherol in mammalian cells in culture

Fraction	Total radioactivity, %
HEp-2	
Purified nuclei	100
0.32 *M* Sucrose + 3 m*M* MgCl$_2$ + 0.2% Triton X-100	18.6
2.0 *M* NaCl soluble	49.3
Residual pellet	31.9
MNB-8	
Purified nuclei	100
0.32 *M* Sucrose + 3 m*M* MgCl$_2$ + 0.2% Triton X-100	21.2
2.0 *M* NaCl soluble	36.7
Residual pellet	42.2

observed, suggesting multiple binding species for vitamin E in the MNB-8 cell line (fig. 6).

The nuclei from both cell lines were purified by 2.2 *M* sucrose ultracentrifugation. Triton X-100 (0.2%) eliminated only 18–21% of the nuclear associated radioactivity. Very significant amount of radioactivity was extracted by high concentration of NaCl suggesting association with nucleoprotein complex (table VI).

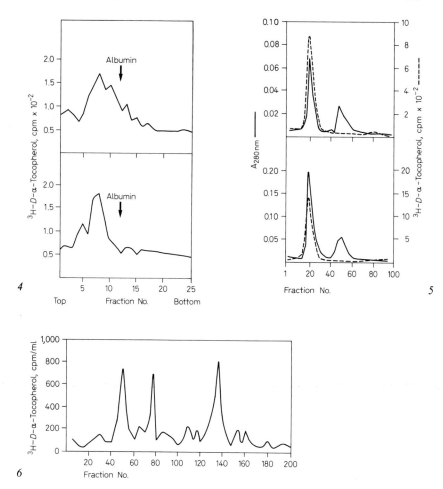

Fig. 4. 5–20% linear sucrose gradient ultracentrifugation of cytosol fractions obtained from HEp-2 and MNB-8 cells incubated with ³H-*D*-α-tocopherol.

Fig. 5. Sephadex G-25 fractionation of cytosol fractions obtained from HEp-2 and MNB-8 cells incubated with ³H-*D*-α-tocopherol.

Fig. 6. Sepharose 6B fractionation of cytosol fraction obtained from MNB-8 cells incubated with ³H-*D*-α-tocopherol.

It was necessary to examine the fate of ³H-*D*-α-tocopherol in the hepatic tissue. Thin-layer chromatography of tissue extracted vitamin E showed that it had the same chromatographic characteristics as that of the authentic *D*-α-tocopherol.

Discussion

In rat liver, our studies were focussed on the site of association of nuclear-bound vitamin E in the intrachromatin domain. All the evidences presented in this study pointed towards its association with chromosomal nonhistone proteins, possibly phosphoproteins. These proteins have very high affinity for DNA. These observations might have important relevance at least in part to its postulated functions at the molecular level, as there are several pieces of evidence that show these specific types of proteins may have important role in the modulation of gene expression [19]. Furthermore, our data has shown that vitamin E appears to affect the transcriptional process as evidenced from hnRNA synthesis. It also has shown that specific classes of hnRNA were preferentially affected depending on the time period of the transcriptional process.

Vitamin E-binding species are not only present in normal mammalian tissue in vivo, such species seem to be present in transformed cells when examined in vitro. In contrast to rat liver, there appeared to be multiple classes of vitamin E binding species in human transformed cells. This is evident from sucrose gradient ultracentrifugation analysis and from gel filtration data. Similar observations have been reported in mouse transformed cells [6]. In addition, it is interesting to note that there is differential behavior by the cells with respect to the uptake of this vitamin and its subsequent distribution among various subcellular components. Significant amounts of vitamin E reached intranuclear sites and appeared to be associated with nucleoprotein complex. It appears that there are perhaps specific classes of chromosomal proteins that are structurally oriented to 'accept' or 'bind' trace lipids with specific affinity and these binding species have very high affinity for DNA. Although the interpretation of these results cannot be done precisely at the present time, these observations might have important relevance with respect to the role of vitamin E in cell metabolism. Future studies will throw more light on this aspect of vitamin E function.

References

1   Dion, P.W.; Bright-See, E.B.; Smith, C.C.; Bruce, W.R.: The effect of dietary ascorbic acid and α-tocopherol on fecal mutagenicity. Mutation Res. *102:* 27–37 (1982).
2   Kayden, et al.: Vitamin E: biochemical, hematological and clinical aspects. Ann. N.Y. Acad. Sci. *393:* 1–506 (1982).

3   Gonzalez, E.R.: Vitamin E relieves cystic breast diseases, alter lipid, hormones. J. Am. med. Ass. *244:* 1077–1078 (1980).

4   Catignani, G.L.; Bieri, J.G.: Rat liver α-tocopherol binding; binding protein. Biochim. biophys. Acta *497:* 349–357 (1977).

5   Guarnieri, C.; Flamigni, F.; Caldrera, C.M.: A possible role of rabbit heart cytosol tocopherol binding in the transfer of tocopherol into nuclei. Biochem. J. *190:* 469–471 (1980).

6   Prasad, K.N.; Gaudreau, D.; Brown, J.: Binding of vitamin E in mammalian cells in culture. Proc. Soc. exp. Biol. Med. *166:* 167–174 (1981).

7   Kitabchi, A.E.; Wimalasena, J.: Specific binding sites of *D*-α-tocopherol in human erythrocytes. Biochim. biophys. Acta *684:* 200–206 (1982).

8   Takahashi, Y.; Uruno, K.; Kimura, S.: Vitamin E-binding proteins in human serum. J. Nutr. Sci. Vitaminol. *23:* 201–209 (1977).

9   Rajaram, O.V.; Fatterpaker, P.; Sreenivasan, A.: Involvement of binding lipoproteins in the absorption and transport of α-tocopherol in the rat. Biochem. J. 140: 509–516 (1974).

10 Patnaik, R.; Nair, P.P.: Studies on the binding of *D*-α-tocopherol to rat liver nuclei. Archs Biochem. Biophys. *178:* 333–341 (1977).

11 Hauswirth, J.W.; Nair, P.P.: Effect of different vitamin E-deficient basal diet on hepatic catalase and microsomal cytochrome P450 and b5 in rats. Am. J. clin. Nutr. *28:* 1087–1094 (1975).

12 Huang, R.C.C.; Huang, P.C.: Effect of protein-bound RNA associated with chick embryo chromatin on template specificity of the chromatin. J. molec. Biol. *39:* 365–378 (1969).

13 Alberga, A.; Massol, N.; Raynard, J.; Baulieu, E.: Estradiol binding of exceptionally high affinity by a nonhistone chromatin fraction. Biochemistry, N.Y. *10:* 3835–3845 (1971).

14 Teng, C.; Teng, C.T.; Allfrey, V.G.: Studies on nuclear acidic proteins. Evidence for their phosphorylation, tissue specificity, selective binding to deoxyribonucleic acid and stimulatory effects on transcription. J. biol. Chem. *246:* 3597–3609 (1971).

15 Bieri, J.G.: Chromatography of tocopherols; in Marinetti, Lipid chromatographic analysis, vol. 2, pp. 459–478 (Dekker, New York 1969).

16 Lowry, O.H.; Rosebrough, N.J.; Farr, A.L.; Randall, R.S.: Protein measurement with the Folin phenol reagent. J. biol. Chem. *193:* 265–275 (1951).

17 Burton, K.: The study of the conditions and mechanisms of the diphenylamine reaction for the colorimetric estimation of deoxyribonucleic acid. Biochem. J. *62:* 315–323 (1956).

18 Ceriotti, G.: Determination of nucleic acids in animal tissues. J. biol. Chem. *214:* 59–70 (1955).

19 Stein, G.W.; Spelsberg, T.C.; Kleinsmith, L.J.: Nonhistone chromosomal proteins and gene regulation. Science *183:* 817–824 (1974).

R. Patnaik, PhD, Department of Medicine,
Divisions of Gastroenterology and
Infectious Diseases, University of Maryland School of Medicine,
Baltimore, MD 21201 (USA)

Prasad (ed.), Vitamins, Nutrition, and Cancer, pp. 118–122 (Karger, Basel 1984)

Vitamin E and Its Effect on Skin Papilloma

Ismail Sadek

Zoology Department, Faculty of Science, Alexandria University, Alexandria, Egypt

Introduction

The role of vitamins in the prevention of neoplasms is becoming increasingly evident. Vitamin A inhibited the carcinogenic effect of 20-methylcholanthrene in the Egyptian toad [11]. Vitamin C (ascorbic acid) also inhibited the carcinogenic effect of DMBA on the skin of *Bufo regularis* [12]. It has been suggested that the presence of antioxidants in food, many of which are added as preservatives, may be related to reduced incidences of human gastric carcinoma [13], inasmuch as antioxidants, of which vitamin E is one, have been shown to have anticarcinogenic properties [14]. Vitamin E has been shown to exert a protective function against chemical carcinogenesis in experimental animals [4]. Also, *Hirooka* et al. [5] stated that vitamin E prevents the progression of early neoplastic lesions to cancers in rats and continuous daily intake of vitamin E appears necessary to maintain chemoprotection against mammary carcinogenesis. Aquasol *DL*-α-tocopheryl acetate induces morphological differentiation in a certain clone (NBP$_2$) of mouse neuroblastoma cells and enhances the growth inhibitory effect of tumor-therapeutic agents on neuroblastoma and rat glioma (C-6) cells in culture [9, 10].

The purpose of the present study is to evaluate the therapeutic effect of vitamin E (*DL*-α-tocopheryl acetate) on skin papillomas induced by DMBA in the Egyptian toad.

Materials and Methods

Toads, *B. regularis,* weighing 50 g each were divided into 3 groups. In the first group (group A, 115 toads) 7,12-dimethylbenz[a]anthracene (Fluka AG, Basel, Switzerland) was applied to the dorsal skin of the toads for 3 months as described by *Sadek and Abdelmegid* [12]. In the second group (group B), 50 toads bearing papillomas were treated with 500 mg/kg/day of vitamin E (*DL*-α-tocopheryl acetate) for 2 weeks by injection into the dorsal lymph sacs. The third group (group C, 50 toads) bearing papillomas was not treated with vitamin E and considered as control.

Results

Skin papillomas were observed in the experimental animals painted with DMBA daily. Skin papillomas ranging in diameter between 2 and 4 mm have been developed in group A in 100 cases out of 115 cases during 3 months (table I). The therapeutic study was started on 50 animals (group B) when the papillomas can be seen spread over the back skin of the animals. Regression of papillomas was observed in 27 of 50 toads of this group. The percent of regression was 54%. Group C, which did not receive vitamin E, shows regression of the papillomas in 5 cases out of 50 cases. The percent of regression was 10%.

Discussion

The study shows that vitamin E increased the regression of established skin papillomas in the Egyptian toad. Vitamin E has strong antioxidant properties [13]. Vitamin E (*DL*-α-tocopherol) inhibited the oral mucosal carcinogenesis in hamsters induced by DMBA [15]. *D*-α-Tocopheryl (vitamin E) acid succinate induces morphological changes and growth inhibition in mouse melanoma (B-16) cells in culture [8]. Also, vitamin E has been shown to decrease carcinogen-induced chromosomal breakage in leukocyte cultures to a similar or even more marked degree than other antioxidants [14], and a vitamin E-enriched diet has also been shown to reduce the incidence of methylcholanthrene-induced tumors in rats [6] and mice [3]. Mice show a reduced production of colorectal tumors, fewer carcinoma, and fewer adenomas with marked atypia when they are fed excess vitamin E [2].

The result of the present investigation suggests that vitamin E could play some role in chemotherapy of skin tumors in the Egyptian toad. The

Table I. Vitamin E and its effect on skin of the Egyptian toad

Weeks	Group A (115 toads) number of toads bearing papilloma	Group B (50 toads)[1]	Group C (50 toads)[1] control
4	15	17	0
8	40	5	2
12	45	5	3
Total	100	27	5

[1] Toads bearing skin papillomas.

exact mechanism by which this regression of tumors occurs is not known but there are numerous possible mechanisms. Antioxidant mechanisms probably neutralize or reduce free radicals, a process which has been described as scavenging of free radicals [23]. The inhibition of polycyclic hydrocarbon tumorigenesis by antioxidants may be related to the ability of antioxidants to prevent the in vivo activation of hydrocarbons to carcinogenic epioxides and/or other electrophilic intermediates [16]. Vitamin E could induce multiple effects during the management of tumors such as cell death [1, 10], differentiation [10], inhibition of cell division [10], potentiation of the effect of tumor-therapeutic agents [9], reduction of the toxic effects of certain chemotherapeutic agents [7, 17, 19, 20], and stimulation of the host's immune system [18]. In general, the antioxidants may protect against chemical carcinogenesis by inhibiting the formation of the carcinogenic electrophile in a number of structurally diverse chemical compounds [21, 22].

It seems also probable that stimulation of the host's immune system is a very dominant force which may regulate the mechanism of action of vitamin E in the Egyptian toad.

Acknowledgments

The help of Prof. *Kedar N. Prasad,* Department of Radiology, School of Medicine, University of Colorado Health Sciences Center, in reviewing this manuscript is appreciated. *DL-α-*Tocopheryl acetate was kindly supplied from Hoffmann-La Roche, Basel, Switzerland.

References

1 Abrams, A.A.: Use of vitamin E in chronic cystic mastitis. New Engl. J. Med. *272:* 1080–1081 (1965).

2 Cook, M.G.; McNamara, P.: Effect of dietary vitamin E on dimethylhydrazine-induced colonic tumors in mice. Cancer Res. *40:* 1329–1331 (1980).

3 Haber, S.L.; Wissler, R.W.: Effect of vitamin E on carcinogenicity of methylcholanthrene. Proc. Soc. exp. Biol. Med. *111:* 774–775 (1962).

4 Harman, D.: Dibenzanthracene-induced cancer: inhibition effect of dietary vitamin E. Clin. Res. *17:* 125–129 (1969).

5 Hirooka, T.; Hatano, T.; Yamamoto, M.: Effect of dietary vitamin E on 7,12-DMBA-induced mammary carcinogenesis. 13th Int. Cancer Congr., 1982, abstr. 155.

6 Jaffe, W.: The influence of wheat-germ oil on the production of tumors in rats by methylcholanthrene. Expl Med. Surg. *4:* 278–282 (1946).

7 Myers, C.E.; McGuire, W.; Young, R.: Adriamycin: amelioration of toxicity by α-tocopherol. Cancer Treat. Rep. *60:* 961–962 (1976).

8 Prasad, K.N.; Ewards-Prasad, J.: Effects of tocopherol (vitamin E) acid succinate on morphological alterations and growth inhibition in melanoma cells in culture. Cancer Res. *42:* 550–555 (1982).

9 Prasad, K.N.; Edwards-Prasad, J.; Ramanujam, J.; Sakamoto, A.: Vitamin E increases the growth inhibitory and differentiating effects of tumor therapeutic agents in neuroblastoma and glioma cells in culture. Proc. Soc. exp. Biol. Med. *164:* 158–163 (1980).

10 Prasad, K.N.; Ramanujam, S.; Gaudreau, D.: Vitamin E induces morphological differentiation and increases the effect of ionizing radiation on neuroblastoma cells in culture. Proc. Soc. exp. Biol. Med. *161:* 570–573 (1979).

11 Sadek, I.A.: Vitamin A and its inhibitory effect as tested on Egyptian toads. Oncology *38:* 23–26 (1981).

12 Sadek, I.A.; Abdelmegid, N.: Ascorbic acid and its effect on the skin of *Bufo regularis.* Oncology *39:* 399–400 (1982).

13 Shamberger, R.J.; Tytko, Willis, C.E.: Antioxidants in cereals and in food preservatives and dedining gastric cancer mortality. Cleve. Clin. Q. *39:* 119–124 (1972).

14 Shamberger, R.J.; Baughman, F.F.; Kalchert, S.L.; Willis, C.E.; Hoffmann, G.C.: Carcinogen-induced chromosomal breakage decreased by antioxidants. Proc. natn. Acad. Sci. USA *70:* 1461–1463 (1973).

15 Shklar, G.: Oral mucosal carcinogenesis in hamsters: inhibition by vitamin E. J. natn. Cancer Inst. *68:* 791–798 (1982).

16 Slaga, T.J.; Bracken, W.M.: The effects of antioxidants on skin tumor initiation and aryl hydrocarbon hydroxylase. Cancer Res. *37:* 1631–1635 (1977).

17 Sonneveld, P.: Effect of α-tocopherol on cardiotoxicity of adriamycin in the rat. Cancer Treat. Rep. *62:* 1033–1036 (1978).

18 Tengerdy, R.P.; Heizerling, R.H.; Mathias, M.M.: Effect of vitamin E on disease resistance and immune responses; in de Duve, Hayaishi, Tocopherol, oxygen and biomembranes. Proc. Int. Symp. on Tocopherol, Oxygen and Biomembranes, Lake Yamanaka 1977, pp. 191–200 (Elsevier/North-Holland Biomedical Press, Amsterdam 1978).

19 Van Vleet, J.F.; Greenwood, L.; Ferrans, V.; Rebar, A.H.: Effect of selenium-vitamin

E on adriamycin-induced cardiomyopathy in rabbits. Am. J. Vitam. Res. *39:* 997–1010 (1978).

20 Wang, Y.M.; Madanat, F.F.; Kimball, J.C.; Gleiser, C.A.; Ali, M.K.; Kaufman, M.W.; Van Eys, J.: Effect of vitamin E against adriamycin-induced toxicity in rabbits. Cancer Res. *40:* 1022–1027 (1980).

21 Wattenberg, L.W.: Inhibition of carcinogenic and toxic effects of polycyclic hydrocarbons by several sulfur-containing compounds. J. natn. Cancer Inst. *52:* 1583–1587 (1974).

22 Wattenberg, L.W.: Inhibition of dimethylhydrazine-induced neoplasia of the large intestine by disulfiram. J. natn. Cancer Inst. *54:* 1005–1006 (1975).

23 Urano, S.; Yomanoi, S.; Hattori, Y.; Matsuo, M.: Radical scavenging: reactions of α-tocopherol. II. The reaction with some alkyl radicals. Lipids *12:* 105–108 (1977).

I. Sadek, MD, Zoology Department, Faculty of Science, Alexandria University, Moharrem Bec, Alexandria (Egypt)

Prasad (ed.), Vitamins, Nutrition, and Cancer, pp. 123–133 (Karger, Basel 1984)

Effect of Vitamin E on Immunity and Disease Resistance

Robert P. Tengerdy[a], *Melvin M. Mathias*[b], *Cheryl F. Nockels*[c]

[a] Department of Microbiology; [b] Department of Food Science and Nutrition, and
[c] Department of Animal Sciences, Colorado State University, Ft. Collins, Colo., USA

Introduction

In the past decade the immunoenhancing effect of vitamin E has been well established and covered in reviews [1–5]. Immunoenhancement has been observed only when vitamin E was supplemented at a level substantially (4–6 times) higher than customarily found in animal diets, or when the vitamin was incorporated into an injectible adjuvant formulation. Since it has been demonstrated that a well balanced nutrition is necessary for the proper functioning of the immune response, a deficiency in any essential nutrient, including vitamin E, would predictably lead to impaired immune functions [1]. This review is, therefore, restricted to the effect of supplemental or pharmacologic doses of vitamin E on immune responses and disease resistance. First examples of immunoenhancement and its possible mechanism will be reviewed, then the correlation between immunoenhancement and disease resistance will be examined.

Immunoenhancement by Vitamin E

The earliest reports on the possible immunoenhancing effect of vitamin E appeared in the 1950s. *Segagni* [6] noted in 1955 that vitamin E-supplemented rabbits produced antibodies earlier to typhoid vaccine, *O*-streptolysin, and Staphylococcus toxoid than rabbits on normal diets, but the peak antibody levels were not higher than those of the controls. *Solano* [7] reported in 1957 that vitamin E, pantothenic acid, riboflavin, *p*-amino-benzoic acid, and nicotinic acid stimulated antibody production in rabbits to vaccines of *Vibrio cholerae, Salmonella typhi,* and to heterologous erythrocytes.

In our laboratory, we started investigations in the 1970s. An illustrative example of our findings is given in table I. The data show the effect of vitamin E as compared to a synthetic antioxidant, *N,N*-diphenyl-*p*-phenyl-ene-diamine (DPPD), on the humoral antibody response of mice to sheep red blood cell immunization. The antibody production was measured in terms of antibody-producing plasma cells (the so-called plaque-forming cells, PFC), or relative amount of antibody secreted into the serum (by hemagglutination – HA – titration that can measure IgM and IgG antibodies separately). The main conclusions from these data are: (1) Vitamin E

Table I. Effect of vitamin E and DPPD on humoral immunity of SRBC immunized mice [data from ref. 8]

Diet[1]	Body weight g	Spleen weight g	PFC per 10^6 cells	HA [2]log titer[2]	
				IgM	IgG
WLB chow	28.0 ± 2.1	0.096 ± 0.021	1,225 ± 85	7.3 ± 0.2	<1
WLB chow + 222 mg DPPD/kg	27.0 ± 2.3	0.123 ± 0.032	5,461 ± 292	7.5 ± 0.9	3.5 ± 0.2
WLB chow 2,035 mg vitamin E/kg	25.6 ± 2.4	0.114 ± 0.024	7,863 ± 295	7.9 ± 0.4	4.1 ± 0.9
Vitamin E-deficient diet[3]	18.5 ± 1.5	0.059 ± 0.007	419 ± 25	6.8 ± 1.2	<1
Vitamin E-deficient diet + 222 mg DPPD/kg	18.3 ± 2.4	0.073 ± 0.010	562 ± 32	6.5 ± 1.2	<1
Vitamin E-deficient diet + 2.0 g vitamin E/kg	26.3 ± 1.9	0.120 ± 0.021	6,520 ± 300	7.5 ± 0.5	3.5 ± 0.2

WLB = Wayne Laboratory Blocks chow.
[1] $p < 0.01$ between controls and treatment groups.
[2] IgM measured by direct HA; IgG after 2-ME reduction.
[3] Nutritional Biochemicals Co., now ICN Pharmaceuticals, Cleveland, Ohio.

at a substantially higher level than available in laboratory diets is necessary for optimal antibody production. (2) This vitamin E requirement can be replaced only partially by DPPD, thus the mode of action is not simply an antioxidant one. (3) The effect is primarily manifested by increased proliferation of plasma cells, as revealed by increased PFC count and spleen weight, and a shift of plasma cells from IgM to IgG production evidenced by hemagglutination titers.

In vitro single cell suspension culturing of sheep red blood cells (SRBC) sensitized mouse spleen cells corroborated the plasma cell proliferative effect of vitamin E and synthetic antioxidants, and went a step further: demonstrated the possibility of vitamin E stimulation of immunocompetent lymphocytes (non-adherent cells) without the cooperation of macrophage like (adherent) cells [9]. Representative data can be seen in table II. 2-Mercaptoethanol (2-ME), and other synthetic antioxidants had a partial stimulatory effect in similar in vitro experiments.

In elegant in vitro studies *Tanaka* et al. [10] and *Corwin and Shloss* [11] demonstrated that vitamin E effectively stimulates B lymphocytes probably through enhanced cooperation of T helper cells, and perhaps bypassing the need for macrophage cooperation. T helper cells were stimulated also by 2-ME in another experiment [12]. On the other hand, no direct stimulation of effector T cells, or cell-mediated immunity has been observed [30]. This also supports the hypothesis about vitamin E cooperative effect, since B cells need cooperation more than T cells do.

Table II. Effect of vitamin E on PFC count of SRBC-stimulated spleen cells in single cell suspension culture [data from ref. 9]

μg[*DL*]-α-tocopherol acetate[1] added per culture	PFC per culture[2]	
	normal spleen cells	non-adherent cells
	18,360	471
1.8	36,990	3,109
5.0	34,471	2,875
50.0	25,786	209

[1] 10^6 normal or column-separated spleen cells were cultured for 5 days before counting.
[2] Solubilized in Emulphor®.

Table III. Correlation between PG levels and mortality in E. coli-infected chickens [data from ref. 17]

Treatment[1]	PG in bursa, µg/g wet tissue[2]			Percent[3] mortality
	$PGF_{2\alpha}$	PGE_2	PGE_1	
Control	71.9 ± 8	22.5 ± 1.9	94.0 ± 14.8	80
Vitamin E	36.2 ± 3.8	21.2 ± 2.7	32.5 ± 6.4	36
Aspirin	39.7 ± 4.6	12.2 ± 1.0	70.0 ± 5.9	42
Vitamin E + aspirin	12.4 ± 3.6	2.9 ± 1.0	23.3 ± 7.7	0
Non-infected control	44.2	27.4	46.6	0

[1] All chickens except noninfected controls were injected with 1×10^9 E. coli. Vitamin E dietary supplement: 300 mg/kg diet; aspirin 50 mg/kg body weight, injected intraperitoneally on the day before infection and daily thereafter.
[2] n = 8. PG radioimmunoassays from bursa taken from sacrificed birds 5 min after infection.
[3] Counted 2 days' postinfection.

These cell cooperative effects of vitamin E point toward possible membrane changes in the affected cells. Although no actual data are available about membrane changes by vitamin E in lymphoid cell populations, such changes may be postulated on the basis of Lucy's [13] hypothesis on the effect of tocopherols on cell membranes.

Another possible explanation for the observed immunoenhancement is the involvement of prostaglandins (PG), known regulators of immunologic processes [14]. Vitamin E, mainly through its antioxidant action, could interfere with the conversion of unsaturated fatty acids to hydroperoxy intermediates, PG, thromboxanes and leukotrienes.

There are indications that vitamin E is involved in the modulation of PG biosynthesis. Machlin [15] observed that serum concentrations of PGE_2 and $PGF_{2\alpha}$ were inversely related to vitamin E concentrations in rat serum. Chan et al. [16] observed a significantly reduced cyclooxygenase activity in vitamin E-deficient rats without a significant change in the $PGE_2/PGF_{2\alpha}$ ratio. In our laboratory, we found that in chickens fed 300 mg/kg diet vitamin E, endogenous PGE_1, PGE_2 and $PGF_{2\alpha}$ levels decreased in the immunopoietic organs, bursa and spleen. When the chickens were infected with pathogenic E. coli, decreased PG levels were accompanied by increased

Table IV. Comparison of *Clostridium perfringens* antitoxin D titers in vitamin E adjuvant and conventionally immunized lambs [data from ref. 20]

Group	Mean antibody titer[1]	
	before vaccination	after vaccination
Vaccinated, control diet	0.312 ± 0.09 (n = 12)	0.513 ± 0.22 (n = 12)
Vaccinated, vitamin E diet	0.332 ± 0.10 (n = 12)	0.725 ± 0.14 (n = 12)
Vitamin E adjuvant, control diet	0.446 ± 0.14 (n = 3)	1.64 ± 0.25 (n = 3)
Vitamin E adjuvant, vitamin E diet	0.354 ± 0.12 (n = 3)	1.046 ± 0.24 (n = 3)

[1] Measured in an ELISA test. Titer expressed in absorbance units at 405 nm and 1:200 serum dilution.

antibody levels and a decreased mortality. A strong indication that PG inhibition contributed to immune enhancement and disease protection was shown by the fact that aspirin, a known PG inhibitor, acted synergistically with vitamin E in depressing PG levels and decreasing mortality from *E. coli* infection. An illustrative example of data is given in table III.

The PG-modulating effect of vitamin E and its role in immunoenhancement cannot be separated from complex interactions between vitamin E, polyunsaturated fatty acids (PUFA), vitamin A, selenium, and other nutritional factors. Interactions have been demonstrated or suggested between vitamin E, selenium, vitamin A, PUFA in immunoregulation [3, 18, 19]. At the heart of these interactions is probably the prevention of peroxidation of linoleic and arachidonic acids leading to membrane stabilization and PG modulation.

A novel mode of administration of vitamin E for maximum immunoenhancement has been found recently in our laboratory. Instead of dietary supplementation, the oily vitamin E may be incorporated into water in oil type adjuvants of vaccines. A popular adjuvant of this type is Freund's adjuvant that contains mineral oil, emulsifier and aqueous solution of antigen. Vitamin E not only replaced the mineral oil in Freund's incomplete adjuvant (FIA), but reduced the hypersensitivity reactions sometimes attendant upon administration of such adjuvants. The practicality of a vitamin E adjuvant vaccine, as a potentially improved vaccine against sheep enterotoxemia caused by *Clostridum perfringens,* is demon-

Table V. Immune response of guinea pigs to adjuvant vaccines of BSA

Vaccine[1]	Mean [2]log HA titer[2]	
	21-day	56-day
BSA	1.8 ± 1.0	4.3 ± 2.0
BSA – vitamin E	6.8 ± 3.0	7.5 ± 3.1
BSA – FIA	4.2 ± 2.3	5.5 ± 2.8
Control	1.0 ± 0.1	1.0 ± 0.1

[1] BSA 1% saline solution; adjuvants: 0.85 ml vitamin E or 0.85 ml mineral oil (FIA), 0.15 ml Arlacel® (emulsifier), 1.0 ml 2% BSA saline solution mixed to stable emulsion.
[2] n = 6; passive hemagglutination test.

strated in table IV. The effect of vitamin E as an adjuvant was much more pronounced than its effect as a dietary supplement. Similar observation was made in experiments with a vitamin E adjuvant vaccine against *B. ovis* induced ram epididymitis [35].

A comparison of vitamin E adjuvant and FIA in immunizing guinea pigs with bovine serum albumin (BSA) is shown in table V. It can be seen that in this experiment the vitamin E adjuvant was slightly superior to FIA. We have no explanation yet for the pronounced immunoenhancement by vitamin E adjuvants. Since the amount of vitamin E administered is modest and a single dose compared to the saturation treatment of dietary supplementation, a local effect is suspected. Since adjuvants generally enhance antibody production by promoting or bypassing cell cooperation, the explanation may be sought along this line.

Correlation between Immunoenhancement and Disease Protection

An elevated antibody level against an infectious agent does not automatically mean increased protection from that agent. It depends on the type and affinity of antibody produced and the interaction of antibody with other components of the complex defensive system of the host. If elevated antibody level promotes increased phagocytosis, a good correlation between humoral immunity and disease protection may be expected.

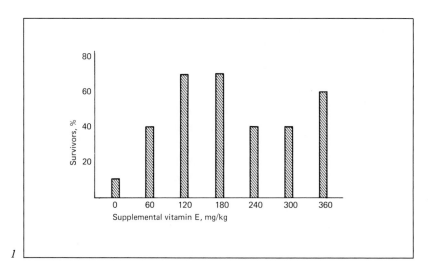

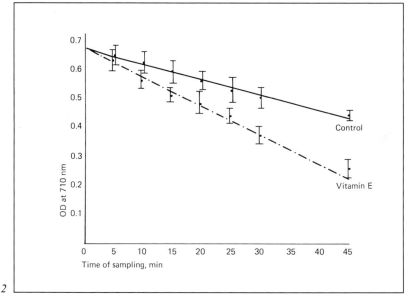

Fig. 1. Protection of immunized mice against *Diplococcus pneumoniae* type I infection by vitamin E. Mice were immunized with 0.5 ng bacterial polysaccharide, and 1 week later challenged with 20,000 organisms. Survivors were counted 5 days later [data from ref. 24].

Fig. 2. Rate of carbon clearance from blood. Mice on control diet and on vitamin E-supplemented diet (180 mg/kg) were used. The means of 4 determinations are shown, the vertical bars representing the standard deviation [data from ref. 24].

In chickens and turkeys infected with *E. coli,* vitamin E induced both increased antibody production and increased phagocytosis [21–23]. In mice infected with *Diplococcus pneumoniae,* vitamin E induced protective immunity as well as promoting increased non-specific phagocytosis. This can be seen in figures 1 and 2.

The non-specific stimulation of phagocytosis by vitamin E is somewhat similar to the non-specific stimulation of the reticuloendothelial system by ubiquinones, especially coenzyme Q_{10} (CoQ_{10}) [25–29]. CoQ_{10} also has a protective role in cancer; it increased the number of survivors in Friend leukemia virus-infected mice and in 3,4,9,10-dibenzpyrene-induced tumors [29]. *Heinzerling* [30] found increased CoQ_{10} levels in the plasma, liver and kidney of *Diplococcus pneumoniae* infected, vitamin E-supplemented mice. Vitamin E is thought to protect the isoprenoid side chain of ubiquinones from oxidation [31, 32]. *Donchenko* et al. [33] reported that injections of vitamin E into rats significantly increased the ubiquinone content in the liver and kidney. These data suggest that the non-specific stimulation of phagocytosis by vitamin E is mediated through ubiquinones by improving the intracellular efficiency of respiratory metabolism.

Increased antibody production did not lead to increased protection in guinea pigs, given supplemental dietary vitamin E or parenteral vitamin E injection, and infected with Venezuelan equine encephalitis virus [34]. In this case, however, immune phagocytosis is not the mechanism of defense against infection.

Conclusions

Vitamin E, supplemented to diets in pharmacologic doses, 4 to 6 times above the currently used levels, enhances humoral antibody production by increasing proliferation of antibody producing B lymphocytes, probably by enhancing cooperation among cells participating in the inductive phase of the immune response and promoting a rapid transition from less efficient IgM antibody production to more efficient IgG antibody production. There is strong suggestive evidence that PG play a regulatory role in this process and that vitamin E modulates PG biosynthesis. No direct enhancement of T cell activity or cell mediated immunity can be attributed to vitamin E. Since cell cooperation is more important in the induction of humoral immunity than cell-mediated immunity, the hypothesis that cooperative effects are the cause of immunoenhancement by vitamin E is supported by all available information.

Vitamin E is a most potent immunoenhancer when administered as a water-in-oil type adjuvant mixed with the antigen. There are only speculations now about the mode of action of vitamin E adjuvants, but since adjuvants generally help or bypass cell cooperative effects, the explanation may not be far from the above expressed hypothesis.

Immunoenhancement has been correlated with increased disease protection in those infections, where immune phagocytosis was the principal mechanism for destroying the infectious agent. In such cases, enhanced antibody production and enhanced metabolic vigor of the phagocytic cells combined for an increased efficiency of bacterial killing. In other cases, with mycobacterial and viral infections, a good correlation between antibody level and disease protection have not been observed.

References

1   Axelrod, A.E.: Nutrition in relation to immunity; in Goodhart, Shils, Modern nutrition in health and disease (Lea & Febiger, Philadelphia 1980).
2   Nockels, C.F.: Protective effects of supplemental vitamin E against infection. Fed. Proc. *38:* 2134–2136 (1978).
3   Sheffy, B.F.; Schultz, R.D.: Influence of vitamin E and selenium on immune response mechanisms. Fed. Proc. *38:* 2139–2141 (1979).
4   Tengerdy, R.: Effect of vitamin E on immune response; in Machlin, Vitamin E, a comprehensive treatise, pp. 429–443 (Dekker, New York 1980).
5   Tengerdy, R.P.; Mathias, M.M.; Nockels, C.F.: Vitamin E, immunity and disease resistance; in Phillips, Baetz, Diet and resistance to disease, pp. 27–42 (Plenum Press, New York 1981).
6   Segagni, E.: Vitamin E effect on vaccination. Minerva pediat. *7:* 985–987 (1955).
7   Solano, G.: Effects of vitamins on antibody production in rabbits to *Vibrio cholerae.* Int. Z. VitamForsch. *27:* 373–375 (1957).
8   Tengerdy, R.P.; Heinzerling, R.H.; Brown, G.L.; Mathias, M.M.: Enhancement of the humoral immune response by vitamin E. Int. Archs Allergy appl. Immun. *44:* 221–227 (1973).
9   Campbell, P.A.; Cooper, H.R.; Heinzerling, R.H.; Tengerdy, R.P.: Vitamin E enhances in vitro immune response by normal and non-adherent spleen cells. Proc. Soc. exp. Biol. Med. *146:* 465–469 (1974).
10 Tanaka, T.; Fujiwara, H.; Torisu, M.: Vitamin E and immunity. I. Enhancement of helper T cell activity. Immunology *38:* 727–730 (1979).
11 Corwin, L.M.; Shloss, J.: Role of antioxidants on the stimulation of the mitogenic response. J. Nutr. *110:* 2497–2505 (1980).

12   Erb, P.; Feldmann, M.: The role of macrophages in the generation of T helper cells. II. The genetic control of the macrophage T cell interaction for helper cell induction with soluble antigens. J. exp. Med. *142:* 460–466 (1975).

13   Lucy, J.A.: Functional and structural aspects of biological membranes: a suggested structural role for vitamin E in the control of membrane permeability and stability. Ann. N.Y. Acad. Sci. *203:* 4–11 (1972).

14   Bourne, H.R.: Immunology; in Ramwell, The prostaglandins, vol. 2, pp. 277–291 (Academic Press, New York 1974).

15   Machlin, L.: Vitamin E and prostaglandins; in deDuve, Hayaishi, Tocopherol, oxygen and biomembranes, pp. 179–189 (Elsevier, New York 1978).

16   Chan, A.C.; Allen, C.E.; Hegarty, P.V.J.: The effects of vitamin E depletion and repletion on PG synthesis in semitendinosus muscle of young rabbits. J. Nutr. *109:* 66–81 (1980).

17   Likoff, R.O.; Guptill, D.R.; Lawrence, L.M.; McKay, C.C.; Mathias, M.M.; Nockels, C.F.; Tengerdy, R.P.: Vitamin E and aspirin depress prostaglandins in protection of chickens against *E. coli* infection. Am. J. clin. Nutr. *34:* 245–251 (1981).

18   Mertin, J.; Meade, C.J.: Importance of the spleen for the immune inhibitory action of linoleic acid in mice. Int. Archs Allergy appl. Immun. *53:* 469–472 (1977).

19   Spallholz, J.E.: Anti-inflammatory, immunologic and carcinostatic attributes of selenium in experimental animals; in Phillips, Baetz, Diet and resistance to disease, pp. 43–61 (Plenum Press, New York 1981).

20   Tengerdy, R.P.; Meyer, D.L.; Lauerman, L.H.; Lueker, D.C.; Nockels, C.F.: Vitamin E enhances humoral antibody response to *Clostridium perfringens,* type D, in sheep. Br. vet. J. *139:* 147–151 (1983).

21   Heinzerling, R.H.; Nockels, C.F.; Quarles, C.L.; Tengerdy, R.P.: Protection of chicks against *E. coli* infection by dietary supplementation with vitamin E. Proc. Soc. exp. Biol. Med. *146:* 174–179 (1974).

22   Julseth, D.R.: Evaluation of vitamin E and disease stress on turkey performance; MS thesis, Fort Collins (1974).

23   Tengerdy, R.P.; Brown, J.C.: Effect of vitamin E and A on humoral immunity and phagocytosis in *E. coli*-infected chicken. Poultry Sci. *56:* 957–962 (1977).

24   Heinzerling, R.H.; Tengerdy, R.P.; Wick, L.L.; Lueker, D.C.: Vitamin E protects mice against *Diplococcus pneumoniae* type I infection. Infect. Immunity *10:* 1292–1298 (1974).

25   Bliznakov, E.; Casey, A.; Premuzic, E.: Coenzyme Q: stimulant of phagocytic activity in rats and immune response in mice. Experientia *26:* 953–956 (1970).

26   Casey, A.C.; Bliznakov, E.G.: Effect and structure-activity relationship of CoQ on phagocytic rate in rats. Chem.-Biol. Interact. *51:* 1–10 (1972).

27   Bliznakov, E.G.: Protective effect of reticulo-endothelial system stimulation; in DiLuzio, The reticuloendothelial system and immune phenomena, pp. 315–332 (Plenum Press, New York 1971).

28   Bliznakov, E.G.; Casey, A.C.: Effect of exogenous ubiquinone-10 on the ubiquinone pool of liver and spleen of mice. Biochim. biophys. Acta *362:* 326–331 (1974).

29   Bliznakov, E.G.: Effect of stimulation of the host defense system by coenzyme Q on dibenzpyrene-induced tumors and infection with Friend leukemia virus in mice. Proc. natn. Acad. Sci. USA *70:* 390–394 (1973).

30 Heinzerling, R.H.: The effect of vitamin E on immunity; PhD thesis, Fort Collins (1974).

31 Folkers, K.: Activity in vivo of ubiquinones and chromols. Vitams Horm. *24:* 525–527 (1966).

32 Olson, R.E.: Anabolism of the coenzyme Q family and their biological activities. Fed. Proc. *24:* 85–92 (1965).

33 Donchenko, H.A.; Dyadychiv, A.; Vounyanko, Y.K.: Change in ubiquinone content in rat tissue with higher concentrations of vitamin E and A. Ukr. Biochem. Zh. *43:* 609–613 (1971).

34 Barber, T.L.; Nockels, C.F.; Jochim, M.M.: Vitamin E enhancement of Venezuelan equine encephalomyelitis antibody response in guinea pigs. Am. J. vet. Res. *36:* 731–734 (1977).

35 Afzal, M.; Tengerdy, R.P.; Ellis, R.P.; Kimberling, C.V.; Morris, C.J.: Protection of rams against epididymitis by a *Brucella ovis* – Vitamin E adjuvant vaccine. Vet. Immunol. Immunopath. (in press).

R.P. Tengerdy, PhD, Department of Microbiology, Colorado State University, Ft. Collins, CO 80523 (USA)

Prasad (ed.), Vitamins, Nutrition, and Cancer, pp. 134–146 (Karger, Basel 1984)

Stimulation of Prognostically Favorable Cell-Mediated Immunity of Breast Cancer Patients by High Dose Vitamin A and Vitamin E[1]

Maurice M. Black[a], *Reinhard E. Zachrau*[a], *Arnold S. Dion*[b], *Monique Katz*[c]

[a] Department of Pathology, New York Medical College, Valhalla, N.Y., USA;
[b] Institute for Medical Research, Camden, N.J., USA;
[c] Department of Radiology, Columbia Presbyterian Hospital, New York, N.Y., USA

As judged by microscopic studies of lymphoreticuloendothelial reactivity [1–3] as well as by in vitro [4–6] and in vivo [7–9] procedures, cell-mediated immunity (CMI) to autologous breast cancer is prognostically favorable. It should be noted that such specific CMI depends on the presence of a tumor-associated immunogen(s) in the cancer tissue and retention of the host's reactivity against such immunogen(s). Thus, the lack of reactivity may reflect loss of specific immunogenicity in the cancer tissue or loss of specific immunity by the host or both.

CMI against autologous breast cancer is regularly demonstrable among patients with preinvasive breast cancer but is uncommon among patients who develop recurrent disease less than 2 years postoperatively [10–12]. It is noteworthy that the CMI-determinant of the preinvasive breast cancer immunogen seems to be similar to the CMI-determinant of the gp55 component of the RIII strain murine mammary tumor virus [13–15]. Accordingly, postoperative measurements of anti-gp55 CMI of breast cancer

[1] Supported in part by Grant No. 5R01 CA25165 of the National Cancer Institute, DHEW, and a Grant from the Cancer Research Institute, Inc., New York, N.Y., USA.

patients provide an index of the type of reactivity which should inhibit the development of second primary breast cancers and the progression of those first breast cancers which retain the gp55-like immunogen. Such measurements indicate that individual breast cancer patients differ in regard to their reactivity to gp55 at particular postoperative intervals. Moreover, patients showing such prognostically favorable CMI may lose this reactivity with increasing postoperative intervals.

Since restoration of anti-gp55 CMI should be prognostically beneficial to patients who have lost such reactivity, it is of interest that some reports indicate that high doses of vitamin A (VA) and vitamin E (VE) may stimulate immunological reactivity [16–19]. Such observations prompted us to examine the effects of VA on CMI responses to gp55 and autologous breast cancer. In a preliminary study we observed that defined doses of VA and VE can stimulate CMI to gp55 and autologous breast cancer in an appreciable proportion of breast cancer patients [20]. We now report similar effects in a larger series of patients treated with VA and in a series of patients treated with VE.

Materials and Methods

The skin window (SW) procedure for measurements of in vivo CMI to autologous breast cancer has been described in detail previously [7]. In essence, it consists of the creation of a microabrasion on the forearm or thigh which is then overlayed with a cryostat section of the target tissue mounted on a 24 × 30 mm glass coverslip. After 28–36 h the coverslip is removed and an imprint prepared from the abraded area. After air-drying, coverslip and imprint are Wright-stained and examined for the type and prominence of mononuclear cell responses as well as representation of basophilic and eosinophilic polymorphonuclear leukocytes.

SW tests against gp55 are performed in the same manner, utilizing coverslips on which a 4-µl drop of phosphate-buffered saline, containing 2 µg gp55, is placed in the center. After air-drying, the coverslips are immersed in a 1:1 mixture of ether and 95% alcohol for 15 min, air-dried again and stored at −20 °C until use. The isolation of gp55 from RIII murine mammary tumor virus has been described elsewhere [21].

Autologous breast cancer tissue was not available for all of the patients tested against gp55. When possible, however, we have performed simultaneous tests against autologous breast cancer and gp55. It should be noted that this study is particularly concerned with the ability of defined doses of VA and VE to stimulate SW reactivity of breast cancer patients to a common target, namely gp55.

From our registry of postoperative breast cancer patients who are in our program of periodic measurements of SW reactivity to gp55 and/or autologous breast cancer, we have identified postoperative patients who were free of demonstrable recurrent disease but were non-responsive to gp55 and, when available, autologous cancer. The patients were invited to participate in a study of the effects of high dose VA and VE on SW reactivity to gp55 and autologous breast cancer. After being given oral and written explanations of the possible untoward effects of the treatment was well as the immediate and long-term goals of the study, they signed an informed consent statement as indication of their wish to participate.

The present study was initiated with VA at daily doses of 300,000 IU for approximately 3 weeks. If such a course of treatment was associated with a negative-to-positive (N-P) change in SW reactivity to gp55, VA administration was discontinued, and the SW responses were monitored at 3- to 4-week intervals for loss of VA-associated reactivity. After loss of reactivity was established, the effects of repeat courses of VA at lower doses were evaluated.

After determining the SW effects of VA on individual patients, similar observations were made in regard to the effect of VE at different dosage levels, ranging from 400 to 1,200 IU. An additional series of patients who had not received VA was also tested for VE-associated SW reactivity.

All patients were questioned repeatedly regarding any untoward signs or symptoms associated with VA and VE therapy. In addition, clinical chemistry profiles were examined for evidence of subclinical abnormalities.

Results

VA-Associated SW Reactivity

As shown in table I, 25 postoperative breast cancer patients who were non-responsive to gp55 were given 300,000 IU VA per day for 18–35 days. 9 of these patients were tested after taking the VA for only 8–14 days. None of the 9 showed reactivity to gp55 at that time. In contrast, 15 (60%) of the 25 patients were responsive to gp55 after 18–35 days of VA therapy. Among patients who had subsequent courses of VA therapy at daily doses of 150,000–200,000 IU, N-P changes in SW reactivity were found in 6/18 patients (33%). However, none of 7 patients treated with daily doses of 100,000 IU VA developed SW reactivity to gp55. It thus appears that VA-associated SW reactivity is dependent on dose and duration of the VA administration. The data in table I also indicate that VA-associated SW reactivity to gp55 began to fade within 1 month and was lost, in most instances, within 3 months after stopping VA administration.

Further evidence of a cause-effect relationship between VA administration and SW reactivity is provided in table II. These data indicate that SW reactivity after second or third courses of VA tend to be similar to the responses associated with a prior course. In short, VA-associated N-P

Table I. High dose VA-associated SW reactivity to RIII-gp55 among postoperative, clinically disease-free breast cancer patients; relationship to daily dose and duration of VA therapy

Daily VA dose, IU	VA therapy duration, days					
	8–14	15–21	22–35	36–60	61–80	15–35
300,000	0/9[1]	5/7	10/18	–	–	15/25 (60)[2]
150,000–200,000	–	2/6	4/12	0/1	–	6/18 (33)
100,000	–	0/3	0/4	–	–	0/7
None[3]	1/2	–	4/8	4/9	1/5	4/8 (50)

[1] Number of gp55-positive tests/total number of tests.
[2] Numbers in parentheses, percentages.
[3] Test of patients who were gp55-positive after prior VA therapy; time intervals in this row = days after termination of VA therapy.

Table II. VA-associated SW reactivity to RIII-gp55 among postoperative, clinically disease-free breast cancer patients who received more than one course of VA therapy; relationship between gp55 reactivity after prior and subsequent therapy courses

Prior VA course[1]	Subsequent VA course(s)[2]		
	SW-positive	SW-negative	total
SW-positive	7	3	10
SW-negative	1	5	6
Total	8	8	16

[1] 300,000 IU VA/day for > 18 days.
[2] 150,000–300,000 IU VA/day for > 18 days.

changes in SW responses to gp55 were reproducible in 7 of 10 tests. Conversely, a positive SW test was found in only 1 of 6 instances where the proceeding treatment was not associated with an N-P change. As indicated by the data in table III, VA may influence SW reactivity over a wide range of postoperative intervals.

Table III. VA-associated[1] SW reactivity of postoperative, clinically disease-free breast cancer patients to RIII-gp55, by postoperative interval

Postoperative interval, months	SW-positive/total number of patients[2]
4–12	0/3
13–24	3/5
25–36	3/4
37–48	0/1
49–60	3/4
> 60	7/10
Total	16/27 (59%)

[1] Following administration of 300,000 IU of VA daily for > 18 days.
[2] All patients non-reactive to RIII-gp55 prior to VA administration.

Table IV. VA-associated SW reactivity against autologous breast cancer in relation to reactivity against RIII-gp55, among postoperative, clinically disease-free patients

Reactivity vs. gp55	Reactivity vs. breast cancer		
	SW-positive	SW-negative	total
SW-positive	16	7 (30)	23 (100)
SW-negative	4	29 (88)	33 (100)
Total	20	36 (64)	56 (100)

In view of the data in tables I and II, it seems unlikely that the observed changes in reactivity in conjunction with VA administration represent random variations. The ability of VA to stimulate SW reactivity to gp55 is an interesting phenomenon. However, it appeared to be of importance to determine the relationship between induced reactivity against gp55 and against autologous breast cancer. As shown in table IV, VA-associated reactivity to gp55 is related to simultaneous reactivity to autologous breast cancer. This relationship is similar to that which we have previously observed for spontaneous reactivity to these targets.

Table V. VE-associated SW reactivity to RIII-gp55 among postoperative, clinically disease-free breast cancer patients; relationship to daily dose and duration of VE therapy

Daily VE dose, IU	VE therapy duration, days				
	8–14	15–21	22–35	36–60	61–80
1,200	1/1[1]	4/4	5/11	3/5	1/1
800	–	–	1/6	–	–
400	–	0/1	–	–	–
None[2]	–	–	1/2	1/2	–

[1] Number of gp55-positive tests/total number of tests.
[2] Tests of patients who were gp55-positive after prior VE-therapy; time interval in this row = days after termination of VE therapy.

VE-Associated SW Reactivity

Of 19 postoperative disease-free breast cancer patients who received 1,200 IU VE/day for more than 18 days, 13 demonstrated a VE-associated N-P change in SW reactivity to gp55. As shown in table V, such a change in reactivity was effected when daily doses of 1,200 IU VE were taken for 14–80 days, but was observed in only 1 of 6 patients who took 800 IU for 22–35 days. As whith the VA-associated positive SW responses, the VE-associated reactivity tended to fade within 1–2 months after termination of the VE administration.

14 of the patients who received VE had been previously tested for VA-associated SW reactivity. As shown in table VI, 7 of 8 patients who showed VA-associated N-P changes in SW reactivity to gp55 were similarly affected by VE. VE-associated N-P changes in SW reactivity were also observed in 4 of 5 patients who had not previously taken VA. In contrast to these findings, of the 6 patients who did not demonstrate an N-P change in SW reactivity to gp55 following VA-therapy, only 1 showed an N-P change after VE treatment. The patient in question was more than 10 years post-mastectomy and clinically free of recurrent disease when first placed on VA therapy. She failed to demonstrate SW reactivity to gp55 after an initial course of 300,000 IU VA daily for 28 days as well as after two subsequent courses of 100,000 IU VA daily for 25 and 22 days, respectively. However, she did show an N-P change in anti-gp55 SW reactivity after taking

Table VI. VE-associated SW reactivity to RIII-gp55 in relation to prior VA-associated anti-gp55 reactivity; postoperative, clinically disease-free breast cancer patients

VA-associated reactivity[1]	VE-associated reactivity[2]		
	SW-positive	SW-negative	total
SW-positive	7 (88)	1	8 (100)
SW-negative	1 (17)	5	6 (100)
No prior VA	4 (80)	1	5 (100)

[1] 150,000–300,000 IU VA daily for > 18 days.
[2] 1,200 IU VE daily for > 18 days.

1,200 IU VE daily for 34 days. This reactivity was not maintained by a subsequent daily intake of 400 IU of VE for 46 days. However, a second course of 1,200 IU VE daily for 26 days resulted again in an N-P change in SW reactivity.

A reverse response pattern was observed in another patient who demonstrated stimulation of SW reactivity to gp 55 after VA but not after VE administration. This patient was non-responsive to gp55 when SW-tested 19 and 22 months postoperatively. No N-P change in SW reactivity occurred after 300,000 IU of VA daily for 12 days nor after a subsequent course of 100,000 IU of VA daily for 21 days. However, a positive response was found after 200,000 IU VA daily for 24 days. Anti-gp55 reactivity was no longer evident 57 days after stopping VA administration. Reactivity was not restored after a course of 1,200 IU VE daily for 29 days. However, it was restored after a second course of 200,000 IU of VA daily. Such reactivity was again lost 26 days later, despite the administration of 1,200 IU VE daily during the 26-day period. Once again, a repeat course of 200,000 IU VA per day for 18 days restored the SW reactivity. It appears from the foregoing data that, although, in most patients, SW reactivity to gp55 is similarly affected by VA and VE, the reactivity of some individuals is selectively affected by one or the other agent.

An additional comparison between VA- and VE-associated SW reactivity to gp55 is provided in table VII. As indicated before, high doses of

Table VII. VA-associated and VE-associated SW reactivity to RIII-gp55; proportion of positive responses and of responses associated with basophilic white blood cells

SW response	VA-associated[1] basophil(+)/total	VE-associated[2] basophil(+)/total
Positive	4/24 (17)[3,4]	11/15 (73)[4]
Negative	0/16	1/6 (17)
Total	4/40 (10)[5]	12/21 (57)[5]

[1] 150,000–300,000 IU VA daily for > 18 days; 27 patients.
[2] 1,200 IU VE daily for > 18 days; 19 patients.
[3] Numbers in parentheses, percentages.
[4] $p < 0.002$; [5] $p < 0.0005$.

both vitamins may induce N-P changes in SW reactivity to gp55. However, it seems that basophilic polymorphonuclear leukocytes are more commonly a component of VE-associated SW responses than of VA-associated responses.

From a nutritional standpoint, β-carotene is a precursor of VA. It would, therefore, be of interest to determine whether β-carotene affects SW reactivity in a similar fashion as VA. Thus far, we have examined this question in only 1 patient. However, in view of the unexpected nature of our findings, they seem worthy of note at this time. This patient had shown an intermediate type of spontaneous SW reactivity to gp55 10 months postoperatively. After taking VA, she showed an increased level of SW reactivity to gp55 and to autologous breast cancer. Such reactivity was maintained for 1 year in association with multiple courses of VA-therapy. On Nov. 5, 1982, she discontinued the VA intake and, when tested on Nov. 30, 1982, she showed moderate SW reactivity to both, gp55 and autologous breast cancer. Subsequently, 180 mg β-carotene daily were taken from Dec. 1, 1982 to Dec. 19, 1982, resulting in a yellow coloration of her skin. However, SW tests on Dec. 21, 1982 and Jan. 18, 1983 were both completely negative to gp55 and autologous breast cancer. It should be emphasized that such a complete lack of reactivity has not been seen in this patient in any of 14 tests performed since the beginning of the first VA therapy course on Nov. 2, 1981. On Jan. 20, 1983 she was again placed on 200,000 IU VA daily for 21 days, followed by 300,000 IU VA per day for 6 days. This treatment resulted in restored SW reactivity to gp55 and autologous breast cancer which was maintained for 43 days after discontinuation of the VA intake. However, only minimal reactivity to gp55 and autologous cancer was seen 70 days after the VA treatment. At this point, the administration of a daily dose of 1,200 IU VE for 16 days was associated with well-defined SW reactivity to both targets. This was confirmed by retesting after 23 days of VE therapy. In this patient, both VA and VE stimulated SW reactivity to gp55 and autologous breast cancer. In contrast, no such effect was associated with β-carotene. Additional studies are needed to determine whether these findings are representative of the general population or are unique for this patient.

Safety of High Dose VA and VE

Careful questioning of all VA-treated patients revealed that approximately one third of these patients experienced mild to moderate dryness of the mouth and some itchiness of the skin while on 300,000 IU VA/day. These symptoms subsided within days after termination of the VA administration. In only 1 patient was the mucosal dryness so pronounced that the daily VA dosage was reduced to 200,000 IU. The latter dose caused only mild dryness which subsided after stopping VA intake. Repeated clinical chemistry studies (SMAC) in this patient did not show any abnormalities. No clinical complaints were reported by our patients who took VE.

Clinical chemistry profiles were routinely monitored for abnormal values which might be associated with high dose vitamin administration. Of all patients monitored, only 1 VA-treated patient showed transient liver enzyme abnormalities. This patient had normal profiles before and after 15 days of treatment with 300,000 IU VA/day. After 28 days of treatment, the serum glutamic-oxaloacetic transaminase (SGOT), serum glutamic-pyruvic transaminase (SGPT) and alkaline phosphatase levels were found elevated to 63, 142 and 278 U/l, respectively (upper limits of normal values: 41, 45 and 115 U/l, respectively). 10 days after stopping the VA intake, SGOT and SGPT levels were back to normal range (21 and 41 U/l, respectively), while the alkaline phosphatase value was 233 U/l. Follow-up profiles, performed 1 and 4 months later, showed all values within normal range. In none of the other patients treated with VA nor in any of the patients taking VE were any significant changes in the clinical chemistry profiles detectable.

Comments

The SW procedure, as used in this study, provides a device for visualizing CMI to specific targets. As such, it can be employed to evaluate the effects of putative immune modulators on reactivity to particular antigens. In addition, the procedure allows for detailed observations regarding the various cell types participating in spontaneous and induced responses to particular antigens.

Our studies to date demonstrate that the oral administration of specific doses of VA for defined periods of time can stimulate SW reactivity to gp55 in a high proportion of clinically recurrence-free postoperative breast cancer patients. While the overall effects of VA and VE on such reactivity are similar, subtle differences are suggested by our findings. Thus, the VE-associated responses more commonly included basophils in the skin window exudates. At present, we have no explanation of the mechanism of such differences in responses. It should be noted, however, that the participation of basophils in SW responses to cancer tissues was reported by *Black and Leis* [7] while *Wolf-Jürgensen* [22] noted basophils in SW tests against other types of antigens.

The finding that VA and VE may stimulate CMI to gp55 should be of practical clinical significance, particularly when such reactivity to gp55 is associated with simultaneous reactivity to autologous breast cancer. Table VIII indicates the potential protective effects of stimulation of CMI against gp55 and autologous breast cancer. Our prior studies suggested that, at any postoperative interval, CMI to gp55 should impede the development and progression of those invasive breast cancers which provoke a positive SW response. As shown in table VIII, immune stimulants are unlikely to benefit those postoperative breast cancer patients who have SW reactivity to gp55 and autologous breast cancer since they have no need for immune stimulation. Immune stimulants are also unlikely to benefit patients having positive responses to gp55 but lacking reactivity to autologous breast cancer. Such patients do not need stimulation of their anti-gp55 CMI and are not likely to be made responsive to autologous cancer tissue lacking gp55-like antigenicity. On the other hand, patients who are non-responsive to gp55 should be at an increased risk of developing second primary breast cancers and metastases from their original cancer. Thus, stimulation of anti-gp55 CMI should reduce the risk of second primaries and also the risk of metastases from those invasive lesions which express gp55-like CMI determinants. If induced reactivity to gp55 has the same biological effects

Table VIII. Influence of high dose VA and VE on SW reactivity to gp55 and autologous breast cancer in relation to spontaneous SW reactivity; clinical implications

SW reactivity		Risk of	
spontaneous gp55/breast cancer	VA-/VE-associated gp55/breast cancer	2nd primary[1]	recurrence[1]
pos./pos.	pos./pos.	low → low	low → low
pos./neg.	pos./neg.	low → low	high → high
neg./pos.[2]	pos./pos.	high → low	?
neg./neg.[3]	pos./pos.	high → low	high → low
neg./neg.[4]	pos./neg.	high → low	high → high

[1] Spontaneous → induced.

[2] It is not certain that there is a prognostically significant breast cancer-associated immunogen which is different from the gp55-like immunogen.

[3] Immunogen present; CMI stimulation protects against metastases as well as second primaries.

[4] Immunogen lacking; CMI stimulation cannot restore anti-breast cancer reactivity and not impede progression of the first breast cancer.

as spontaneous reactivity, then high doses of VA and VE should be of value as immunotherapeutic agents, particularly in an adjuvant setting.

The mechanism whereby high doses of VA and VE increase CMI to gp55 is not clear. Certainly it is not the result of a correction of a vitamin deficiency-associated immune deficiency. All of the patients were well-nourished, healthy appearing individuals at the time of testing. Moreover, their CMI to gp55 was not increased by the daily administration of 50,000–100,000 IU VA or 400–800 IU VE for 3–4 weeks. Furthermore, even among patients showing an N-P change in reactivity after high doses of VA and VE, such reactivity tended to fade when the respective doses were reduced. These observations suggest that the cellular and molecular effects of high doses of VA and VE are different from the physiological effects of VA and VE. It further appears that the stimulation of a prognostically favorable type of CMI in breast cancer patients requires doses in excess of those which have been recently suggested for use in so-called intervention studies, namely daily doses of 10,000–25,000 IU VA and of 400–600 IU VE. It seems, therefore, unlikely that the latter doses of VA or VE will result in an immunologically mediated reduction in breast cancer incidence.

In any case, we suggest that intervention studies of the influence of defined doses of vitamins on the risks of particular types of cancer should include measurements of prognostically significant CMI before and after the vitamin treatment. The failure to do so will make it difficult, if not impossible, to determine whether there is an immunological component to the observed effect.

References

1 Black, M.M.; Speer, F.D.: Immunology of cancer. Surgery Gynec. Obstet. *109:* 105–116 (1959).

2 Cutler, S.J.; Black, M.M.; Mörk, T.; Harvey, S.; Freeman, C.: Further observations on prognostic factors in cancer of the female breast. Cancer *24:* 653–667 (1969).

3 Black, M.M.; Barclay, T.H.C.; Hankey, B.F.: Prognosis in breast cancer utilizing histologic characteristics of the primary tumor. Cancer *36:* 2048–2055 (1975).

4 Black, M.M.; Leis, H.P., Jr.; Shore, B.; Zachrau, R.E.: Cellular hypersensitivity to breast cancer. Assessment by a leukocyte migration procedure. Cancer *33:* 952–958 (1974).

5 Akiyoski, T.; Nakamura, Y.; Kawaguchi, M.; Tsuji, H.: Cellular hypersensitivity to autologous tumor extract in patients with breast carcinoma. Jap. J. Surg. *8:* 236–241 (1978).

6 Cannon, G.B.; Dean, J.H.; Herberman, R.B.; Keets, M.; Alford, C: Lymphoproliferative responses to autologous tumor extracts as prognostic indicators in patients with resected breast cancer. Int. J. Cancer *27:* 131–138 (1981).

7 Black, M.M.; Leis, H.P., Jr.: Human breast carcinoma. III. Cellular responses to autologous breast cancer: skin window procedure. N.Y. St. J. Med. *70:* 2583–2588 (1970).

8 Black, M.M.; Leis, H.P., Jr.: Cellular responses to autologous breast cancer tissue: correlation with stage and lymphoreticuloendothelial reactivity. Cancer *28:* 263–273 (1971).

9 Black, M.M.; Leis, H.P., Jr.: Cellular responses to autologous breast cancer tissue: sequential observations. Cancer *32:* 384–389 (1973).

10 Black, M.M.; Zachrau, R.E.: Antitumor immunity in breast cancer patients: biologic and therapeutic implications. J. reprod. Med. *23:* 21–32 (1979).

11 Black, M.M.; Chabon, A.B.: In situ carcinoma of the breast; in Somers, Pathology annual, pp. 185–210 (Appleton Century Crofts, New York 1969).

12 Black, M.M.: Cellular and biologic manifestations of immunogenicity in precancerous mastopathy. Natn. Cancer Inst. Monogr. *35:* 73–82 (1972).

13 Black, M.M.; Zachrau, R.E.; Shore, B.; Dion, A.S.; Leis, H.P., Jr.: Cellular immunity to autologous breast cancer and RIII-murine mammary tumor virus preparations. Cancer Res. *38:* 2068–2076 (1978).

14 Black, M.M.: Structural, antigenic and biological characteristics of precancerous mastopathy. Cancer Res. *36:* 2596–2604 (1976).

15 Black, M.M.; Kwon, S.: Precancerous mastopathy: structural and biological considerations. Path. Res. Pract. *166:* 491–514 (1980).
16 Cohen, B.E.; Gill, F.; Cullen, P.R.; Morris, P.J.: Reversal of postoperative immunosuppression in man by vitamin A. Surgery Gynec. Obstet. *149:* 658–662 (1979).
17 Patek, P.; Collin, J.L.; Yogeeswaran, G.; Dennert, G.: Antitumor potential of retinoic acid: stimulation of immune-mediated effectors. Int. J. Cancer *24:* 624–628 (1979).
18 Beisel, W.R.: Single nutrients and immunity. Am. J. clin. Nutr. *35:* suppl., pp. 417–468 (1982).
19 Bellag, W.: Vitamin A and retinoids: from nutrition to pharmacotherapy in dermatology and oncology. Lancet *i:* 860–863 (1983).
20 Black, M.M.; Zachrau, R.E.; Dion, A.S.; Katz, M.: Vitamin A stimulation of specific cell-mediated immunity in breast cancer patients. Fed. Proc. *42:* 1197 (1983).
21 Dion, A.S.; Williams, C.J.; Pomenti, A.A.: The major structural proteins of murine mammary tumor virus: techniques for isolation. Analyt. Biochem. *82:* 18–28 (1977).
22 Wolf-Jürgensen, P.: Basophilic leukocytes in delayed hypersensitivty. Experimental studies in man using the skin window technique (Munksgaard, Copenhagen 1966).

M.M. Black, MD, Department of Pathology, New York Medical College,
Valhalla, NY 10595 (USA)

Prasad (ed.), Vitamins, Nutrition, and Cancer, pp. 147–158 (Karger, Basel 1984)

Role of Tocopherol and Cholesterol in Myeloproliferative Diseases[1]

Harriet S. Gilbert

The Polly Annenberg Levee Division of Hematology, Department of Medicine,
Mount Sinai School of Medicine of the City University of New York,
New York, N.Y., USA

Introduction

Myeloproliferative disorders (MPD) are a group of chronic syndromes resulting from monoclonal dysplasia of the pluripotential hematopoietic stem cell. The syndromes, which include polycythemia vera (PV), myeloid metaplasia (MyM), essential thrombocythemia (ET), and chronic myelocytic leukemia (CML), are low-grade malignancies characterized by increased proliferation of bone marrow with intact maturation of hematic cell progeny, extramedullary blood production, reactive fibrosis of the bone marrow, and a high incidence of transition to high-grade malignancies, such as acute leukemia and cancer of nonhematic organs. We have described a state of chronic hypocholesterolemia in MPD in which total cholesterol, low density lipoprotein (LDL) cholesterol, and high density lipoprotein (HDL) cholesterol are reduced as a result of increased lipoprotein turnover [1–4]. Studies of patients treated with myelosuppressive therapy or splenectomy revealed that cholesterol levels are inversely related to proliferative disease activity, in particular to the degree of splenomegaly.

Erythrocyte membrane structure and function are known to be influenced by alterations in circulating lipids, exemplified by the hypocholesterolemia of abetalipoproteinemia that produces abnormal membrane lipid composition and decreased membrane fluidity [5]. Abetalipoproteinemic erythrocytes display marked sensitivity to oxidative stress which has been

[1] Supported in part by Grants CA 31656 and RR 71 from the National Institutes of Health, and Grants from Hoffmann-La Roche, Inc. and the Jack Martin Fund.

attributed to both altered membrane lipid composition and decreased antioxidant capacity resulting from a concomitant deficiency of tocopherol. PNH, another clonal disorder of the pluripotential hematic stem cell, has been shown to predispose erythrocytes to peroxidation susceptibility in the absence of recognized causes of abnormal membrane autoxidation [6], suggesting that this phenomenon may be an expression of the underlying clonal dysplasia that characterizes MPD. Similarities between MPD and other diseases that display abnormal erythrocyte membrane lipid peroxidation prompted an assessment of peroxidation susceptibility in these syndromes. Measurements of malonyldialdehyde (MDA) generation in response to an oxidant challenge revealed a significant increase in lipid peroxidation in MPD [7]. Biochemical studies of MPD erythrocytes revealed that this abnormality was present despite increased concentrations of erythrocyte reduced glutathione (GSH) [8]. MDA and GSH have been identified as mutagens [9, 10] and their presence in increased amounts in MPD could play a role in the development of further malignant transformation. We undertook studies to evaluate the tocopherol status of patients with MPD and to determine the effect of supplementation on tocopherol levels and MDA production by MPD erythrocytes.

Materials and Methods

Patient Population. The study sample consisted of control subjects and patients with MPD (60% with PV, 40% with MyM). Control subjects were hematologically normal and were seen for routine medical care or management of arteriosclerotic heart disease, hypertension, or osteoarthritis. MPD was diagnosed by history, physical examination, and laboratory testing using criteria previously described [11–13]. Patients were untreated at the time of testing, except for 3 who were receiving hydroxyurea. None had received phlebotomy for at least 1 month. The research was carried out according to the principles of the Declaration of Helsinki and approved by the Research Administrative Committee of the Mount Sinai Medical Center. Blood samples were obtained at the time of venipuncture for diagnostic testing with informed consent of the subject.

Lipid Peroxidation Assay. Red blood cells (RBC) were prepared for assay of lipid peroxidation by a modification of the methods of *Stocks* et al. [14], as described by *Snyder* et al. [15]. RBC susceptibility to lipid peroxidation was determined by MDA formation using the addition technique of *Stocks and Dormandy* [16], in which RBC suspensions prepared as described above were incubated with H_2O_2 for 2 h at 37 °C with constant shaking. The final composition of the incubation mixture was 5 mmol/l glucose, 5 mmol/l H_2O_2, and 2 mmol/l sodium azide in phosphate-buffered saline, pH 7.4. In the initial screening studies of the normal and MPD populations incubations were performed in a 25-ml flask using an incubation volume of 10 ml. For subsequent studies related to the biochemical properties of the RBC, the assay method was modified to make possible the use of smaller quantities of blood, as described by *Harm* et al. [17]. The incubation volume was reduced to 2 ml and incubations were performed in 16 × 100-mm test tubes. This modification resulted in proportionately higher yields of MDA for all samples, but the relationship between MDA generation of normal and MPD blood was not affected. MDA was assayed as TBA-reactive material forming a complex with absorption at 532 nm and expressed as nmol MDA/g Hb.

Biochemical Studies. GSH was measured by the method of *Beutler* [18] using DTNB as the sulfhydryl reagent. Glutathione stability was determined as described by *Dacie and Lewis* [19]. The effect of GSH on lipid peroxidation was studied by depleting RBC of GSH by incubation of whole blood suspensions with NEM at final concentrations varying from 10 to 50 mmol/l for 10 min at 0 °C, as described by *Beutler* [20]. Treated cells were washed and assayed as described above. Plasma lipids and lipoproteins were measured as described previously [1].

Tocopherol and Free Cholesterol Assays. α-Tocopherol, β- and γ-tocopherol, and free cholesterol were measured by high-performance liquid chromatography by modification of the method of *Bieri* et al. [21; and *Stump, Roth, Gilbert,* unpublished observation]. The chromatograph was a Hewlett-Packard 1084B, equipped with a programmable, variable wavelength detector with stopped-flow scan capability and autosampler and integrator. The column was a 25 cm × 4.6-mm ID ODS Reversible (5 μm particle size) from Regis Chemical (Morton Grove, Ill.). A 5 cm × 4.6-mm ID guard column packed with Pelliguard LC-18 from Supelco (Bellefonte, Pa.) was attached before the analytical column. Elution was performed with methanol-water (96:4) at a flow rate of 1.05 ml/min, at 30 °C. The eluant was monitored at 265 nm for α-tocopheryl quinone, at 292 nm for β- and γ-tocopherol, α-tocopherol, and α-tocopheryl acetate and at 215 nm for cholesterol.

Sample Preparation. Whole blood was drawn into heparinized, evacuated tubes (Becton-Dickinson, Rutherford, N.J.). RBC were separated from plasma by centrifugation and washed 3 times with 0.9% saline solution with removal of the buffy coat. A solution containing 0.5% pyrogallol and 0.9% sodium chloride was added to the washed cells, bringing the hematocrit to between 30 and 40%. An aliquot containing the equivalent of 0.35 ml of packed RBC was transferred to a 20-ml screw-capped centrifuge tube. While vortexing the red cell suspension, 2.0 ml of a methanol solution containing 10 μg/ml internal standard (α-tocopheryl acetate) and 1.0% pyrogallol were slowly added. The methanol solution was kept at −20 °C prior to use and added cold. The mixture was then extracted with 4.0 ml petroleum ether by vortexing for 45 s. The petroleum ether layer was transferred to a 12-ml conical centrifuge tube and the solvent evaporated at 30 °C with a gentle stream of dry nitrogen. The residue was dissolved in 200 μl methanol-ethanol (4:1), the tube placed in a sonicator for 10 min, and then vortexed to insure complete dissolution. 80 μl of this solution was injected onto the chromatograph for analysis. Plasma was prepared by placing 1.0 ml in a 20-ml screw-capped centrifuge tube, 1.0 ml of a methanol solution containing 100 μg/ml internal standard (α-tocopheryl acetate) was added, and the sample was extracted with 4.0 ml of petroleum ether by vortexing for 30 s. The solvent was evaporated as described, the residue dissolved in 400 μl of methanol-ethanol (4:1) and 80 μl injected onto the chromatograph.

Cholesterol, α-tocopherol, and the sum of β- and γ-tocopherol were quantified from a standard curve of their peak height ratios versus α-tocopheryl acetate. In plasma the β- and γ-isomers comprise approximately 2 and 10% of the total tocopherol, respectively [22]. Their molar absorptions at 292 nm differ by only 5% [23] so the error in calculating their sum by comparing their combined absorption to that of a γ-tocopherol standard is less than 1 %. Since γ- and β-tocopherol coelute on an octadecylsilyl column, the sum of these two isomers was calculated by this procedure. Standards for RBC were prepared by adding 0.9–3.6 µg γ-tocopherol, 3.1–12.5 µg α-tocopherol, and 280–1,150 µg cholesterol in four increments to equal volumes of RBC. For plasma, 3.5–14.2 µg γ-tocopherol, 12.5–50.0 µg α-tocopherol and 350–1,400 µg cholesterol were added in four increments to equal aliquots of plasma. α-Tocopherol quinone was calculated from the ratio of the absorbance at 265 nm of a chromatographed standard compared to the absorbance of the internal standard α-tocopheryl acetate measured at 292 nm. A linear relationship was found between the peak height ratios (standard/internal standard) and the concentration ratios (standard/internal standard) for each of the compounds. No detectable α-tocopherol was formed from the internal standard during the extraction.

Incubation of Erythrocytes with α-Tocopherol. RBC were prepared from heparinized blood by centrifugation, removal of buffy coat and plasma, washing thrice with phosphate-buffered saline containing 5 mM glucose. α-Tocopherol was dissolved in N,N-dimethylacetamide, added at varying concentrations, and incubated with RBC for 3 h at 37 °C. Control incubations were performed with N,N-dimethylacetamide. Incubated RBC were prepared for tocopherol determinations and lipid peroxidation assays as described above.

Statistical Methods. Comparisons between values for normal subjects and patients with MPD were performed using Student's t test for nonpaired data. Samples were tested for normality by means of the Kolmogorov-Smirnov test. An F-test for equality of variances was performed, and the t statistic calculated for equal or unequal variances, as appropriate. Paired t tests were used to compare results obtained on RBC from the same subject. Differences between groups were considered significant when p was less than 0.05. Linear regression was determined by the method of least squares.

Results

Cholesterol, Tocopherol, and Glutathione Concentrations. The presence of low total cholesterol in MPD was confirmed and shown to be accompanied by significant reductions in plasma free cholesterol and relatively less reduction in plasma α-tocopherol (table I). Plasma α-tocopherol and free cholesterol were significantly correlated in both normal and MPD populations (r = 0.662, p < 0.001). Erythrocyte free cholesterol and α-tocopherol were normal and did not reflect alterations in plasma levels. Studies of erythrocyte GSH metabolism revealed elevated GSH levels and normal GSH stability in MPD (table II).

Oral α-Tocopherol Supplementation. The effect of daily oral supplementation with 800–1,200 IU *DL*-α-tocopherol was evaluated in 7 patients with MPD. Although significant increases in plasma and erythrocyte α-tocopherol concentrations were produced (table III), in vitro erythrocyte

Table I. Cholesterol and tocopherol levels in plasma and RBC of normals and patients with MPD

Variable	Normal (n = 26)	MPD (n = 22)	p*
Plasma			
Total cholesterol, mg/dl	192 ± 31[1]	134 ± 31	< 0.001
Free cholesterol, μg/ml	629 ± 138	534 ± 121	0.02
α-Tocopherol, μg/ml	10.2 ± 2.4	8.9 ± 2.5	0.08
β- and γ-tocopherol, μg/ml	1.6 ± 0.9	1.5 ± 0.6	> 0.3
RBC			
Free cholesterol, mg/ml	1.3 ± 0.1	1.3 ± 0.1	> 0.3
α-Tocopherol, μg/ml	2.8 ± 0.6	2.9 ± 0.6	> 0.3
β- and γ-tocopherol, μg/ml	0.5 ± 0.3	0.5 ± 0.3	> 0.3

* Student's t test.
[1] Mean ± SD.

Table II. Erythrocyte glutathione in myeloproliferative disease

Variable	Controls (n = 14)	MPD (n = 20)	p value
GSH, μmol/g Hb	7.7 ± 1.3	9.5 ± 2.1	< 0.02
GSH stability[1]	8.2 ± 7	6.4 ± 6	n.s.

Values are expressed as mean ± SD.
[1] Percent lost at 1 h.

Table III. The effect of daily oral administration of 800–1,200 IU vitamin E in 7 patients with myeloproliferative disease

Variable	Off vitamin E	On vitamin E
Plasma α-tocopherol, μg/ml	9.5 ± 1.5	22.7 ± 6.5
Erythrocyte α-tocopherol, μg/ml packed cells	3.2 ± 0.54	6.8 ± 0.43
MDA formation, nmol/g Hb	1,069 ± 216	1,078 ± 310

Values expressed as mean ± SD.

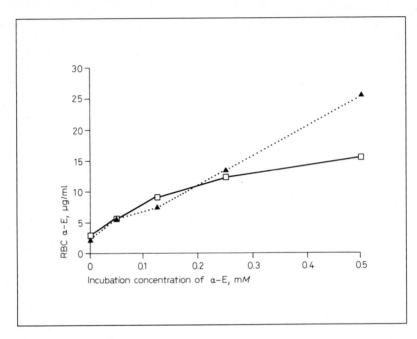

Fig. 1. Effect of incubation with α-tocopherol on erythrocyte α-tocopherol content. Mean values of cells from 9 normal subjects (triangles) and 11 patients with MPD (squares) are plotted. Uptake by normal cells was linear (RBC concentration = 2.3 + 0.46 × incubation concentration; r = 0.997, p < 0.001). Uptake by MPD cells was linear only up to a 0.25 mM incubation concentration, then plateaued (RBC concentration = 4.6 + 0.24 × incubation concentration; r = 0.955, p < 0.001). Erythrocyte α-tocopherol concentrations achieved in MPD were significantly less than normal when cells were incubated with 0.5 mM α-tocopherol (15.7 ± 3.4 versus 25.9 ± 8.4, p < 0.001).

susceptibility to lipid peroxidation remained markedly abnormal and was unaffected by a 2-fold increase in erythrocyte α-tocopherol levels.

In vitro α-Tocopherol Loading. In vitro studies were conducted to determine the relation between RBC α-tocopherol concentrations and lipid peroxidation susceptibility and to establish if, and at what concentration, reduction of MDA generation would be observed. Figure 1 shows RBC concentrations after incubation of normal and MPD RBC with concentrations of α-tocopherol from 0.05 to 0.5 mM (equivalent to plasma concentrations of 21.5–215 μg/ml). Linearity of α-tocopherol uptake is demon-

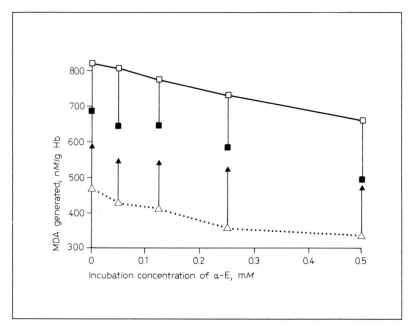

Fig. 2. The effect of in vitro α-tocopherol loading of erythrocytes on MDA generation. Mean levels in 9 normals (triangles) and 11 patients with MPD (squares) are shown. Lipid peroxidation was significantly increased in MPD at all concentrations of α-tocopherol. Although MPD RBC incubated with 0.5 mM α-tocopherol showed a decrease in lipid peroxidation, MDA generation was still significantly greater than that of unloaded normal cells (p < 0.02).

strated at lower concentrations, with an impairment of concentrating ability by MPD erythrocytes at high tocopherol concentrations.

In vitro erythrocyte tocopherol loading protects against lipid peroxidation of both normal and MPD cells (fig. 2). However, MPD erythrocytes generate more MDA at all concentrations of α-tocopherol and loading of MPD RBC failed to restore lipid peroxidation to normal. Figure 3 demonstrates that 0.05 mM α-tocopherol fails to inhibit lipid peroxidation of MPD RBC, as compared with significant inhibition of normal RBC, but is an effective inhibitor at higher concentrations. Erythrocyte α-tocopherol concentrations comparable to those achieved by in vivo oral supplementation have no significant inhibitory effect on MDA generation, but higher concentrations produce significant inhibition (fig. 4).

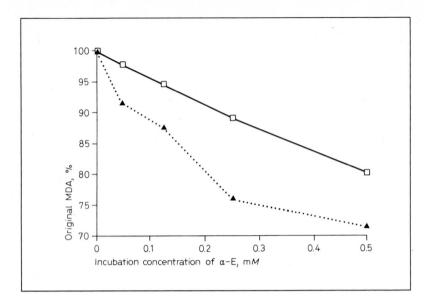

Fig. 3. The relationship between erythrocyte incubation concentration of α-tocopherol during in vitro loading and MDA generation. Values were normalized for 9 normals (triangles) and 11 patients with MPD (squares) and results expressed as percent of MDA generation by unloaded erythrocytes. Comparison between doses by paired t test showed a significant decrease in MDA generation by normal cells at incubation concentrations of 0.05 mM α-tocopherol (p < 0.025). In contrast, inhibition of MDA generation by MPD erythrocytes was not significantly at this concentration, but was observed at incubation concentrations of 0.125 mM and greater. The antioxidant effect of α-tocopherol was significantly greater in normal than MPD cells at all concentrations.

Discussion

These studies have demonstrated that hypocholesterolemia in MPD has an effect on plasma tocopherol concentrations, but does not reduce RBC cholesterol or tocopherol content. Despite normal tocopherol concentrations and increased GSH levels, the erythrocytes of MPD display increased susceptibility to lipid peroxidation. Oral supplementation with doses of α-tocopherol that doubled RBC α-tocopherol content did not reduce MDA generation by MPD erythrocytes. The effect of vitamin E supplementation to increase antioxidant capacity in diseases characterized by increased erythrocyte peroxidation susceptibility and chronic hemolysis has been the subject of several investigations which have generated consid-

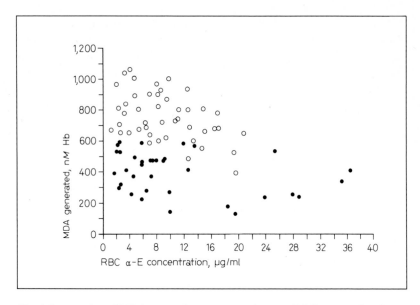

Fig. 4. Scatter plot of MDA generation versus erythrocyte (RBC) α-tocopherol concentration after in vitro loading of normal (closed circles) and MPD (open circles) cells. α-Tocopherol and MDA generation were determined in RBC from 9 normals and 11 patients with MPD incubated without additions and with 4 concentrations of α-tocopherol ranging from 0.05 to 0.5 mM. Each point represents one assay. Inhibition of peroxidation was not significant at RBC α-tocopherol concentrations corresponding to those achieved by in vivo loading (6.8 ± 0.43 µg/ml packed RBC).

erable interest and conflicting results [24]. Efficacy has been evaluated by in vitro changes in erythrocyte peroxidation susceptibility, by clinical improvement measured in terms of transfusion requirement, and by determinations of erythrocyte survival.

The relationship between RBC tocopherol content and MDA generation in the in vitro assay of lipid peroxidation must be well-defined if evaluation of efficacy is to be based on this criterion. Our simultaneous measurements of extra-erythrocyte tocopherol levels, erythrocyte tocopherol concentrations, and MDA generation have provided quantitative data for the relationships between these variables in normal and peroxidation-susceptible RBC. Although under physiological conditions partitioning of tocopherol into RBC was observed in the presence of decreased plasma tocopherol, under loading conditions the α-tocopherol concentration of normal and MPD RBC was directly related to the extra-erythrocyte α-tocopherol concentration. Incubation of normal RBC with tocopherol at concentrations equivalent to those found in plasma of subjects supplemented with 800–1,200 IU DL-α-tocopheryl acetate resulted in doubling of RBC tocopherol and significant reduction in MDA generation. In contrast, MDA generation by MPD erythrocytes was not significantly reduced until RBC tocopherol concentrations were increased 4- to 5-fold. The results of our in vitro studies explain the failure to reduce MDA generation with the oral supplementation regimen we employed in the 7 MPD patients. They also indicate that the erythrocyte is undersaturated with tocopherol and provide evidence for the premise that administration of higher doses of vitamin E will result in further elevation of RBC tocopherol.

The discrepancy in tocopherol loading between normal and MPD RBC at high tocopherol concentrations is of interest, although the levels at which this occurred were far greater than those encountered in vivo. At physiological and pharmacological tocopherol concentrations loading of tocopherol by MPD erythrocyte appeared to be intact. The mechanisms responsible for maintaining RBC tocopherol concentration have not been elucidated. *Kitabchi* et al. [25] have demonstrated specific, saturable binding sites for α-tocopherol which have properties expected of a biologically significant receptor. The integrity of these receptors and their role in decreased loading at high tocopherol concentrations in MPD erythrocytes remains to be evaluated.

MDA is toxic to RBC by virtue of its capacity to cross-link with amino groups of phospholipids and peptides. The action of MDA on erythrocytes produced significant alterations in erythrocyte deformability [26]. Increased susceptibility to in vitro lipid peroxidation is believed to be associated with MDA production in vivo. Since MDA is mutagenic, chronic exposure to increased tissue MDA levels could represent a risk to MPD patients. Although GSH normally functions in vivo as an antioxidant, its extracellular oxidation under certain in vitro conditions has been shown to induce lipid peroxidation [27]. The increased GSH of MPD erythrocytes fails to protect these cells against lipid peroxidation and may even have a paradoxical oxidant effect [8]. The recent report that glutathione is positive in the Ames test at concentrations found in mammalian tissues [10] suggests that an additional risk factor in MPD may be conferred by chronically elevated erythrocyte GSH levels.

Our in vitro studies indicate that inhibition of MDA formation can be produced if sufficient erythrocyte tocopherol concentrations are attained.

The in vivo studies show that MPD patients absorb and load tocopherol into erythrocytes when given oral supplementation, suggesting that further evaluation of tocopherol supplementation using higher dosage regimens is warranted to determine the feasibility of reaching RBC tocopherol concentrations that have an antioxidant effect in vitro. If attainable and free of toxicity, the effect of such regimens on the anemia of MPD and the incidence of malignant transformation should be determined.

Acknowledgements

The author thanks *Eugene F. Roth,* Jr., MD, *Henry Ginsberg,* MD, and *Decherd D. Stump,* MS, for their collaboration in these studies and *Caroline Chin, Tung Han,* and *Margaret O'Connor* for their expert technical assistance. The CLINFO Data Management and Analysis System was employed in these studies.

References

1 Gilbert, H.S.; Ginsberg, H.; Fagerstrom, R.; Brown, W.V.: Characterization of hypocholesterolemia in myeloproliferative disease: relation to disease manifestations and activity. Am. J. Med. *71:* 595–602 (1981).

2 Gilbert, H.S.; Ginsberg, H.: Hypocholesterolemia as a manifestation of disease activity in chronic myelocytic leukemia. Cancer *51:* 1428–1433 (1983).

3 Ginsberg, H.; Gilbert, H.S.; Gibson, J.C.; Le, N.-A.; Brown, W.V.: Increased low-density-lipoprotein catabolism in myeloproliferative disorders. Ann. intern. Med. *96:* 311–316 (1982).

4 Ginsberg, H.; Goldberg, I.J.; Wang-Iverson, P.; Gitler, E.; Le, N.-A.; Gilbert, H.S.; Brown, W.V.: Increased catabolism of native and cyclohexanedione modified low density lipoprotein in subjects with myeloproliferative diseases. Arteriosclerosis *3:* 233–241 (1983).

5 Cooper, R.A.; Durocher, J.R.; Leslie, M.H.: Decreased fluidity of red cell membrane lipids in abetalipoproteinemia. J. clin. Invest. *60:* 115–121 (1977).

6 Mengel, C.E.; Kann, H.E., Jr.; Meriwether, W.D.: Studies of paroxysmal nocturnal hemoglobinuria erythrocytes: increased lysis and lipid peroxide formation by hydrogen peroxide. J. clin. Invest. *46:* 1715–1723 (1967).

7 Gilbert, H.S.; Roth, E.F., Jr.: Increased lipid peroxidation of erythrocytes in myeloproliferative disorders (Abstract). Blood *60:* 21a (1982).

8 Gilbert, H.; Roth, E.F., Jr.: Failure of increased erythrocyte glutathione content to protect against lipid peroxidation in myeloproliferative disease: a paradoxical role for glutathione in membrane lipid peroxidation (Abstract). Clin. Res. *31:* 312A (1983).

9 Mukai, F.H.; Goldstein, B.D.: Mutagenicity of malonaldehyde, a decomposition product of peroxidized polyunsaturated fatty acids. Science *191:* 868–869 (1976).

10   Glatt, H.; Protic-Sabijic, M.; Oesch, F.: Mutagenicity of glutathione and cysteine in the Ames test. Science *220:* 961–962 (1983).

11   Gilbert, H.S.: The spectrum of myeloproliferative disorders. Med. Clins N. A. *57:* 355–393 (1973).

12   Gilbert, H.S.: Definition, clinical features and diagnosis of polycythemia vera. Clin. Haematol. *4:* 263–290 (1975).

13   Gilbert, H.S.: Agnogenic myeloid metaplasia; in Conn, Conn, Current diagnosis, pp. 496–500 (Saunders, Philadelphia 1977).

14   Stocks, J.; Kemp, M.; Dormandy, T.L.: Increased susceptibility of red blood cell lipids to autoxidation in haemolytic states. Lancet *i:* 266–269 (1971).

15   Snyder, L.M.; Sauberman, N.; Condara, H.; Dolan, J.; Jacobs, J.; Szymanski, I.; Fortier, N.L.: Red cell membrane response to hydrogen peroxide-sensitivity in hereditary xerocytosis and in other abnormal red cells. Br. J. Haemat. *48:* 435–444 (1981).

16   Stocks, J.; Dormandy, T.L.: The autoxidation of human red cell lipids induced by hydrogen peroxide. Br. J. Haemat. *20:* 95–111 (1971).

17   Harm, W.; Fortier, N.L.; Lutz, H.U.; Fairbanks, G.; Snyder, L.M.: Increased lipid peroxidation in hereditary xerocytosis. Clinica chim. Acta *99:* 121–128 (1979).

18   Beutler, E.: Red cell metabolism: a manual of biochemical methods, pp. 112–114 (Grune & Stratton, New York 1975).

19   Dacie, J.V.; Lewis, S.M.: Practical haematology; 5th ed., pp. 221–222 (Churchill-Livingstone, Edinburgh 1975).

20   Beutler, E.: Red cell metabolism: a manual of biochemical methods, pp. 115–117 (Grune & Stratton, New York 1975).

21   Bieri, J.H.; Tolliver, T.J.; Catignani, G.L.: Simultaneous determination of α-tocopherol and retinol in plasma or red cells by high pressure liquid chromatography. Am. J. clin. Nutr. *32:* 2143–2149 (1979).

22   De Leenher, A.P.; De Bevere, V.O.R.C.; Claeys, A.E.: Measurement of α, β-, and γ-tocopherol in serum by liquid chromatography. Clin. Chem. *25:* 425–428 (1979).

23   Baxter, J.G.; Robeson, C.D.; Taylor, J.D.; Lehman, R.W.: Natural α, β, and γ-tocopherols and certain esters of physiological interest. J. Am. chem. Soc. *65:* 918–924 (1943).

24   Bieri, J.G.; Corash, L.; Hubbard, V.S.: Medical uses of vitamin E. New Engl. J. Med. *308:* 1063–1071 (1983).

25   Kitabchi, A.E.; Wimalasena, J.: Specific binding sites for *D*-α-tocopherol on human erythrocytes. Biochim. biophys. Acta *684:* 200–206 (1982).

26   Pfafferott, D.; Meiselman, J.; Hochstein, P.: The effect of malonyldialdehyde on erythrocyte deformability. Blood *59:* 12–15 (1982).

27   Hunter, F.E.; Scott, A.; Hoffstein, P.E.; Gebicki, J.M.; Weinstein, J.; Schneider, A.: Studies on the mechanism of swelling, lysis, and disintegration of isolated liver mitochondria exposed to mixtures of oxidized and reduced glutathione. J. biol. Chem. *239:* 614–621 (1964).

H.S. Gilbert, MD, Professor of Medicine, Mount Sinai School of Medicine,
19 East 98th Street, New York, NY 10029 (USA)

Prasad (ed.), Vitamins, Nutrition, and Cancer, pp. 159–165 (Karger, Basel 1984)

Serum Alpha-Tocopherol Levels in Relation to Serum Lipids and Lipoproteins after Oral Administration of Vitamin E[1]

R.S. London, G.S. Sundaram, S. Manimekalai, L. Murphy, M.A. Reynolds, P. Goldstein

Department of Obstetrics and Gynecology, Sinai Hospital of Baltimore, Baltimore, Md., USA

Introduction

Numerous prospective studies have been planned for the next decade to determine the possible role of supplemental vitamin E (tocopherol) in the reduction of cancer risk. It is anticipated that compliance to the treatment regimen will be monitored by some biologic measure of tocopherol, but at present there is no consensus regarding how best to monitor serum tocopherol concentrations in human studies. Different indices of serum tocopherol concentrations have been used, but the relation between these indices (i.e. cholesterol, lipoprotein, etc.) and administered doses of tocopherol is not clear.

The current study was designed to investigate the relations between the dose of synthetic D,L-α-tocopherol administered and ratios of serum tocopherol concentrations to serum total cholesterol and lipoprotein-cholesterol fractions.

[1] This study was supported in part by a grant from the Biochemical Division of Hoffmann-La Roche, Inc., Nutley, N.J.

Materials and Methods

65 patients, 18–45 years of age, were enrolled in this protocol after informed consent was obtained. All patients had regular menstrual intervals, confirmed mammary dysplasia, and no other known underlying medical pathology. Beginning 4 weeks prior to therapy, and continuing until the completion of the study, patients abstained from vitamin supplements, hormones or any prescription drugs which would interfere with metabolism and/or absorption of α-tocopherol.

Patients were randomly administered placebo or α-tocopherol (free alcohol form) in divided doses of 150, 300 or 600 IU/day for a 2-month period. Neither the patients nor the investigators were aware of which treatment was administered. Pre- and post-therapy luteal phase fasting blood samples were drawn for assays of tocopherol, cholesterol and lipoprotein cholesterol concentrations. Side effects were monitored at each visit.

Serum tocopherol concentrations were determined by a spectrophotometric method [1]. Lipoprotein cholesterol concentrations were measured using precipitation with dextran sulfate and $MgCl_2$, and sequential ultracentrifugation [2]. The following measurements were obtained before and after treatment: total serum cholesterol, very low density lipoprotein (VLDL), low density lipoprotein (LDL), and high density lipoproteins (HDL_2 and HDL_3).

The relationship of oral tocopherol dose to each serum parameter was examined using a partial correlation [3], from which differences among patients in height, weight, age and pretreatment concentration were controlled. Since the pretreatment concentration of each serum parameter was partialed out in the analysis, these correlations provide a measure of the relationship of oral tocopherol dose to the change in the serum parameter from before to after therapy. Thus, each correlation provides a sensitive statistical test of the effect of orally administered tocopherol on a given serum parameter.

Results

The distribution of serum α-tocopherol concentrations before treatment in our patients is shown in figure 1. The levels range from 0.5 to 1.5 mg/dl, and agree well with those found by other investigators [4]. The mean ± SEM concentrations of serum tocopherol before and after oral tocopherol therapy are shown in table I, with the adjusted mean concentrations shown graphically in figure 2. A significant effect of oral tocopherol dose on serum concentrations was found, as indicated by the partial correlation, $r = 0.56$, $p < 0.001$. This positive correlation reflects that post-therapy serum tocopherol concentrations increased as a function of increasing oral dose.

The mean ± SEM values of the ratio of serum tocopherol to total cholesterol before and after oral tocopherol therapy are shown in table II. A significant positive correlation emerged between oral tocopherol dose and

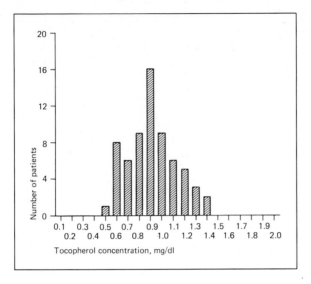

Fig. 1. Distribution of pretreatment serum tocopherol levels in 65 women (ages 18–45).

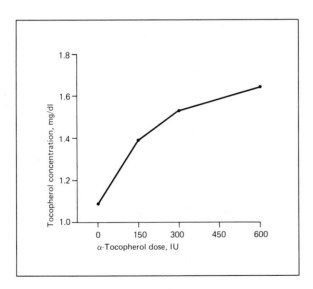

Fig. 2. Post-therapy means adjusted for patients' age, weight, height and pre-therapy tocopherol concentrations.

Table I. Concentrations of serum tocopherol before and after oral tocopherol therapy

Treatment	Pre-therapy	Post-therapy
Placebo	1.04 ± 0.030	1.15 ± 0.034
150 IU	0.90 ± 0.032	1.35 ± 0.066
300 IU	0.97 ± 0.033	1.53 ± 0.053
600 IU	0.97 ± 0.028	1.63 ± 0.066

Values reported are mean concentration ± SEM.

Table II. Ratio of serum tocopherol/total cholesterol before and after oral tocopherol therapy

Treatment	Pre-therapy	Post-therapy
Placebo	0.0058 ± 0.00037	0.0063 ± 0.00081
150 IU	0.0052 ± 0.00038	0.0064 ± 0.00052
300 IU	0.0053 ± 0.00036	0.0067 ± 0.00045
600 IU	0.0053 ± 0.00029	0.0077 ± 0.00051

Values reported are mean ± SEM.

post-therapy values of this serum parameter ($r = 0.31$, $p < 0.001$). This correlation also reflects that post-therapy values of the ratio increased as a function of increasing oral tocopherol dose.

Table III shows the mean ± SEM values of the ratio of serum tocopherol to LDL cholesterol before and after therapy. As with the preceding serum parameters, oral tocopherol dose was positively correlated with post-therapy values, indicating that the higher the orally administered dose, the higher the values of the ratio ($r = 0.37$, $p < 0.004$).

The mean ± SEM values of the ratio of serum tocopherol to HDL_2-cholesterol before and after therapy are shown in table IV. A significant effect of oral tocopherol dose on this ratio was found, as indicated by the partial correlation, $r = 0.33$, $p < 0.006$. The positive correlation indicates

Table III. Ratio of serum tocopherol/LDL cholesterol before and after oral tocopherol therapy

Treatment	Pre-therapy	Post-therapy
Placebo	0.012 ± 0.0012	0.011 ± 0.0009
150 IU	0.010 ± 0.0010	0.012 ± 0.0013
300 IU	0.013 ± 0.0018	0.012 ± 0.0007
600 IU	0.011 ± 0.0008	0.015 ± 0.0010

Values reported are mean $\pm$ SEM.

Table IV. Ratio of serum tocopherol/HDL$_2$ cholesterol before and after oral tocopherol therapy

Treatment	Pre-therapy	Post-therapy
Placebo	0.034 ± 0.0046	0.030 ± 0.0029
150 IU	0.029 ± 0.0026	0.033 ± 0.0041
300 IU	0.025 ± 0.0031	0.034 ± 0.0053
600 IU	0.031 ± 0.0033	0.045 ± 0.0054

Values reported are mean $\pm$ SEM.

that the higher the oral tocopherol dose, the higher the post-therapy value of this ratio.

Finally, there was no significant effect of oral tocopherol on the ratio of serum tocopherol to either VLDL or HDL$_3$ cholesterol (rs $= -0.01$ and 0.10, ps > 0.05, respectively).

Discussion

As monitored by serum tocopherol concentrations, the alcohol form of α-tocopherol was well absorbed at doses of 150–600 IU/day; this dose regimen correlated significantly with serum levels. This finding suggests that in individuals with a 'normal' lipid and lipoprotein milieu, compliance to vitamin E 'intervention' studies (i.e. chemoprevention type prospective programs) may be followed by simple measurement of serum tocopherol concentrations. It is well established that tocopherol concentrations in serum vary with the cholesterol levels [5, 6], certain lipoproteins [7], and in certain pathologic states [8]. This fact may be related to the fact that tocopherol is transported in the blood by lipoproteins [9], or that cholesterol is bound to the lipoproteins. Because of the intimate association of tocopherol to the lipid/lipoprotein components of plasma, and the observation that tocopherol correlates well with LDL [7], we studied the ratios of serum tocopherol to a number of different lipoprotein fractions and cholesterol, using sophisticated techniques to measure lipoprotein concentrations. Our findings confirm those of previous observations, that response to oral tocopherol may be monitored as a ratio of tocopherol concentration to total cholesterol, LDL or HDL_2. However, in this investigation those correlations were not as significant as with dose and serum concentration alone.

One other observation may be noted as a result of this study. Tocopherol concentrations vary with age [10], and perhaps sex (as expressed in relation to cholesterol) [6]. However, much of the literature dealing with serum tocopherol levels as influenced by dietary supplements or manipulation does not use appropriate statistical techniques to control for what appear to be relevant confounding variables – for instance age, weight, sex, pretreatment concentrations, etc. All future studies dealing with tocopherol supplements should be designed with appropriate statistical methods to control for these types of variables.

Conclusions

The free alcohol tocopherol form of vitamin E appears to be well absorbed at doses from 150 to 600 IU/day with no side effects. When confounding variables are controlled, response to exogenous tocopherol may be monitored as a ratio of tocopherol to total cholesterol, LDL or HDL_2. In experimental paradigms in healthy individuals, serum tocopherol concentrations seem to adequately reflect patients' compliance to therapy. It does not seem necessary to measure lipid or lipoprotein-cholesterol parameters solely to obtain tocopherol/lipid ratios in clinical studies using 'healthy' individuals, as long as appropriate statistical methods are utilized to control for confounding variables.

References

1 Bieri, J.G.; Teets, L.; Belavady, B.; Andrews, E.L.: Serum vitamin E levels in a normal adult population in the Washington, D.C. Area. Proc. Soc. exp. Biol. Med. *117:* 131 (1964).

2 Sundaram, G.S.; London, R.; Manimekalai, S.; Nair, P.P.; Goldstein, P.: Alpha tocopherol and serum lipoproteins. Lipids *16:* 223–227 (1981).

3 Nie, N.; Hall, C.; Jenkins, J.; Steinbrenner, K.; Bent, D.: Statistical methods for the social sciences (McGraw-Hill, New York 1975).

4 Farrell, P.: Deficiency states, pharmacologic effects and nutrient requirements; in Vitamin E: a comprehensive treatise (Dekker, New York 1980).

5 Pelkonen, R.: Plasma vitamin A and E in the study of lipid and lipoprotein metabolism in coronary artery disease. Acta med. scand. *174:* suppl., pp. 1–101 (1963).

6 Lehmann, J.; Marshall, M.; Slover, H.; Iacono, J.: Influence of dietary fat level and dietary tocopherol on plasma tocopherols of human subjects. J. Nutr. *107:* 1006–1015 (1977).

7 Davies, T.; Keller, J.; Losowsky, M.: Interrelation of serum lipoprotein and tocopherol levels. Clinica chim. Acta *24:* 431–436 (1969).

8 Muller, D.P.R.; Harries, J.T.: Vitamin E studies in children with malabsorption. Biochem. J. *112:* 28P (1969).

9 McCormick, E.; Cornwell, D.G.; Brown, J.R.: Studies on the distribution of tocopherol in human serum lipoproteins. J. Lipid Res. *1:* 221–228 (1960).

10 Hoppner, K.; Phillips, W.; Murray, T.; Campbell, J.: Data on serum tocopherol levels in a selected group of Canadians. Can. J. Physiol. Pharmacol. *48:* 321–323 (1970).

R.S. London, MD, Department of Obstetrics and Gynecology,
Sinai Hospital of Baltimore, Inc., Baltimore, MD 21215 (USA)

Other Vitamins and Nutrients

Prasad (ed.), Vitamins, Nutrition, and Cancer, pp. 166–179 (Karger, Basel 1984)

Prevention of Radiation Transformation in vitro

Ann R. Kennedy

Laboratory of Radiobiology, Department of Cancer Biology, Harvard University, School of Public Health, Boston, Mass., USA

Introduction

There are now many reports that agents can modify the induction of radiation or chemical carcinogen-induced transformation in vitro; these studies have recently been reviewed [1]. Many of our previous studies on modifying agents for transformation have given information about the mechanism involved in the malignant transformation of cells [2–17], but little information on the effects of agents which could possibly be used as human cancer chemopreventive agents. We have now studied several possible chemopreventive agents, including retinoids, ascorbic acid and protease inhibitors, for their ability to affect radiation-induced transformation in C3H10T½ cells, and those results will be discussed here. Many of our previous experiments with protease inhibitors have already been published [3–5, 10, 12, 14, 16].

It has previously been shown that vitamin A analogues, known as retinoids, will inhibit carcinogenesis in various systems [18] as well as malignant transformation in vitro induced by X-irradiation [19, 20] and chemical carcinogens [21, 22]. There have been, however, a number of recent reports suggesting that the retinoids may also act as tumor-promoting agents rather than as inhibitors of carcinogenesis [23, 24]. Of particular importance is the evidence that retinoids can promote carcinogenesis when simulated sunlight (which includes the UVB and UVA regions of 313 nm and 360 nm, respectively) is used as the initiating agent [24] since retinoids are widely used in skin creams for acne and thus could promote UV light- (or sunlight-) induced human skin cancer. We report here studies performed on the interactions between three major wavelengths of UV light (UVA,

UVB, and UVC) and two retinoids in the induction of malignant transformation in vitro using C3H10T½ cells. These experiments were performed specifically to determine whether retinoids could act as promoting agents for UV light-induced transformation in vitro.

There are now several reports that ascorbic acid can suppress chemical carcinogen (3-methylcholanthrene)-induced transformation in vitro [25–28]. The effects of ascorbic acid on carcinogenesis in vivo have been reviewed [29], and are at present controversial, with some data suggesting that ascorbic acid can act as a cocarcinogen to enhance carcinogenesis by 3-methylcholanthrene [30]. There are also now many reports that protease inhibitors suppress carcinogenesis in vivo [31–41] as well as transformation in vitro [3–5, 10, 12, 14, 16, 42–44]. The effects of protease inhibitors on carcinogenesis and transformation in vitro have recently been reviewed [1].

The experiments to be reported here on retinoids, protease inhibitors and ascorbic acid have been performed with the C3H10T½ (clone 8) transformation assay system, developed by *Reznikoff* et al. [45, 46], which has been used extensively in our laboratory for studies of radiation-induced transformation in vitro. Previous studies on radiation transformation indicate that transformation is a two-step process: the first step is a frequent alteration occurring in a large fraction of irradiated cells, while the second step, that of malignant transformation, is a rare event which occurs randomly during cellular proliferation (with an approximate frequency of 10^{-6} per cell per generation) [8, 9, 47–49]. In the typical radiation transformation experiment, a sufficient number of cells are seeded into Petri dishes such that approximately 300 viable cells result (considering the plating efficiency of the cells and the toxicity of the treatment); these cells then proliferate until confluence is reached at 10 days to 2 weeks postirradiation (at approximately 2×10^6 cells/dish). The dishes then remain in confluence for approximately 4 weeks until transformed foci, overlying the confluent monolayer, can be scored. Radiation transformation of C3H10T½ cells is shown schematically in figure 1. It is during the growth phase of the culture, when the second step in transformation occurs randomly, that tumor-promoting agents, such as 12-*O*-tetradecanoylphorbol-13-acetate (TPA), can enhance transformation [6]. Similarly, agents such as protease inhibitors suppress transformation when present during the growth phase of cultures [12, 14]. Neither protease inhibitors nor TPA need to be present continuously during cellular proliferation to have their modifying effects on transformation; the addition of such modifying agents to cultures can be delayed

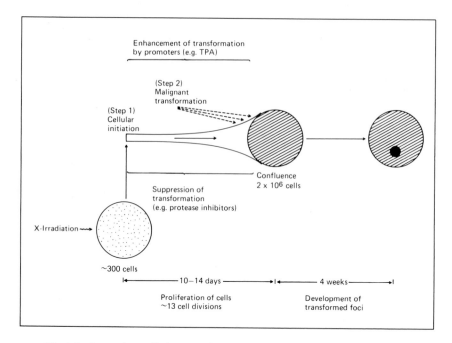

Fig. 1. In the routine radiation transformation experiment utilizing C3H10T½ cells, a sufficient number of cells are seeded such that, considering the plating efficiency and toxicity of the radiation exposure, approximately 300 viable cells result. With doses of 400–600 rad, all of the surviving cells have undergone 'step 1' of the transformation process (see text). The cells proliferate until confluence is reached about 10–14 days postirradiation. Malignant transformation, or step 2 of the transformation process, is a rare event which can occur at any point during cellular proliferation, at a constant probability per mitosis [48, 49]. As 'step 2' in transformation occurs as a function of cell division, it is most likely to occur when the most cells are dividing, or just before confluence is reached [48, 49]. It is during the growth phase of the culture that tumor promoters act to enhance and protease inhibitors can suppress the yield of transformed foci, which ultimately develop overlying the confluent monolayer of cells. The irradiated cells remain in confluence for about 4 weeks, at which time transformed foci can be scored.

until many days postirradiation [6, 12, 14]. We have previously observed that a 1-day treatment of the protease inhibitor antipain at 5 days postirradiation is sufficient to significantly suppress radiation transformation, which suggests that antipain is capable of irreversibly blocking an ongoing cellular process initiated by the radiation exposure and related to the induction of malignant transformation [14].

Although other possible human cancer chemopreventive agents do have some effect on the process of in vitro transformation, the protease inhibitors are clearly the most effective of the agents we have studied in their ability to suppress carcinogen-induced transformation in vitro. In this paper, the efficiency of various protease inhibitors will be compared in terms of their ability to suppress X-ray-induced transformation or the TPA enhancement of transformation in vitro.

Materials and Methods

Details of experimental techniques for radiation transformation experiments using C3H10T½ cells have been described elsewhere [1–17]. Stock cultures were maintained in 60-mm Petri dishes and were passed by subculturing at a 1:20 dilution every 7 days. The cells used were in passages 9–14. They were grown in a humidified 5% CO_2 atmosphere at 37 °C in Eagle's basal medium supplemented with 10% heat-inactivated fetal bovine serum and gentamycin. Cells were exposed to X-rays or UV light 24 h after seeding. Plating efficiencies were determined from 3 plates seeded with a cell density one fifth that of the plates used for the transformation assay; these cultures were terminated at 10 days. The various treatment toxicities were considered in the design of the experiments such that all dishes used for the transformation assay contained approximately 300 viable cells per dish. Types 2 and 3 foci were scored as transformants.

For UVC (254 nm) light exposure experiments, the cells were irradiated by a bank of 5 GE G8T5 tubes as previously described [50]. In the UVA light exposure experiments, the cells were irradiated through saline for 60 s using two 4-foot long Sylvania lamps (FR40T12/PUVA) with peak emission in the UVA range at 360 nm and a dose of 2.67×10^{-4} W/cm². For UVB light exposure experiments, the cells were irradiated through saline for 4 min using two 4-foot long Sylvania lamps (F40T12/2021) with peak emission in the UVB range of 313 nm and a dose of 0.58×10^{-4} W/cm².

The retinoid used, the trimethylmethoxyphenyl analogue of N-ethylretinamide (RO-11-1430) was donated by Hoffmann-La Roche (Nutley, N.J.). This retinoid was selected as it was reported to inhibit C3H10T½ cell transformation in vitro induced by X-irradiation [19]. The retinoid was initially dissolved in dimethyl sulfoxide (DMSO) and diluted such that the final concentration in the medium was 0.5 μg/ml. Retinoid treatment was begun 48 h after UV light treatment and added to cultures every time the media was changed during the 6-week transformation assay.

The dose of UVC (254 nm) light chosen for this study was 130 erg/mm², a dose previously shown to be in the plateau region of the dose response curve for the induction of malignant transformation in vitro by 254 nm UV light [50]. In addition, doses of UVA and UVB which induced transformed foci were selected for the interaction studies with retinoids. It is apparent from the data in tables I and II that the retinoid RO-11-1430 can suppress UV light-induced transformation in vitro. In each case, the fraction of dishes containing transformed foci in dishes exposed to both RO-11-1430 and UVC, UVB, or UVA light was decreased when compared to similar irradiated cultures which did not receive retinoid treatments. This was a statistically significant decrease in retinoid treated cultures only for the results using UVA light with the retinoid.

Table I. Effect of retinoid, RO-11-1430, on the induction of UVC (254 nm) light-induced transformation in C3H10T½ cells

Group	Treatment	Exper-iment No.	Plating efficiency %	Surviving cells per dish	Total surviving cells	Fraction of dishes[1]	Total
A	Controls (no treatment)	1	45.0	450	4,500	0/10	0/20
		2	48.0	360	3,600	0/10	
B	130 erg/mm^2 (UV light, 254 nm)	1	0.4	400	6,800	2/17 = 0.12	9/47 = 0.19
		2	0.3	218	6,480	7/30 = 0.23	
C	130 erg/mm^2 (UV light, 254 nm) + RO-11-1430 (0.5 µg/ml)	1	0.3	320	5,120	0/16	4/45 = 0.09
		2	0.3	255	7,395	4/29 = 0.14	

[1] Fraction of dishes used which contained transformants (types 2 and 3 foci); statistical analysis (χ^2 analysis with Yates' continuity correction): group B versus C, $p > 0.05$.

Table II. Effect of a retinoid, RO-11-1430, on the induction of UVA (360 nm) and UVB (313 nm) light-induced transformation in C3H10T½ cells

Group	Treatment	Plating efficiency %	Surviving cells per dish	Total surviving cells	Fraction of dishes[1]
A	Control	30.0	300	5,100	0/17
B	UVB (4 min)	23.0	345	3,795	3/11 = 0.27
C	UVB (4 min) + RO-11-1430 (0.5 µg/ml)	9.0	135	1,755	0/13
D	UVA (1 min)	23.0	345	7,590	10/22 = 0.45
E	UVA (1 min) + RO-11-1430 (0.5 µg/ml)	7.0	105	945	0/9
F	RO-11-1430 (0.5 µg/ml)	6.0	90	1,980	0/22

[1] Fraction of dishes used which contained transformants (types 2 and 3 foci); statistical analysis: group B versus C, $p > 0.05$ (Fisher exact test); group D versus E, $p < 0.05$ (χ^2 analysis with Yates' continuity correction or Fisher exact test).

It has been reported that RO-11-1430 can suppress X-ray-induced transformation in vitro when present for 96 h postirradiation [19]. To determine whether this retinoid could suppress radiation transformation when present for only 1 day postirradiation, beginning either immediately postirradiation or at day 5 postirradiation, an experiment similar in design to those reported by *Harisiadis* et al. [19] was performed. As shown in table III, a 24-hour treatment with RO-11-1430 does not have a significant suppressive effect on X-ray-induced transformation in vitro.

Our experiment with ascorbic acid additions to irradiated cultures (600 rad) was performed in the same manner as the chemical carcinogen-induced transformation experiments described by *Benedict* et al. [25]. Purified ascorbic acid was obtained from Dr. *William Benedict* and added to cultures daily (5 days per week) at 5 μg/ml, a concentration of ascorbic acid shown to be inhibitory to 3-methylcholanthrene-induced transformation in vitro [25]. As shown in table IV, there were no significant ascorbic acid suppressive effects on X-ray induced transformation for any of the treatment protocols.

Protease inhibitors are very effective inhibitors for the suppression of radiation transformation in vitro; much of our work with protease inhibitors has previously been pub-

Table III. Effect of 0.5 μg/ml RO-11-1430, a retinoid, on X-ray induced transformation in vitro

Treatment	Experiment No.	Plating efficiency[1] %	Total viable cells	Total foci observed		Fraction of dishes used which contained transformed foci		
				type 3	types 2+3	type 3	types 2+3	total[2]
I 600 rad	1	4.1	9,430	19	31	4/23	17/23	39/51 = 0.76
	2	4.7	13,160	22	35	11/28	22/28	
II 600 rad + RO-11-1430, beginning immediately post-irradiation and continued for 24 h	1	7.1	15,620	19	33	4/22	15/22	32/49 = 0.65
	2	4.6	12,420	14	21	9/27	17/27	
III 600 rad + RO-11-1430, added to cultures for 24 h at 5 days post-irradiation	1	4.2	10,080	18	38	7/24	21/24	36/52 = 0.69
	2	4.9	13,720	16	25	8/28	15/28	

[1] Controls = 12.8%, experiment 1; and 25.0%, experiment 2.
[2] Statistical analysis: χ^2 analysis with Yates' continuity correction: group I versus II or III, $p > 0.05$.

lished [3–5, 10, 12, 14, 16]. A comparison of the efficiency of the various protease inhib-itors we have used, for the suppression of X-ray-induced transformation in vitro or the enhancement of radiation transformation in vitro, is shown in table V, where a + indicates a statistically significant suppressive effect, as determined by a χ^2 analysis of the data, for the various protease inhibitors studied.

Discussion

Our studies with various potential cancer chemopreventive agents have shown that only some of the agents tested have the ability to affect the induction of transformation in vitro by ionizing radiation, with protease inhibitors clearly being the most effective agents we have studied.

Table IV. Effect of 5 µg/ml ascorbic acid on X-ray-induced transformation in vitro[1]

Treatment group	Plating efficiency %	Total surviving cells	Total foci observed		Fraction of dishes used which contained transformed foci	
			type 3	types 2+3	type 3	types 2+3
1 Controls – no treatment	45.0	2,835	0	0	0/7	0/7
2 Ascorbic acid treatments throughout assay	38.9	5,600	0	3	0/16	3/16 = 0.19
3 600 rad	4.4	17,600	8	28	4/40 = 0.10	21/40 = 0.53
4 600 rad + ascorbic acid, beginning immediately post-irradiation with treatment throughout assay	2.9	10,730	7	37	0/37	22/37 = 0.59
5 600 rad + ascorbic acid, beginning immediately post-irradiation and continued until day 23 post-irradiation	3.4	13,260	9	32	4/39 = 0.10	21/39 = 0.54
6 600 rad + ascorbic acid, beginning on day 23 post-irradiation and continued throughout assay	4.4	19,800	9	35	6/45 = 0.13	23/45 = 0.51

[1] Ascorbic acid was added to cultures daily – 5 days/week.

The retinoid RO-11-1430 has the ability to inhibit transformation in vitro induced by three different wavelengths of UV light (UVA, UVB, UVC) when added to cultures at weekly intervals throughout the transformation assay. Although the peak emissions for the UVA and UVB light lamps used in our experiments were 360 and 313 nm, respectively, both of these exposure conditions involved a small component of shorter wavelength UV light, which is known to be more efficient for the production of biological effects (such as the induction of malignant transformation) [51]. In a previous study of ours in which we observed that fluorescent light could transform C3H10T½ cells, transformation was abolished when irradiations were carried out through Petri dish covers, which blocked the transmission of shorter wavelengths in the fluorescent light emission spectrum [51].

Table V. Suppressive effects of protease inhibitors on X-ray transformation and the enhancement of transformation by TPA

Inhibitor	Proteases inhibited	Suppression of	
		X-ray transformation	TPA enhancement of X-ray transformation
Antipain	papain, trypsin, thrombokinase, cathepsins A and B, plasmin and plasminogen activator	++	+++
Elastatinol	elastase	–	–
Leupeptin	plasmin, trypsin, papain, cathepsin B, plasminogen activator	++	±
Chymostatin	chymotrypsin (papain, cathepsin B)	+++	+++
Soybean trypsin inhibitor	trypsin, thromboplastin, plasmin, elastase	–	++
Bowman-Birk inhibitor	chymotrypsin, trypsin	++	–
FOY-305 (N,N–Dimethylcarbanoyl-methyl-4-(4-guanidino-benzoyloxy)-phenylacetate) methansulfonate	trypsin, plasmin, kallikrein, thrombin	–	+

Thus, it is possible that all three wavelengths of UV light used in the studies reported here resulted in biologic damage of a similar type, and it is not surprising that the suppressive effect of RO-11-1430 on the induction of transformation was consistent at each UV wavelength area analyzed.

It has been reported that RO-11-1430 is capable of inhibiting transformation induced by ionizing radiation when present for 96 h postirradiation [19]. We have observed here, however, that RO-11-1430 has no effect on radiation transformation when present for only 24 h either immediately following the X-ray exposure or at 5 days postirradiation. These results suggest that this retinoid acts to suppress X-ray-induced transformation in a different manner from the protease inhibitor antipain, which does significantly suppress radiation transformation when present for 24 h either immediately after or at 5 days postirradiation.

We have observed that a different retinoid, 13-*cis*-retinoic acid, when added to cultures at weekly intervals throughout the transformation assay, significantly enhances the yield of transformants resulting from UV light exposures in C3H10T½ cells and thus acts as a weak promoting agent in this system [*Long and Kennedy*, unpublished data]. Our in vitro results showing enhancement of UV light-induced transformation in vitro by this retinoid are analogous to the experiments performed in mouse skin with UV light and retinoic acid in which the retinoid acted to enhance mouse skin carcinogenesis [24]. It has previously been reported that 13-*cis*-retinoic acid does not affect 3-methylcholanthrene-induced transformation in C3H10T½ cells, while several other retinoids, like RO-11-1430, do suppress chemical carcinogen-induced transformation in vitro [22]. These results clearly show that retinoids, depending on their structures, can have very different effects on carcinogen-induced transformation in vitro. There are now many other types of experiments which have shown that retinoids can act both as tumor promoting agents and as suppressive agents for carcinogenesis in vivo and in vitro [18–24].

The available data suggest that radiation and chemical carcinogen-induced transformation of C3H10T½ cells occurs by the same or very similar pathways [1, 8, 9, 47–49, 52] and in general, the same modifying agents appear to affect transformation induced by both physical or chemical carcinogens in the same way [reviewed in ref. 1]. Thus, it is not clear why ascorbic acid failed to suppress radiation transformation in vitro while it clearly has a suppressive effect on methylcholanthrene-induced transformation in vitro [25–28]. There are, however, several chemical agents which can modify chemical carcinogen-induced transformation in vitro by altering metabolism of the chemical carcinogen [reviewed in ref. 1] and, thus, would not be expected to affect radiation transformation in the same way.

The most effective of the possible cancer preventive agents which we have studied are the protease inhibitors, which have the ability to completely abolish radiation transformation as well as the enhancement of transformation by TPA when present postirradiation. The protease inhibitors we have studied appear to affect the induction of transformation in vitro in different ways, however, suggesting that more than one protease may be important in the malignant transformation of cells. The protease inhibitors antipain and chymostatin affect both X-ray-induced transformation as well as the enhancement of transformation by TPA; leupeptin and the Bowman-Birk inhibitor affect X-ray-induced transformation, while soybean trypsin inhibitor and FOY-305 affect only the enhancement of X-ray transformation by TPA. Chymostatin and the Bowman-Birk protease inhibitor are among the most effective of the protease inhibitors we have studied, with the ability to suppress X-ray transformation at dose levels at which other protease inhibitors are not effective (when given as weekly additions to cultures). There are other protease inhibitors, such as elastatinol, which do not suppress X-ray-induced transformation in vitro or the TPA enhancement of transformation (see table V). The mechanism by which some protease inhibitors suppress radiation transformation is unknown. We have hypothesized that protease inhibitors can irreversibly block an ongoing cellular process, begun by the radiation exposure and related to the induction of malignant transformation [14]. Other possible mechanisms for their effects on transformation have recently been reviewed [1, 12].

The suppressive effect of protease inhibitors on malignant transformation appears to be a general one and not specific for X-ray induced transformation of C3H10T½ cells. We have shown that protease inhibitors suppress steroid hormone- (e.g. 17β-estradiol [10] and cortisone [unpublished data]) induced transformation of C3H10T½ cells, and other investigators have observed that protease inhibitors suppress chemical carcinogen-induced transformation of C3H10T½ cells [43] and hamster embryo cells [44]. We have shown that antipain and leupeptin suppress X-ray-induced transformation in 3T3 cells [3] and that antipain and the Bowman-Birk inhibitor suppress X-ray-induced transformation [53] of normal human diploid (1522) cells [Sheela and Kennedy, unpublished data]. Other evidence that protease inhibitors will be effective in human cells comes from our studies with cells from patients with Bloom's syndrome, an autosomal recessive genetic disease in which there is an increased susceptibility to

cancer. We have shown that the protease inhibitors, antipain, soybean trypsin inhibitor and the Bowman-Birk inhibitor, suppress the high spontaneous levels of chromosome aberrations and sister chromatid exchanges
occurring in the cells of patients with Bloom's syndrome; these chromosome abnormalities are thought to be related to the high cancer incidence
occurring in Bloom's syndrome patients [54]. The fact that the Bowman-
Birk inhibitor is effective, at non-toxic dose levels, at suppressing chromosome abnormalities in Bloom's syndrome cells is particularly exciting since
we have proposed that this protease inhibitor could be an effective human
cancer chemopreventive agent [16]. We have previously shown that, when
ingested in the diet, the Bowman-Birk inhibitor reaches the colon in an
active form [16]. In addition, we have reported that this inhibitor very
effectively suppresses X-ray-induced transformation in vitro [16]; thus, the
Bowman-Birk protease inhibitor from soybeans appears to be a very promising chemopreventive agent for human cancer.

Acknowledgments

I thank Dr. *Walter Troll* and the US Japan Cooperative Cancer Research Program for
the protease inhibitors antipain, leupeptin, elastatinol and chymostatin, Dr. *Jon Yavelow*
and Dr. *Walter Troll* for the Bowman-Birk inhibitor, and Dr. *Tsuyohiko Mori* and the
ONO Pharmaceutical Co., Ltd. (Osaka, Japan) for the FOY-305 protease inhibitor used in
our studies.

I thank Dr. *Sheila Long* for performing the UVA and UVB cell irradiations and
Marilyn Collins and *Babette Radner* for expert technical assistance in the studies presented
here. This research was supported by NIH Grants CA-22704 and ES-00002.

References

1   Kennedy, A.R.: Promotion and other interactions between agents in the induction of
    transformation in vitro in fibroblasts; in Slaga, Mechanisms of tumor promotion,
    vol. III, pp. 13–55 (CRC, West Palm Beach, Fla. 1984).
2   Kennedy, A.R.; Mondal, S.; Heidelberger, C.; Little, J.B.: Enhancement of X-ray
    transformation by 12-*O*-tetradecanoyl-phorbol-13-acetate in a cloned line of C3H
    mouse embryo cells. Cancer Res. *38:* 439–443 (1978).
3   Kennedy, A.R.; Little, J.B.: Protease inhibitors suppress radiation-induced malignant
    transformation in vitro. Nature, Lond. *276:* 825–826 (1978).
4   Little, J.B.; Nagasawa, H.; Kennedy, A.R.: DNA repair and malignant transforma-
    tion: effect of X-irradiation, TPA and protease inhibitors on transformation and
    sister chromatid exchanges in mouse 10T½ cells. Radiat. Res. *79:* 241–255 (1979).
5   Kennedy, A.R.; Little, J.B.: Radiation transformation in vitro: modification by expo-

sure to tumor promoters and protease inhibitors; in Radiation biology in cancer research, pp. 295–307 (Raven Press, New York 1980).

6   Kennedy, A.R.; Murphy, G.; Little, J.B.: The effect of time and duration of exposure to 12-O-tetradecanoyl-phorbol-13-acetate (TPA) on X-ray transformation of C3H10T½ cells. Cancer Res. *40:* 1915–1920 (1980).

7   Kennedy, A.R.; Little, J.B.: Actinomycin D suppresses radiation transformation in vitro. Int. J. Radiat. Biol. *38:* 465–468 (1980).

8   Kennedy, A.R.; Little, J.B.: An investigation of the mechanism for enhancement of radiation transformation in vitro by TPA. Carcinogenesis *1:* 1039–1047 (1980).

9   Kennedy, A.R.; Little, J.B.: High efficiency, kinetics and numerology of transformation by radiation in vitro; in Burchenal, Oettgen, Cancer: achievements, challenges and prospects for the 1980s, vol. 1, pp. 491–500 (Grune & Stratton, New York 1981).

10 Kennedy, A.R.; Weichselbaum, R.R.: Effects of 17β-estradiol on radiation transformation in vitro; inhibition of effects by protease inhibitors. Carcinogenesis *2:* 67–69 (1981).

11 Little, J.B.; Kennedy, A.R.: Promotion of X-ray transformation in vitro; in Hecker et al. Carcinogenesis *7:* 243–257 (1982).

12 Kennedy, A.R.; Little, J.B.: Effects of protease inhibitors on radiation transformation in vitro. Cancer Res. *41:* 2103–2108 (1981).

13 Kennedy, A.R.; Weichselbaum, R.R.: Effects of dexamethasone and cortisone with X-irradiation on the malignant transformation on C3H10T½ cells. Nature, Lond. *294:* 97–98 (1981).

14 Kennedy, A.R.: Antipain, but not cycloheximide, suppresses radiation transformation when present for only one day at five days post-irradiation. Carcinogenesis *3:* 1093–1095 (1982).

15 Little, J.B.; Kennedy, A.R.; Nagasawa, H.: Involvement of free radical intermediates in oncogenic transformation and tumor promotion in vitro; in Nygaard, Simic, Radioprotectors and anticarcinogens, pp. 487–493 (Academic Press, New York 1983).

16 Yavelow, J.; Finlay, T.H.; Kennedy, A.R.; Troll, W.: Bowman-Birk soybean protease inhibitor as an anticarcinogen. Cancer Res. *43:* 2454–2459 (1983).

17 Kennedy, A.R.; Troll, W.; Little, J.B.: Role of free radicals in the initiation and promotion of radiation transformation in vitro. Carcinogenesis (submitted).

18 Sporn, M.B.; Newton, D.L.: Chemoprevention of cancer with retinoids. Fed. Proc. *38:* 2528–2534 (1979).

19 Harisiadis, L.; Miller, R.C.; Hall, E.J.; Borek, C.: A vitamin A analogue inhibits radiation-induced oncogenic transformation. Nature, Lond. *274:* 486–487 (1978).

20 Miller, R.C.; Geard, C.R.; Osmak, R.S.; Rutledge-Freeman, M.; Ong, A.; Mason, H.; Napholz, A.; Perez, N.; Harisiadis, L.; Borek, C.: Modification of sister chromatid exchanges and radiation-induced transformation in rodent cells by the tumor promoter 12-O-tetradecanoyl-phorbol-13-acetate and two retinoids. Cancer Res. *41:* 655–659 (1981).

21 Merriman, R.L.; Bertram, J.S.: Reversible inhibition by retinoids of 3-methyl-cholanthrene-induced neoplastic transformation of C3H10T½ clone 8 cells. Cancer Res. *39:* 1661–1666 (1979).

22 Bertram, J.S.: Structure-activity relationships among various retinoids and their

ability to inhibit neoplastic transformation and to increase cell adhesion in the C3H/10T½ Cl 8 cell line. Cancer Res. *40:* 3141–3146 (1980).

23   Shroder, E.W.; Black, P.H.: Retinoids: tumor preventers or tumor enhancers? J. natn. Cancer Inst. *65:* 671–674 (1980).

24   Forbes, P.D.; Urbach, F.; Davies, R.E.: Enhancement of experimental photocarcinogenesis by topical retinoic acid. Cancer Lett. *7:* 85–89 (1979).

25   Benedict, W.F.; Wheatley, W.L.; Jones, P.A.: Inhibition of chemically induced morphologic transformation and reversion of the transformed phenotype by ascorbic acid in C3H10T½ cells. Cancer Res. *40:* 2796–2801 (1980).

26   Benedict, W.F.; Wheatley, W.L.; Jones, P.A.: Differences in anchorage-dependent growth and tumorigenicities between transformed C3H/10T½ cells with morphologies that are or are not reverted to a normal phenotype by ascorbic acid. Cancer Res. *42:* 1041–1045 (1982).

27   Gol-Winkler, R.; De Clerck, Y.; Gieler, J.E.: Ascorbic acid effect on methylcholanthrene-induced transformation in C3H10T½ clone 8 cells. Toxicology *17:* 237–239 (1980).

28   Rosin, M.P.; Peterson, A.R.; Stich, H.F.: The effect of ascorbate on 3-methylcholanthrene-induced cell transformation in C3H10T½ mouse-embryo fibroblast cell cultures. Mutation Res. *72:* 533–537 (1980).

29   Cameron, E.; Pauling, L.; Leibowitz, B.: Ascorbic acid and cancer: a review. Cancer Res. *39:* 663–681 (1979).

30   Banic, S.: Vitamin C acts as a cocarcinogen to methylcholanthrene in guinea pigs. Cancer Lett. *11:* 239–242 (1981).

31   Troll, W.; Klassen, A.; Janoff, A.: Tumorigenesis in mouse skin: inhibition by synthetic inhibitors of proteases. Science *169:* 1211–1213 (1970).

32   Hozumi, M.; Ogawa, M.; Sugimura, T.; Takeuchi, T.; Umezawa, H.: Inhibition of tumorigenesis in mouse skin by leupeptin, a protease inhibitor from Actinomycetes. Cancer Res. *32:* 1725–1729 (1972).

33   Troll, W.: Blocking tumor promotion by protease inhibitors; in Magee et al., Fundamentals in cancer prevention, pp. 41–55 (University Park Press, Baltimore 1976).

34   Troll, W.; Wiesner, R.; Shellabarger, C.J.; Holtzman, S.; Stone, J.P.: Soybean diet lowers breast tumor incidence in irradiated rats. Carcinogenesis *1:* 469–472 (1980).

35   Troll, W.; Belman, S.; Wiesner, R.; Shellabarger, C.J.: Protease action in carcinogenesis; in Holtzer, Tschesche, Biological functions of proteinases, pp. 165–170 (Springer, Berlin 1979).

36   Troll, W.; Weisner, R.; Belman, S.; Shellabarger, C.J.: Inhibition of carcinogenesis by feeding diets containing soybeans. Proc. Am. Ass. Cancer Res. *20:* 265 (1979).

37   Fukui, Y.; Takamura, C.; Yamamura, M.; Yamamoto, M.: Effect of leupeptin on carcinogenesis of rat mammary tumor induced by 7,12-dimethylbenz[a]-anthracene; in 34th Annu. Meet., 1975. Proc. Japan Cancer Ass., p. 20.

38   Yamamoto, R.S.; Umezawa, H.; Takeuchi, T.; Matsushima, T.; Hara, K.; Sugimura, T.: Effect of leupeptin on colon carcinogenesis in rats with azoxymethane. Proc. Am. Ass. Cancer Res. *15:* 38 (1974).

39   Yamamura, M.; Nakamura, N.; Fokui, Y.; Takamura, C.; Yamamoto, M.; Minato, Y.; Tamura, Y.; Fujii, S.: Inhibition of 7,12 DMBA-induced mammary tumorigenesis by a synthetic protease inhibitor, *N,N*-dimethylamino (*p-p'*-guanidino-benzoyloxy)benzilcarbonyloxyglycolate. Gann *69:* 749–752 (1978).

40 Nomura, T.; Hata, S.; Enomoto, T.; Tanaka, H.; Shibata, K.: Inhibiting effects of antipain on urethane induced lung neoplasia in mice. Br. J. Cancer *42:* 624–626 (1980).

41 Berenblum, I.; Burger, M.; Knyszynski, A.: Inhibition of radiation-induced lymphatic leukemia in C57BL mice by 195 alpha-2-globulin (α_2-MG) from human blood serum. Radiat. Res. *60:* 501–505 (1974).

42 Borek, C.; Miller, C.; Pain, C.; Troll, W.: Conditions for inhibiting and enhancing effects of the protease inhibitor antipain on X-ray-induced neoplastic transformation in hamster and mouse cells. Proc. natn. Acad. Sci. USA *76:* 1800–1803 (1979); corrections, etc., Proc. natn. Acad. Sci. USA *76:* 6699 (1979).

43 Kuroki, T.; Drevon, C.: Inhibition of chemical transformation in C3H10T½ cells by protease inhibitors. Cancer Res. *39:* 2755–2761 (1979).

44 DiPaolo, J.A.; Amsbaugh, S.C.; Popescu, N.C.: Antipain inhibits *N*-methyl-*N'*-nitro-*N*-nitrosoguanidine-induced transformation and increases chromosomal aberrations. Proc. natn. Acad. Sci. USA *77:* 6649–6653 (1980).

45 Reznikoff, C.A.; Bertram, J.S.; Brankow, D.W.; Heidelberger, C.: Quantitative and qualitative studies on chemical transformation of cloned C3H mouse embryo cells sensitive to postconfluence inhibition of cell division. Cancer Res. *33:* 3239–3249 (1973).

46 Reznikoff, C.A.; Brankow, D.W.; Heidelberger, C.: Establishment and characterization of a cloned line of C3H mouse embryo cells sensitive to postconfluence inhibition of cell division. Cancer Res. *33:* 3231–3238 (1973).

47 Kennedy, A.R.; Fox, M.; Murphy, G.; Little, J.B.: Relationship between X-ray exposure and malignant transformation in C3H10T½ cells. Proc. natn. Acad. Sci. USA *77:* 7262–7266 (1980).

48 Kennedy, A.R.; Cairns, J.; Little, J.B.: The timing of the steps in transformation of C3H10T½ cells by X-irradiation. Nature, Lond. *307:* 85–86 (1984).

49 Kennedy, A.R.; Little, J.B.: Evidence that a second event in X-ray-induced oncogenic transformation in vitro occurs during cellular proliferation. Radiat. Res. (in press).

50 Chan, G.L.; Little, J.B.: Induction of oncogenic transformation in vitro by ultraviolet light. Nature, Lond. *264:* 442–444 (1976).

51 Kennedy, A.R.; Ritter, M.A.; Little, J.B.: Fluorescent light induces malignant transformation in mouse-embryo derived cells. Science *207:* 1209–1211 (1980).

52 Fernandez, A.; Mondal, S.; Heidelberger, C.: Probabilistic view of the transformation of cultured C3H/10T½ mouse embryo fibroblasts by 3-methylcholanthrene. Proc. natn. Acad. Sci. USA *77:* 7272–7276 (1980).

53 Sheela, S.; Kennedy, A.R.: X-Ray induced transformation of human foreskin fibroblasts. Carcinogenesis (submitted).

54 Kennedy, A.R.; Radner, B.; Nagasawa, H.: Protease inhibitors suppress chromosome abnormalities in cells from patients with Bloom's syndrome. Proc. natn. Acad. Sci. USA *81* (1984).

A.R. Kennedy, DSc, Laboratory of Radiobiology, Department of Cancer Biology, Harvard University, School of Public Health, Boston, MA 02115 (USA)

Prasad (ed.), Vitamins, Nutrition, and Cancer, pp. 180–194 (Karger, Basel 1984)

Inhibition of Prostaglandin E$_2$ Synthesis Controls Tumor Growth and Metastases Mediated by Dietary Fats[1]

G.M. Kollmorgen[a], *M.M. King*[b], *S.D. Kosanke*[c], *Cuong Do*[a]

[a] Cancer Research Program, Oklahoma Medical Research Foundation;
[b] Biomembrane Research Program, Oklahoma Medical Research Foundation;
[c] Department of Pathology, College of Medicine, University of Oklahoma Health Sciences Center, Oklahoma City, Okla., USA

Introduction

Recent evidence indicates that most cancers have external causes and, in principle, these cancers should be preventable [1]. External causes include substances in the air we breathe, the water we drink, the food we eat, and the environment in which we live and work. Other evidence indicates that many types of experimental cancers are 'initiated' by a carcinogen and that their subsequent growth, development, and metastases are influenced by 'promoters' [2, 3]. While the influence of vitamins and minerals may be largely restricted to the initiation phase of tumor development, the majority of evidence indicates that dietary fats act primarily during the promotional phase of tumor development [1, 4]. Even though certain dietary factors may allow tumor initiation to proceed normally, other dietary factors may prevent subsequent tumor growth and development by inhibiting the process of tumor promotion. Hence, dietary factors which act on one stage of tumor development must be considered in light of other factors which influence tumorigenesis during other stages of tumor development. In addition, tumor cells induced by the same carcinogen in the

[1] This investigation was supported by PHS Grant No. CA 33705 awarded to *G.M.K.* and CA 34143 to *M.M.K.* by the National Cancer Institute, DHHS.

same animal tend to display considerable heterogeneity. Consequently local environmental factors may inhibit the growth of some tumor cells while stimulating the growth of other tumor cells. In addition, tumor-host relationships may vary considerably from system to system and be further influenced by time, age, sex, reproductive status, and hormones produced by the host.

Other studies suggest that a variety of cells, derived from the immune system, act directly or indirectly via their products to influence tumor growth. For example, rats treated with antilymphocyte serum after exposure to DMBA had a higher tumor incidence [5] and their tumors were more invasive [6] compared to the non-treated controls. Conversely, rats treated with immune stimulants [7, 8] were protected against DMBA-induced mammary tumors.

It is now clear that the function of some cells within the immune system is regulated by prostaglandin E_2 (PGE_2). PGE_2 can be secreted by macrophages/monocytes and by tumor cells. Attempts have been made to correlate PGE_2 production by mammary tumor cells with their ability to invade and metastasize [9, 10]. Other evidence indicates that PGE_2 inhibits the function of natural killer cells [11, 12] which may act as a surveillance network designed to destroy abnormal cells.

PGE_2, which acts as a local hormone, is synthesized by nearly all cells within the body. While the immediate precursor is arachidonic acid, the ultimate precursor is linoleic acid. Linoleic acid is a major constituent of corn oil (about 60%).

Since diets containing high levels of corn oil (20%) influence the development, incidence and multiplicity of DMBA-induced mammary adenocarcinoma in rats [20], studies were designed to determine if the promotional effects of polyunsaturated dietary fats were, at least in part, mediated via the immune system. Specifically, studies were done to determine relationships between dietary fat content, rate of tumor growth, and quantity of PGE_2 synthesis by cultured normal spleen cells.

Materials and Methods

Rats

Sprague-Dawley female rats were obtained from Charles River (Portage, Mich.) and Wistar-Furth, inbred, female rats were obtained from Harlan Sprague-Dawley (Madison, Wisc.). All rats arrived as weanlings and were housed in a temperature- and humidity-controlled facility with a 12-hour light/dark cycle.

Diets

Weanling rats were fed either Purina laboratory chow (St. Louis, Mo.), or semipurified diets containing 2, 5, 10 or 20% stripped corn oil (table I) prepared by ICN Life
Sciences, Inc. (Cleveland, Ohio). These diets were stored in sealed, plastic containers, in
the dark and maintained at 4 °C. Diets were analyzed for fatty acid content and total fat
content before use. Results from these analyses indicated that neither the fatty acid content

Table I. Constituents of diets

	20% fat diet			10% fat diet		
	g/100 g diet	calories	% of total calories	g/100 g diet	calories	% of total calories
Casein	24.40	97.60	21.17	22.15	88.60	21.36
DL-Methionine	0.60	2.40	0.52	0.54	2.16	0.52
Fat[1]	20.00	180.00	39.05	10.00	90.00	21.72
Vitamins[2]	1.22	4.88	1.06	1.10	4.40	1.06
Salts[3]	4.88	0.00	1.06[4]	4.40	0.00	1.06[4]
Choline	0.12	0.48	0.11	0.11	0.44	0.11
Alphacel	4.88	0.00	1.06[4]	4.40	0.00	1.06[4]
Sucrose	43.90	175.60	38.09	57.30	229.20	55.26
Totals	100.00	460.96	100.00	100.00	414.80	100.03

	5% fat diet			2% fat diet		
	g/100 g diet	calories	% of total calories	g/100 g diet	calories	% of total calories
Casein	20.92	83.68	21.38	20.00	80.00	21.16
DL-Methionine	0.52	2.08	0.53	0.50	2.00	0.53
Fat[1]	5.00	45.00	11.50	2.00	18.00	4.76
Vitamins[2]	1.05	4.20	1.07	1.00	4.00	1.06
Salts[3]	4.15	0.00	1.06[4]	4.00	0.00	1.06[4]
Choline	0.11	0.44	0.11	0.10	0.40	0.11
Alphacel	4.25	0.00	1.09[4]	4.00	0.00	1.06[4]
Sucrose	64.00	256.00	65.41	68.40	273.60	72.38
Totals	100.00	391.40	100.00	100.00	378.00	100.00

[1] Stripped corn oil (Eastman).
[2] AIN-76 vitamin mix.
[3] AIN-76 salt mix.
[4] Expressed as g/total calories.

nor the total fat content were altered under these conditions during the storage period. While caloric density varied slightly from diet to diet, each rat consumed approximately 70 kcal/rat/day and the nutrient:caloric ratios of all constituents except fat and sucrose were similar in each diet.

Metastatic Mammary Tumor Cells

A mammary tumor was induced in a Wistar-Furth, inbred, female rat after exposure to 40 mg of DMBA [13]. This tumor was minced and cells dissociated by vigorous aspiration. It was then injected into other Wistar-Furth, inbred, female rats, and grew both as a primary tumor at the site of injection, and as metastatic tumors in adjacent lymph nodes. This tumor, designated as DMBA-4, typically metastasized into lymph nodes, lung, and liver [13, 14]. These cells were serially transplanted into 21-day-old Wistar-Furth, inbred, female rats and were kindly supplied by Dr. *Untae Kim* (Buffalo, N.Y.). Approximately 5×10^3 viable tumor cells (in 0.2 ml phosphate-buffered saline, pH = 7.0) were injected into the fat pad of the sixth mammary gland which is adjacent to the right inguinal lymph node. Viability was determined using trypan blue exclusion.

Cultured Mammary Tumor Cells

Cultured rat mammary adenocarcinoma tumor cells (designated R_2T_2) were obtained from an explant of mammary adenocarcinoma taken from a rat exposed to DMBA, and fed the 20% fat diet. These cells grew as a monolayer when cultured in Medium 199 (powdered medium, Earl's unmodified salts) supplemented with 10% fetal calf serum, penicillin (5 U/ml) and streptomycin (5 µg/ml). These cells were grown in loosely capped plastic flasks, which were maintained in a CO_2 incubator at 37 °C and the pH was controlled at about 7.0 with 8% CO_2 in air. Cells attached quickly after transfer and had a doubling time of 24 $\pm$ 2.6 h. Indomethacin and PGE_2 were solubilized in ethanol and were added to cells during log growth. Control cells were grown in medium containing the same concentration of alcohol. Cultures were exposed to drugs for 48 h before the cells were removed with trypsin (0.05%), counted, and tested for viability using trypan blue exclusion.

In vivo Treatment with Indomethacin

Indomethacin was dissolved in 95% ethanol (8 mg indomethacin/ml ethanol). This was diluted with 400 ml of drinking water (tap water). Final concentration of indomethacin in drinking water was 20 mg/l, and the final concentration of ethanol in drinking water was 0.25%. Control rats were given only 0.25% ethanol in their drinking water. Water was supplied ad libitum, changed and measured daily, and it was determined that indomethacin-treated rats consumed between 2.19 and 2.41 mg of indomethacin/kg of body weight/day.

Analyses of Serum Fatty Acids

Lipids were extracted according to the method of *Folch* et al. [15]. Briefly, 2-ml serum samples were added to a 50-ml separatory funnel containing 10 volumes of cold chloroform:methanol (2:1 v/v). The serum was extracted with vigorous shaking for 3 min, then allowed to stand at room temperature for 30 min. A one-fifth volume of 0.5% NaCl and an internal standard (methyl arachidate) equal to approximately 10% of the total lipids being extracted was added and the mixture was reextracted as above.

The two-phase extraction system was held in the dark overnight at 4 °C for extraction and phase separation. The lower chloroform layer was transferred to a round bottom flask, the flask connected to a vacuum rotary-evaporative system and evaporated to dryness. Absolute ethanol was added to the flask (1–2 ml) to remove residual water, and again evaporated to dryness.

Fatty acid methyl esters were prepared from the lipid samples by the method of *Morrison and Smith* [16]. The chloroform was evaporated from the sample and 1 ml BF$_3$:MeOH added. The sample was boiled 15 min in tightly capped test tubes with Teflon-lined caps. After cooling, 1 ml water and 2 ml chromato-quality hexane were added, and the mixture extracted using 90 s vigorous shaking with a Vortex lab mixer. The layers were allowed to separate, the hexane layer removed and two additional hexane extractions performed, each being removed and combined with the first. The combined hexane extractions were evaporated to dryness under vacuum, and the fatty acid methyl esters assayed at 190 °C on a Tracor 222 gas-liquid chromatograph, using a 10% SP-2330 column with N$_2$ as carrier, at a flow rate of 40 ml/min. Differences in the amounts of fatty acids were determined with the Student's t test.

Autopsies

Wistar-Furth rats with metastatic tumors were killed when they were 50 days old. Untreated rats fed 20% fat diets became moribund at this time. Lymph nodes (right and left inguinal, right and left axillary, lumbar, mesenteric and thymus) were removed, weighed and prepared for histological evaluation. All lymph nodes were scored for the presence of tumor cells as follows: 0 (containing no tumor cells), +1 (containing up to 25% tumor cells), +2 (containing between 25 and 50% tumor cells), +3 (containing between 50 and 75% tumor cells), and +4 (containing more than 75% tumor cells). Quantitative analysis of metastatic involvement in lymph nodes was done by: (a) determining which lymph nodes contained no tumor cells and which lymph nodes contained tumor cells, (b) estimating the average tumor cell content (by reading at least 5 different slides) of lymph nodes which contained tumor cells, and (c) measuring the mass (in grams) of each involved lymph node.

Assays for PGE$_2$ on Cultured Spleen Cells

Spleens were taken from 50-day-old Wistar-Furth non-tumor bearing rats since these tumor cells were found to metastasize to the spleen. Sprague-Dawley rats were exposed to DMBA when they were 50 days old. Treatment with indomethacin began when rats were 64 days old. Spleens were taken when rats were 80 days old. Single cell suspensions were prepared from spleens and placed in plastic Petri dishes containing RPMI 1640 medium supplemented with 10% fetal calf and 10% autologous serum (20% total serum). Cells were cultured in 10 ml of medium (about 17.0×10^6 cells/ml) for 24 h with the pH controlled at 7.0. The percentage of monocytes (esterase positive) which attached to the substrate varied between 21 and 24% and was not influenced by diet or treatment with indomethacin. Control dishes contained only medium and serum. When incubation was complete, supernates were removed and suspended cells were eliminated with centrifugation. 3-ml samples of supernate were acidified, extracted with ethyl acetate and dried under nitrogen [17]. The dried extracts were dissolved in 1 ml of benzene:ethyl acetate:methanol (70:30:5) and applied to a 2-gram silicic acid column that had been previously equilibrated with benzene:ethyl acetate (70:30). Neutral lipids were first eluted in 10 ml of benzene:ethyl acetate (70:30), PGA-PGB were eluted in 10 ml of ethyl acetate, and PGE_1 and PGE_2 with an additional 15 ml of ethyl acetate:methanol (93:7). The reproducibility of this elution procedure was assayed using ^3H-labeled PGE_2. The fraction containing PGE_2 was dried under nitrogen, resuspended in 1 ml of ethanol, and an 0.8-ml aliquot counted in a liquid scintillation counter to determine percent recovery of the initial ^3H-PGE_2.

A 0.1 ml sample of the resuspended PGE_2 fraction was assayed after appropriate dilution with 0.1 M sodium phosphate buffer (pH 7.6). In each assay, a highly specific antibody for PGE_2 (Institut Pasteur, Paris) was added to either the unknowns or to standard quantities of PGE_2 (0–100 pg) in the presence of ^3H-PGE_2 (about 7,000 cpm). The validity and reliability of the antibody has been documented previously [18]. The PGE_2 antibody has 3.2% cross-reactivity with PGE_1 and negligible (less than 0.2%) cross-reactivity with PGA_1, PGA_2, $PGF_{1\alpha}$, $PGF_{2\alpha}$, PGB_2, and the 15-keto- and 15-keto-13-14-dihydro-metabolites of PGE_1 and PGE_2 and 6-keto-$PGF_{1\alpha}$. Incubation was done at 4 °C for 8 h, then bound antibody and free PGE_2 were separated by adding 1 ml of dextran-coated charcoal (25 mg dextran, 250 mg charcoal, in 100 ml of phosphate buffer). Each assay was done in triplicate and statistical analyses done using the Student's t test.

Results

As shown in table II, the average daily water consumption per rat was not influenced by dietary fat. Consequently, the quantity of indomethacin ingested on a daily basis was similar in all dietary groups. The average daily indomethacin consumption (mg/kg of body weight) varied from 2.19 to 2.41. As we reported earlier [19], carcass weights were not influenced by differences in dietary fat.

Table II. Average daily indomethacin consumption per rat in Sprague-Dawley female rats

Dietary fat content, %	Water consumption, l	Indomethacin consumption	
		mg	mg/kg body weight/day
2	0.0248	0.4960	2.36
5	0.0236	0.4720	2.19
10	0.0241	0.4820	2.25
20	0.0265	0.5300	2.41

Sprague-Dawley female rats were given water ad libitum containing indomethacin (20 mg/l). Average daily water consumption per rat was calculated on a daily basis for a period of 4 weeks starting when rats were 78 days old. Each group consisted of 10 rats.

The data shown in table III clearly illustrate that the rate of tumor growth was influenced by dietary fat. When rats were fed a 2% fat diet, nearly all of the tumor growth occurred in the right inguinal lymph node (adjacent to the site of tumor cell injection). However, when rats were fed a 20% fat diet, there was a significant ($p \leqslant 0.05$) increase in the rate of tumor growth in the right inguinal node as well as in all other lymph nodes ($p \leqslant 0.05$) compared to rats fed the 2% fat diet. When only the right inguinal node was considered, only rats fed the 20% fat diet had a significantly greater tumor mass ($p \leqslant 0.05$) compared to all other dietary groups. When all lymph nodes were considered, rats fed diets containing either 10 or 20% fat had significantly greater tumor masses ($p \leqslant 0.05$) compared to rats fed diets containing either 2 or 5% fat. Hence, the threshold for a fat effect probably lies somewhere between 5 and 10% dietary fat. When rats were treated with indomethacin, the rate of tumor growth was significantly inhibited in all dietary groups ($p \leqslant 0.05$) and was not dependent on dietary fat.

Data shown in table IV illustrates that PGE_2 production by spleen cells increased as the dietary fat content increased. This was true for both Wistar-Furth and Sprague-Dawley rats which were not given tumor cells or were

Table III. Weight of tumor-bearing lymph nodes in control and indomethacin-treated rats

Dietary fat content, %	Right inguinal lymph node		All lymph nodes[1]	
	untreated	indomethacin-treated	untreated	indomethacin-treated
2	9.3 ± 2.1	6.0 ± 0.58	10.0 ± 1.1	6.0 ± 0.67
5	10.2 ± 1.9	5.1 ± 0.61	12.0 ± 1.4	6.0 ± 0.60
10	12.6 ± 1.3	5.9 ± 0.38	21.0 ± 2.3	7.0 ± 0.71
20	22.4 ± 3.6	5.3 ± 0.49	30.0 ± 3.4	8.0 ± 0.90

[1] All rats were killed and autopsied on day 50 when control rats on the 20% fat diet become moribund. Lymph nodes which contained tumor cells included the following: right and left inguinal, right and left axillary, mesenteric, lumbar, and thymus. Each group consisted of 7 or 10 rats. Weights of lymph nodes (g) are expressed as the mean value per group ± 1 standard deviation.

Table IV. PGE$_2$ in supernates of spleen cells from rats fed different quantities of dietary fat

Dietary fat content %	Wistar-Furth rats, no tumors, not exposed to DMBA		Sprague-Dawley rats, no tumors, not exposed to DMBA		Sprague-Dawley rats exposed to DMBA 30 days previously	
	controls	treated with indomethacin	controls	treated with indomethacin	controls	treated with indomethacin
2	12.4±1.1	3.6±0.29	6.3±0.51	1.95±0.041	23.10±1.98	7.18±0.67
5	15.0±1.5	4.2±0.32	–	–	–	–
10	20.2±1.9	4.4±0.36	–	–	–	–
20	23.1±2.1	5.4±0.52	15.9±1.12	4.93±0.52	48.80±5.21	29.80±2.78

Mean values ± 1 standard deviation are expressed in terms of ng PGE$_2$ per 3.5 ml of 24-hour spleen cell supernates. All rats were fed diets from time of weaning (21 days old). Sprague-Dawley rats were given 10 mg of DMBA at 50 days of age. Wistar-Furth rats were killed when they were 50 days old and Sprague-Dawley rats were killed when they were 80 days old. Each dietary group consisted of 20 rats; 10 were treated with indomethacin (3.0 mg/kg of body weight/day) and 10 were untreated.

Table V. Growth of tumor cells in lymph nodes of Wistar-Furth rats

Lymph nodes	Percent of nodes containing tumor cells		Average tumor cell content of lymph nodes		Average mass of lymph nodes containing tumor cells, g	
	un-treated	indomethacin-treated	un-treated	indomethacin-treated	un-treated	indomethacin-treated
Right inguinal	100	100	3.56	2.91	13.56±0.47	6.07±0.15*
Lumbar nodes	88	88	2.58	2.15	5.12±0.13	2.64±0.06*
Thymus	54	44	1.54	1.34	1.41±0.04	1.30±0.04
Right axillary	54	40	1.65	1.52	1.80±0.06	0.69±0.02*
Mesenteric nodes	32	20	1.28	0.99	0.98±0.09	0.73±0.13
Left axillary	4	4	0.63	0.38	0.09	0.04
Left inguinal	4	0	0.38	0.00	0.20	–

5×10^3 tumor cells (suspended in 0.2 ml of phosphate-buffered saline) were injected into the right inguinal node area when rats were 21 days old. All rats were killed and autopsied on day 50 when the control rats became moribund. There were 25 rats in both the untreated and indomethacin-treated groups (* $p \leq 0.05$).

Table VI. Effects of indomethacin and PGE_2 on the growth of cultured R_2T_2 rat mammary tumor cells

Drug concentration, mol	Indomethacin	PGE_2
10^{-6}	110 ± 0.08	64 ± 0.52
10^{-7}	102 ± 0.75	98 ± 0.12
10^{-8}	98 ± 0.62	102 ± 0.13
10^{-9}	101 ± 0.91	97 ± 0.09
10^{-10}	96 ± 0.78	100 ± 0.11

Rat mammary tumor cells (R_2T_2) were cultured in medium 199 supplemented with 10% fetal calf serum, penicillin (5 U/ml) and streptomycin (5 µg/ml). Indomethacin and PGE_2 were added to cells in log growth and were present for 48 h before cells were counted and examined for viability. A minimum of 10^5 cells was counted at each drug concentration. Results are expressed as a percentage of control values (cells grown in the absence of drugs, but exposed to the same alcohol concentration).

not exposed to DMBA. When similar rats in these groups were treated with indomethacin, PGE_2 production was inhibited and was essentially the same in all dietary groups. PGE_2 production in indomethacin-treated Wistar-Furth rats correlates well with the rate of tumor growth in these rats as shown in table III. Exposure to DMBA also increased PGE_2 production in Sprague-Dawley rats fed either 2 or 20% fat. While indomethacin inhibited PGE_2 production in both dietary groups, inhibition was more pronounced in the low fat group.

The observation that indomethacin inhibited tumor growth and PGE_2 synthesis in rats fed the semipurified diets containing 5% fat was also apparent when rats were fed chow diets which contain about 5% fat. Data shown in table V indicates that maximum inhibition of tumor growth was noted in the right inguinal lymph node, adjacent to the site of tumor cell injection. These data emphasize that the effects of indomethacin were not limited to the control of tumor growth which was mediated by high levels of dietary fat.

Indomethacin did not affect the growth of mammary tumor cells in culture. As shown in table VI, indomethacin concentrations of 10^{-6} to 10^{-10} *M* had no influence on the growth or viability of these cells when compared to similar cells grown in the absence of drug. In addition, physi-

Table VII. Concentration of fatty acids in serum of Wistar-Furth rats fed different quantities of dietary fat

Dietary fat content, %	Oleic acid 18:1	Linoleic acid 18:2	Total fatty acids[1]
2	2,945 ± 148	575 ± 28.8	8,464 ± 419
5	2,225 ± 107	927 ± 48.3	8,386 ± 431
10	1,130 ± 57.6	1,861 ± 93.5	7,832 ± 398
20	693 ± 39.2	2,274 ± 114	7,838 ± 401

Based on the following fatty acids: 14:0, 16:0, 16:1, 18:0, 18:1, 18:2, 20:4, 22:4, 22:6 and 24:1.
[1] The concentration of fatty acids is expressed in terms of μg/ml serum/kg of body weight. Diets were started when rats were 21 days old and rats were killed when they were 50 days old. There were 20 rats in each dietary group. 10 rats in each dietary group were treated with indomethacin and 10 rats in each group were untreated, and served as controls. Treatment with indomethacin did not affect total fatty acid concentrations and concentrations of individual fatty acids except for oleic acid and linoleic acid as shown above.

ological concentrations of PGE_2 did not affect the growth of cultured mammary tumor cells. The inhibition of growth observed using $10^{-6} M$ PGE_2 has no physiological significance, since this concentration of PGE_2 has not been reported in any body tissues or fluids.

Dietary fat and/or treatment with indomethacin did not influence the total serum concentration of fatty acids as measured by 10 different fatty acids (table VII). The only influence of dietary fat, in both untreated and indomethacin-treated rats, was that linoleic acid increased significantly ($p \leqslant 0.01$) and oleic acid decreased significantly ($p \leqslant 0.01$) as the dietary fat content increased from 2 to 20%.

Discussion

The observation that dietary fat stimulated the growth of metastatic tumors is consistent with other data indicating that primary tumors, induced with DMBA, grew more rapidly when rats were fed high levels of unsaturated fat [20]. While studies reported in this paper were not designed to define a threshold for a 'fat effect', these data suggest that such a threshold must exist when the dietary fat content (by weight) is between 5 and

10% of the total diet. Based on caloric intake, this threshold must lie between 12 and 22% of total calories consumed. However, two additional points must be emphasized. First, while dietary fat may promote tumor growth, there is no evidence to indicate that dietary fat can or does initiate tumor growth. Second, there is no reason to believe that a threshold requires the exclusive use of unsaturated fat. In fact other investigators reported that tumor incidence was similar when rats were fed diets containing either 3% unsaturated fat (sunflower seed oil) and 7% saturated fat (coconut oil) or 10% unsaturated fat (sunflower seed oil) [4].

While the mechanisms by which dietary fat influence tumor growth remain elusive, it seems likely that factors other than hormones are involved [21, 22]. For example, both high levels of dietary fat and hypophysectomy stimulate prolactin production. However, hypophysectomized rats fed low fat diets did not attain the tumor incidence characteristic of rats fed high fat diets [21]. While our own studies show a very good correlation between dietary fat content, rate of tumor growth, and levels of PGE_2 synthesis by spleen cells, cause-and-effect relationships have not yet been established. However, the observation that indomethacin inhibited both PGE_2 synthesis and rate of tumor growth strongly suggests that prostaglandins and perhaps other metabolic products of the cyclooxygenase and/or lipoxygenase pathways are involved in regulating tumor growth.

Other observations suggest that indomethacin does not act directly on tumor cells. First, the growth of cultured mammary tumor cells, as shown in table VI, was not influenced by concentrations of indomethacin ranging from 10^{-6} to 10^{-10} M. Second, in other studies [23] indomethacin was not effective in inhibiting tumor growth in mice which were not immunocompetent. Hence, an indirect effect of indomethacin is much more likely. In addition, PGE_2 at physiological concentrations did not influence the growth of cultured mammary tumor cells. The observation that PGE_2 at 10^{-6} M inhibited tumor growth has no physiological significance since, as mentioned above, this concentration of PGE_2 has not been reported to exist in any body tissues or fluids. However, it is necessary to be cautious in extrapolating these data to other tumor cells or tumor-host systems. Sensitivity to PGE_2 and other products of the cyclooxygenase pathway may vary considerably within the same tumor and even more so when comparing tumors of different origin. *Foecking* et al. [24] reported that DMBA-induced mammary tumors in Sprague-Dawley female rats regressed after bilateral ovariectomy. Regressing tumors released more PGE_2 per gram of tissue compared to growing tumors. However, it is not known from these data if PGE_2

was produced by infiltrating host cells or by tumor cells. It is possible that the properties of tumor cells and the infiltration of host cells were dramatically influenced by ovariectomy.

Other data support the hypothesis that PGE_2 synthesis by mammary tumor cells correlates with the metastatic potential of these cells. *Fulton* et al. [9] measured PGE_2 production in mouse mammary neoplasms which ranged from non-metastatic to highly metastatic. While the non-metastatic cells produced low levels of PGE_2, the highly metastatic cells produced high levels of PGE_2. Since these studies were done on cultured mammary tumor cells, host infiltrative cells (especially macrophages) were not involved.

While our data indicate that PGE_2 synthesis by mononuclear cells from spleen increased as the dietary fat content increased, the production of PGE_2 by other cells, particularly mammary tumor cells, may also be increased by dietary fat. No attempt was made to measure PGE_2 synthesis in lymph nodes containing tumor cells. Lymph nodes also varied considerably in the amount of infiltrating lymphocytes and macrophages. Hence, it would be difficult to determine the source of PGE_2 in these heterogeneous cell populations. However, *Rolland* et al. [10] assayed for PGE_2 in freshly excised human breast cancers, in both primary and metastatic lesions. They suggested that elevated levels of PGE_2 production could be used as a marker of high metastatic potential of neoplastic cells in breast cancer. *Pelus and Bockman* [25] reported that peritoneal macrophages from tumor-bearing mice released significantly more PGE_2 compared to macrophages from control mice. All other properties of macrophages tested in these two groups of mice were similar. On the other hand, *Harvey* et al. [26] concluded that circulating levels (venous blood) of PGE did not correlate with the non-specific immunosuppression seen in cancer patients. Hence, PGE_2 concentration in the immediate environment of the tumor may be more indicative of tumor growth, invasion, or metastases compared to PGE_2 concentrations in body fluids.

Other evidence indicates that tumor cells not only produce PGE_2 themselves, but they also induce PGE_2 production in monocytes/macrophages [27]. *Goodwin* et al. [28] reported that PHA-stimulated cultures of mononuclear cells from patients with Hodgkin's disease produced about 4-fold more PGE_2 compared to mononuclear cells from normal controls. PGE_2 production was significantly decreased when glass-adherent cells were removed from mononuclear cell preparations taken from patients with Hodgkin's disease.

Regardless of the source of PGE_2, it is clear that physiological concentrations of PGE_2 inhibited cellular immune responses. For example, PGE_2 concentrations of $10^{-8} M$ or less inhibited responses to mitogens [29], E-rosette formation [30], the generation of cytotoxic cells in mixed lymphocyte culture [31], T cell cytotoxicity [31], natural killer activity [12, 32], and antibody-dependent cytotoxicity [33]. In addition, spleen lymphocytes from rats fed 20 % unsaturated fat diets responded poorly to concanavalin A in culture when compared to lymphocytes from rats fed 2 % fat diets [34].

Several different lines of evidence indicate that growth of DMBA-induced tumors was influenced by the host's immune system. Rats treated with antilymphocyte serum developed a higher incidence of DMBA-induced mammary tumors [5] and these tumors were more invasive compared to those in untreated rats [6]. On the other hand, *Weislow* et al. [7] were able to protect rats against DMBA-induced mammary tumor by immunizing with a mouse xenotropic type C virus. *Kollmorgen* et al. [8, 35, 36] used the methanol extraction residue of bacillus Calmette-Guérin in Sprague-Dawley female rats, fed low fat diets, to either prevent or treat mammary tumors induced by DMBA.

Other studies indicated that indomethacin enhanced immune responses [37] or prevented tumor-induced immune suppression [27]. However, the effects of indomethacin on other products derived from the cyclooxygenase pathway and on products derived from the lipoxygenase pathway need to be carefully analyzed before inhibitors of these pathways can be considered for addition to clinical therapeutic protocols.

References

1 Executive Summary of the Report of the Committee on Diet, Nutrition and Cancer. Cancer Res. *43:* 3018–3023 (1983).

2 Fischer, S.M.; Slaga, T.J.: Modulation of prostaglandin synthesis and tumor promotion; in Powles et al., Prostaglandins and cancer. 1st Int. Conf., pp. 255–264 (Liss, New York 1982).

3 Bresnick, E.: Prostaglandin response in mouse skin to tumor promoters; in Powles et al., Prostaglandins and cancer. 1st Int. Conf., pp. 255–264 (Liss, New York 1982).

4 Carroll, K.K.; Davidson, M.B.: The role of lipids in tumorigenesis; in Arnott et al., Molecular interactions of nutrition and cancer, pp. 237–245 (Raven Press, New York 1982).

5 Vandeputte, M.: Immunosuppression and cancer. Ann. Inst. Pasteur *122:* 677–683 (1972).

6 Gardner, H.A.; Kellen, J.A.: Facilitation of DMBA-induced tumor invasion by anti-lymphocyte serum. J. clin. Hematol. Oncol. *7:* 843–848 (1977).

7   Weislow, O.S.; Allen, P.T.; Shepherd, R.E.; Twardzik, D.R.; Fowler, A.K.; Hellman, A.: Protection against 7,12-dimethylbenz[α]anthracene-induced rat mammary carcinoma by infection with mouse xenotropic type C virus. J. natn. Cancer Inst. *61:* 123–129 (1978).

8   Kollmorgen, G.M.; Sansing, W.; Fischer, G.; Cunningham, D.; Longley, R.; Lehman, A.; King, M.; McCay, P.: A possible role of MER in protection against DMBA-induced tumors in rats fed different diets; in Crispen, Neoplasm immunity: experimental and clinical, pp. 17–35 (Elsevier/North-Holland, Amsterdam 1980).

9   Fulton, A.; Rios, A.; Loveless, S.; Heppner, G.: Prostaglandins in tumor-associated cells; in Powles et al., Prostaglandins and cancer. 1st Int. Conf., pp. 701–703 (Liss, New York, 1982).

10 Rolland, P.H.; Martin, D.M.; Jacquemier, J.; Rolland, A.M.; Toga, M.: Prostaglandin in human breast cancer: evidence suggesting that an elevated prostaglandin production is a marker of high metastatic potential for neoplastic cells. J. natn. Cancer Inst. *64:* 1061–1070 (1980).

11 Kollmorgen, G.M.; Longley, R.E.; Kosanke, S.D.; Carpenter, M.P.: Dietary fat stimulates mammary tumor growth and inhibits immune responses; in Meyskens, Prasad, 1st. Int. Conf. on the Modulation and Mediation of Cancer by Vitamins (Karger, Basel 1983).

12 Brunda, M.J.; Herberman, R.B.; Holden, H.T.: Inhibition of murine natural killer cell activity by prostaglandins. J. Immun. *124:* 2682–2687 (1980).

13 Kim, U.: The metastatic pattern and properties of tumor cells; in Proc. 1st Int. Conf. on Carcinogenesis, Immunology and Transplantation. Transplant. Proc. (in press, 1983).

14 Kim, U.: Characteristics of metastasizing and non-metastasizing tumors and their interaction with the host immune system in the development of metastasis; in Hellmann, Hilgard, Eccles, EORTC Metastasis Group Int. Conf. on Clinical and Experimental Aspects of Metastasis, pp. 210–214 (Nijhoff, The Hague 1981).

15 Folch, J.; Lees, M.; Stanley, G.H.S.: A simple method for the isolation and purification of total lipids from animal tissues. J. biol. Chem. *226:* 497–509 (1957).

16 Morrison, W.R.; Smith, L.M.: Preparation of fatty acid methyl esters and dimethylacetals from lipids with boron tri-fluoride-methanol. J. Lipid Res. *5:* 600–608 (1964).

17 Stahl, R.A.K.; Ahmad, A.A.; Block, D.L.; Lee, J.B.: Stimulation of rabbit renal PGE_2 biosynthesis by dietary sodium restriction. Am. J. Physiol. *237:* F344 (1979).

18 Dray, F.; Charbonnet, B.: Dosage radioimmunologique des prostaglandines F_2 et E_1 dans le plasma périphérique de l'homme normal; in Seminaire les prostaglandines, p. 133 (INSERM, Paris 1973).

19 Kollmorgen, G.M.; King, M.M.; Kosanke, S.D.; Do, C.: Dietary fat and indomethacin influence growth of transplantable mammary tumors in rats. Cancer Res. *43:* 4714–4719 (1983).

20 King, M.M.; Bailey, D.M.; Gibson, D.D.; Pitha, J.V.; McCay, P.B.: Incidence and growth of mammary tumors induced by 7,12-dimethylbenz[α]anthracene as related to the dietary content of fat and antioxidant. J. natn. Cancer Inst. *63:* 657–663 (1979).

21 Ip, C.; Yip, P.; Bernardis, L.L.: Role of prolactin in the promotion of dimethylbenz[α]anthracene-induced mammary tumors by dietary fat. Cancer Res. *40:* 374–378 (1980).

22 Chan, P.C.; Didato, F.; Cohen, L.A.: High dietary fat, elevation of rat serum prolactin and mammary cancer. Proc. Soc. exp. Biol. Med. *149:* 133–135 (1975).

23 Strausser, H.R.; Humes, J.L.: Prostaglandin synthesis inhibition: effect on bone changes and sarcoma tumor induction in BALB/c mice. Int. J. Cancer *15:* 724–730 (1975).

24 Foecking, M.K.; Panganamala, R.V.; Abou-Issa, H.; Minton, J.P.: Modulation of prostaglandins in hormone dependent mammary carcinoma; in Powles et al., Prosta-glandins and cancer. 1st Int. Conf., pp. 657–662 (Liss, New York 1982).

25 Pelus, C.; Bockman, R.: Increased prostaglandin synthesis by macrophages from tumor-bearing mice. J. Immun. *123:* 2118–2125 (1979).

26 Harvey, H.A.; Allegra, J.C.; Demen, L.M.; Loderer, J.R.; Brenner, D.E.; Trautlein, J.J.; White, D.S.; Gillin, M.A.; Lipton, A.: Immunosuppression and human cancer: role of prostaglandins. Cancer *39:* 2362–2364 (1977).

27 Plescia, O.J.; Smith, A.H.; Grinwich, K.: Subversion of immune system by tumor cells and role of prostaglandins. Proc. natn. Acad. Sci. USA *72:* 1848–1851 (1975).

28 Goodwin, J.S.; Messner, R.P.; Bankhurst, A.D.; et al.: Prostaglandin producing sup-pressor cells in Hodgkin's disease. New Engl. J. Med. *297:* 963–968 (1977).

29 Goodwin, J.S.; Messner, R.P.; Peake, G.T.: Prostaglandin suppression of mitogen-stimulated leukocytes in culture. J. clin. Invest. *62:* 753–760 (1974).

30 Erten, U.; Emre, T.; Cavdar, A.O.; Turker, R.K.: An in vitro study of the effect of PGE_2 and $F_{2\alpha}$ on E-rosette-forming activity of normal lymphocytes. Prostaglandins Med. *5:* 255–258 (1980).

31 Darrow, T.L.; Tomar, R.H.: Prostaglandin-mediated regulation of the mixed lym-phocyte culture and generation of cytotoxic cells. Cell. Immunol. *56:* 172–183 (1980).

32 Roder, J.C.; Klein, M.: Target-effector interaction in the natural killer cell system. J. Immun. *123:* 2785–2790 (1979).

33 Garovoy, M.R.; Strom, T.B.; Kaliner, M.; Carpenter, C.B.: Antibody dependent lym-phocyte-mediated cytotoxicity mechanism and modulation by cyclic nucleotides. Cell. Immunol. *20:* 197–204 (1975).

34 Kollmorgen, G.M.; Sansing, W.A.; Lehman, A.A.; Fischer, G.; Longley, R.E.; Alex-ander, S.S., Jr.; King, M.M.; McCay, P.B.: Inhibition of lymphocyte function in rats fed high-fat diets. Cancer Res. *39:* 3458–3462 (1979).

35 Kollmorgen, G.M.; King, M.M.; Lehman, A.A.; Fischer, G.; Longley, R.E.; Daggs, B.J.; Sansing, W.A.: The methanol extraction residue of bacillus Calmette-Guérin protects against 7,12-dimethylbenz[α]anthracene-induced rat mammary carcinoma (40693). Proc. Soc. exp. Biol. Med. *162:* 410–415 (1979).

36 Kollmorgen, G.M.; King, M.M.; Roszel, J.F.; Daggs, B.J.; Longley, R.E.: The influence of dietary fat and non-specific immunotherapy on carcinogen-induced rat mammary adenocarcinoma. Vet. Path. *18:* 82–91 (1981).

37 Pelus, L.M.; Strausser, H.R.: Indomethacin enhancement of spleen-cell responsive-ness to mitogen stimulation in tumorous mice. Int. J. Cancer *18:* 653–660 (1976).

M.M. King, PhD, Biomembrane Research Program,
Oklahoma Medical Research Foundation, 825 NE 13th Street,
Oklahoma City, OK 73104 (USA)

Prasad (ed.), Vitamins, Nutrition, and Cancer, pp. 195–211 (Karger, Basel 1984)

Relationship of Ethanolic Beverages and Ethanol to Cancers of the Digestive Tract[1]

Selwyn A. Broitman

Departments of Pathology and Microbiology, Boston University School of Medicine, Boston, Mass., USA

Currently, major limitations exist in obtaining reliable data on alcohol consumption, as consumption is underreported in this country, and others, owing to the tax liability of alcoholic beverages. Based upon tax-paid withdrawals in the USA, each individual of drinking age, 14 or older, is credited with an average apparent consumption of 2.61 gallons of absolute ethanol [30]. Since only about two thirds of the population (60% of women and 77% of men) consume alcohol [1] (table I), the quantity consumed only by 'drinkers' is 4.21 gallons of absolute ethanol per year. However, 11% of the adult population or 16.7% of the drinkers in the USA are alcohol abusers and consume approximately 50% of the alcoholic beverages [2]. In these men and women, alcoholic beverages contribute to approximately 29.1 and 40.3%, respectively, of their total caloric intake. In the remaining segment of the drinking population, alcoholic beverages account for approximately 5.8% in men and 8.1% in women of kilocalories consumed. It should be emphasized that at best these figures represent the minimum quantities of alcoholic beverages consumed. Alcoholic beverages prepared for personal use but with Government sanction, those consumed by the military and other governmental organizations and those prepared and/or imported illegally are *not* included. Thus, the consumption of alcoholic beverages accounts for a considerable portion of calories in a substantial segment of the population who are alcohol abusers and a smaller but significant percentage in the majority of the adult population in the USA.

[1] Supported in part by the National Large Bowel Cancer Project, National Cancer Institute, National Institutes of Health, Bethesda, Md. – Grant CA 16750.

Table I. Estimated apparent consumption of ethanol (kcal) by alcohol 'abusers' and average drinkers in USA in 1978

Alcohol 'abusers'
16.7% of the drinking population consume approximately 50% of alcoholic beverages in the USA or 12.60 gal absolute ethanol/year (264,000 kcal)

Percent of diet as absolute ethanol, kcal[1]
     Men   29.1%
     Women 40.3%

Average drinker
83.3% of the drinking population consume 2.53 gal absolute ethanol/year (53,130 kcal)

Percent of diet as absolute ethanol, kcal
     Men   5.8%
     Women 8.1%

---

[1] Estimates of the percentage of kilocalories obtained from ethanol are based upon an average consumption by men of 2,500 kcal/day and by women of 1,800 kcal/day. Consequently, values obtained for women may be artifactually somewhat greater than for men.

For purposes of definition, an alcohol abuser may be regarded as an individual consuming approximately 30% or more of his/her caloric intake as ethanol. Of necessity, this represent a somewhat simplistic and arbitrary decision. However, such a dietary regimen would have, with time, a serious impact on the nutritional status of the individual and this in turn may well be a factor in the association of ethanol consumption with cancers at certain sites. The description of 'alcohol abuser' in most of the early epidemiologic reports to be considered were made on clinical grounds, generally in association with an admission of 'excessive' consumption of ethanolic beverages by the patient. In some of the more recent epidemiologic studies estimates of ethanol intake have been provided and the term 'alcohol abuser' has been applied in accord with the definition stated above.

Epidemiologically, the consumption of alcoholic beverages has been linked to the occurrence of cancers of various tissue sites. However, there may be differing contributions to cancer causality associated with certain alcoholic beverages which may be distinct from the effects of ethanol per se. Therefore, consideration of the effects of alcohol and alcoholic beverages as a risk factor in cancer development are viewed from a number of perspectives: (a) effects associated with specific alcoholic beverages, (b) effects of ethanol in the ethanol abuser, (c) synergy between ethanol consumption and cigarette smoking in cancers at certain sites, and (d) effects of ethanol in the 'moderate' drinker.

Specific Alcoholic Beverages

There is little, if any, firm epidemiologic evidence linking ethanol consumption per se in moderate drinking populations to cancer at any site. However, a number of reports are available implicating specific alcoholic beverages as a risk factor in cancers at certain sites in populations generally not regarded as alcohol abusers. *Kono and Ikeda* [43], utilizing per capita consumption of various types of alcoholic beverages and standard mortality ratios in the 46 prefectures of Japan, found only suggestive correlations between cancer of the esophagus in males and both whiskey and shochu consumption; cancer of the rectum in males and wine consumption; cancer of the prostate and shochu consumption.

An association which has been observed by some, but not all, investigators is that of beer consumption and intestinal cancer. In Britain, *Stocks* [85] observed a significant association among 166 males with intestinal cancer and beer drinking. In 314 male colorectal cancer patients, *Wynder and Shigematsu* [101] showed a significantly higher proportion of beer drinkers versus one control group, but no differences with a second control group. In a Dublin cohort study, an association between beer consumption and colorectal cancer was noted [17]. *Bjelke* [8] reported a dose-response relationship for the risk of colorectal cancer and the frequency of beer and liquor consumption in a prospective study of 12,000 middle-aged Norwegian men. A steeper dose-response gradient was exhibited with beer than with liquor consumption. *Breslow and Enstrom* [10] and *Enstrom* [19] demonstrated a statistically significant association between beer drinking (based on tax data and cancer incidence data of the National Cancer Institute, 1950–1957, in 41 of the United States) and rectal cancer. A similar association was noted between annual per capita consumption of beer and rectal cancer in 24 countries [10]. *Vitale* et al. [91], also using an international sample and apparent consumption estimates of ethanol from beer, wine, and distilled spirits, demonstrated a correlation coefficient of 0.78 for beer consumption colon cancer in 19 countries. Poor correlations were obtained with total ethanol consumption, distilled spirit consumption or wine consumption and colon cancer.

Conversely, case control studies of intestinal cancer in Finland, Kansas and Norway by *Pernu* [66], *Higginson* [27], and *Bjelke* [7], respectively, showed no significant relationship with beer drinking. Nevertheless, there appears to be a statistical association between beer drinking and colorectal cancers in some countries and in some locales within countries, but not others. An association internationally between colorectal cancer and beer consumption, but not ethanol from other sources, implies that if a relationship exists, it is related to the beverage consumed, possibly the location brewed and/or the brewing procedure but not to ethanol consumption per se.

Specific Alcoholic Beverages and Esophageal Cancer

In a very early and remarkable observation *Lamy* [46] reported on the association of absinthe consumption in French chronic alcoholics and esophageal cancer. In other early observations in China [45, 104], pai-kan, a locally prepared distillate of 60% ethanol, was incriminated as a causal factor in esophageal cancer; cancer at this site comprised approximately half of the gastrointestinal tract cancers. In the Normandy region of France – where the morbidity and mortality from alcohol-related diseases is exceptionally high – individuals consuming home-distilled apple brandy exhibited a greater risk of esophageal cancer than non-drinkers [88]. The risk was further increased by smoking [87, 89]. In Zambia, cancer of the esophagus is common, and in western Kenya esophageal cancer accounts for about 25% of all cancer deaths in men. *Cook* [14] and *Cook and Collis* [15] showed an association of esophageal cancer with consumption of beer prepared from maize; in adjacent areas of Africa where beer is produced from bananas, millet or sorghum, esophageal cancer was noted to be rare.

These observations indicate the possibility that certain locally prepared alcoholic beverages have a causal relationship to esophageal cancer. In the majority of studies cited – where it could be determined – esophageal cancer occurred in the alcohol 'abuser' presumably without the cooperativity of cigarette smoking. In at least one study, however, it was noted that cigarette smoking enhanced the risk of esophageal cancer above an increased risk associated with excessive consumption of apple brandy. It is speculated at this time that carcinogens inherent in such locally prepared beverages in conjunction with nutritional restriction imposed by alcohol abuse may be etiological factors in the development of esophageal cancer in these populations.

Alcohol Abuse and Cancers of the Head and Neck

An association of cancer at various sites in individuals who are alcohol abusers has been appreciated for some time. In 1937 *Piquet and Tison* [67] observed that 95% of their patients with esophageal cancer were alcohol abusers. In a study of 4,000 French patients, *Schwartz* et al. [78, 79] and *Schwartz* [77] showed a significant correlation between the mean daily alcohol consumption and the frequency of cancers of the tongue, hypopharynx, and larynx. The majority of individuals with cancers at these sites were heavy drinkers. In 1964 the World Health Organization [97] concluded, on the basis of surveyed literature, that excessive consumption of alcoholic beverages was associated with cancer of the mouth, larynx and esophagus. In the USA case control studies conducted since that time have established that excessive alcoholic beverage consumption increases the risk of incurring cancer of the oral cavity, excluding the lip [11, 35, 37, 72, 90, 99], glottis and supraglottis, extrinsic larynx [59, 75, 76, 90, 98], and esophagus [33, 98]. Additionally, patients with tongue cancer who drink excessively and smoke had a higher mortality rate due to tumors than individuals with tongue cancers who neither smoke nor drink [32]. Salient features of these studies have been summarized in the congressional report [35].

A number of correlational analyses using ethanol consumption derived from per capita estimates of apparent consumption or dietary interview data indicated a direct association with the incidence of and/or mortality of esophageal cancer in western countries [10, 12, 28, 42, 53, 54, 74]. Esophageal cancer mortality was also shown to exhibit high correlations with mortality rates from cirrhosis and alcoholism [52, 88].

Synergy between Alcohol Consumption and Cigarette Smoking in Cancers of the Head and Neck

Alcohol abusers are more often than not, smokers. *Flamant* et al. [20] stressed the interaction between excessive alcohol consumption and smoking for cancers of the oral cavity and the esophagus. Since then, *Keller and Terris* [35], *Wapnick* et al. [94], *Rothman and Keller* [72], and *Martinez* [56] confirmed these findings supporting a cooperative role between tobacco and alcohol in cancers of the oral cavity, the larynx, and esophagus. *Roth-*

man and Keller [72] estimate that avoidance of alcohol and tobacco in males could effect a theoretical reduction of 76% of these cancers. In women alcohol abusers and smokers, development of cancer of the tongue and buccal cavity occurred 15 years earlier than in women who neither drank nor smoked [3]. *Flamant* et al. [20] suggested that alcohol abuse may be more important in the development of esophageal cancer than smoking, but smoking may be more closely related to cancers of the mouth and pharynx.

It is difficult to ascertain if alcohol abuse per se in the absence of smoking (other than with specific beverages cited above) enhances the risk of cancers of the oral cavity, pharynx, larynx, and esophagus. Synergistic effects of alcohol on the risk of cancer at these sites are noted in smokers consuming 45 ml or more of ethanol per day [75]. Cancer at sites correlating best with past ethanol consumption rather than tobacco exposure include the floor of the mouth, supraglottis, hypopharynx, and esophagus [64, 82, 84]. Since these sites are directly exposed to ethanol, *Kissin* [38] suggested a direct local effect of ethanol rather than a systemic one. The synergistic effects of alcohol and tobacco in oral cavity cancer have been estimated to be 2.5 times the expected effect of tobacco and alcohol alone [71]. Several other environmental factors have been described which may relate to esophageal cancer development and include geographic, ethnic, and dietary factors [68, 73, 78, 83]. Case control studies by *Graham* et al. [26] illustrated that the interaction of tobacco and alcohol in cancers of the oral cavity was apparent only in those individuals with clinical evidence of inadequate dentition.

Rothman and Keller [72] and *McCoy and Wynder* [58] detected a modest but increased risk in cancers of the upper respiratory tract due to ethanol alone. *Williams and Horn* [96] also reported an increased risk for cancers at this site with ethanol consumption when smoking was controlled. Other reports as well indicated a dose-response of ethanol consumed, with increasing risk of upper respiratory tract cancer [96, 99, 102].

Because of the apparent synergy between excessive ethanol consumption and tobacco exposure, *McCoy and Wynder* [58] state, it is difficult to conclude equivocally that ethanol consumption per se is a risk factor for cancer of the upper alimentary tract and upper respiratory tract. The occurrence of cancer at these sites independent of excessive alcohol consumption and smoking implies that excessive alcohol consumption alone may augment other processes, i.e. impaired nutritional status, associated with the development of cancer at these sites (see below).

Alcohol Abuse and Hepatoma

MacDonald [55] called attention to the relationship between excessive alcohol consumption and hepatoma in a Boston population. In a similar population at the same institution, *Purtilo and Gottlieb* [69] studied 98 individuals with hepatoma; of these, about one half were alcohol abusers. They concluded that clinical alcoholism contributed to hepatoma development via cirrhosis. In studies of the association between aflatoxin ingestion in African patients with hepatoma, *Keen and Martin* [34] concluded that cirrhosis resulting from aflatoxin was an intermediary event leading to hepatoma. African patients with hepatoma exhibited heptitis-associated antigen (HAA) [93]. Hepatitis B antigenemia is frequently found in individuals with hepatocellular carcinoma [81, 93, 103]. Hepatoma is commonly found in individuals with preexisting cirrhosis. Although not proven, it appears that hepatic injury leading to cirrhosis – induced by alcoholism, aflatoxin ingestion, hepatitis antigen – may be a precursor lesion leading to the development of hepatoma.

Whether alcohol ingestion per se may be a hepato-carcinogen leading directly to the development of hepatoma without intervening cirrhosis is not known. *Lieber* et al. [49] and *Keller* [36] have provided a small number of patients where hepatocellular carcinoma occurred in individuals without cirrhosis. To date, however, the numbers of patients are inadequate to indicate if this event occurs with a significantly greater frequency in individuals who are alcohol abusers compared to those who are not.

Effects of Alcohol in the 'Moderate' Drinker

Currently, a major difficulty in assessing the relationship of moderate ethanol consumption to cancers of the head and neck concerns data collection on ethanol consumption. The social stigma associated with excessive ethanol consumption, the time frame during which recall data is requested, verification of the subject's drinking habits by family member and other variables, frequently yield ethanol consumption estimates that are greatly understated. In a recent study [2], self-reported consumption accounted for 40–60% of beverage sales; beverage sales, which reflect only tax-paid purchases, provide in turn only the minimum estimate of consumption. Survey research methods in general yield lower estimates than do methods utilizing apparent consumption. Also, the failure of most survey instruments to assess alcohol consumption on atypical as well as typical days leads to underreporting alcohol consumption. Thus, epidemiologic studies purporting to show an increased risk for cancers of the head and neck associated with 'moderate' consumption of ethanol must be interpreted in the light of these serious limitations of data collection.

Possible Mechanisms for the Association of Alcohol Consumption and Cancers of the Digestive Tract

Currently, there is relatively little experimental data to indicate a mechanism for the association of ethanol consumption to cancer at various sites in the digestive tract. A number of possibilities have been advanced [18, 49, 58, 75, 86, 91, 92], and include the following: (1) Ethanol or ethanolic beverage constituents or contaminants as carcinogens, co-carcinogens or promoters. (2) Ethanol as a solvent for carcinogens. (3) Enhanced bioactivation of carcinogens due to ethanol consumption. (4) Immunosuppression imposed by excessive ethanol consumption. (5) Nutritional inadequacies imposed by excessive ethanol consumption.

There is no experimental evidence to date to indicate that alcohol per se can function as a carcinogen or a promoter. Studies in mice, rats, and Chinese hamsters, human lymphocytes and HeLa cells in vitro reviewed by *Obe and Ristow* [62] showed no effect of ethanol on chromosomes. Sister chromatid exchange (SCE) studies in human lymphocytes also yielded negative results with ethanol [63]. However, aldehydes (formaldehyde, from methanol, an alcoholic beverage contaminant, and acetaldehyde, an ethanol metabolite) showed dose-dependent increases in SCE in human lymphocytes [61, 70]. The relationship between SCE and carcinogenesis is currently controversial; nevertheless, the genotoxic effect of acetaldehyde detected with this assay raises the index of suspicion that this intermediate could contribute to carcinogenesis. *Korsten* et al. [44] showed that blood acetaldehyde levels following i.v. ethanol infusion were much higher in the alcohol abuser than in non-alcoholic controls.

Various products produced conjointly with ethanol in the fermentation or distillation process of ethanolic beverage production have been shown to act as carcinogens experimentally. Congeners – fusel oils [24] and nitrosamines [50] – have been reported to induce esophageal and gastric tumors experimentally. A variety of polycyclic hydrocarbons, including benzo[α]pyrene and benzanthracene, are also commonly found [25, 57]. Agents such as asbestos used in the clarification of beverages can often be detected as contaminants of alcoholic beverages [5, 6, 23, 95]. An association of certain alcoholic beverages such as beer with colorectal cancer, and certain locally prepared beverages with esophageal cancer suggests a possibility that carcinogens are inherent in these beverages.

The solvent properties of ethanol have been suggested as a possible mechanism for facilitating the transport of carcinogens across membranes [21]. Ethanol molecules are intercalated in bilayer membranes between lipids. Such an effect expands membranes and increases fluidity, altering membrane function. Since ethanol's effects on membrane function are time-dose dependent, *Freund* [21] suggested the possibility that moderate social use of ethanol could either suppress or enhance tumor induction. Conversely, chronic or excessive ethanol consumption could have effects on tumorigenesis different from those of moderate users of ethanol. Experimental data to validate this hypothesis is yet to be obtained.

Ethanol feeding in experimental animals has been reported to enhance bioactivation of carcinogens. Liquid ethanol diets, when fed to rats, increased the cytochrome P-450 content and activity as well as the activity of microsomal benzo[α]pyrene hydroxylase in the proximal small bowel mucosa. The latter enzymatic change was associated with increased mutagenic activity of benzo[α]pyrene by the Ames test [80]. In a similar experiment by the same group, *Garro* et al. [22] reported an increase in dimethyl nitrosamine (DMN) demethylase activity of hepatic microsomes and a parallel increase in the mutagenicity of DMN. Ethanol consumption in hamsters increased hepatic nitrosopyrrolidine α-hydroxylase activity and augmented the mutagenic activation of nitrosopyrrolidine [58]. Similarly, lung microsomes from ethanol-fed rats exhibited increased activity in converting tobacco pyrolysate to mutagenic compounds compared to controls [49]. Thus, chronic ethanol ingestion, by its ability to induce enzymes concerned with drug metabolism in various tissues, also appears effective in augmenting the activation of certain mutagens. These studies imply that ethanol could function as a co-carcinogen. Not available, however, are studies concerned with the effects of ethanol on the enzymatic detoxification of potential mutagen/carcinogens.

A wide array of immunologic abnormalities have been described in individuals who are alcohol abusers and transient effects have been noted in normal individuals given a single dose of ethanol. Cell-mediated humoral immunity has been known for some time to be impaired in chronic alcoholics [91]. Hepatic disease as a consequence of alcohol abuse is associated with impaired T and B cell function [48]. In normal individuals given alcohol, leukocyte mobilization was found to be decreased [9]. Elucidating the effects of alcohol on host immunocompetence per se is an extremely complex problem. While alcohol alone may have immediate effects on certain parameters of immune function, the effects of disease related to alcoholism also has an impact on immune function. Recently, *Beisel* et al. [4] identified a diverse assortment of immune system abnormalities as they related to single nutrient deficiencies. Since the alcohol abuser is likely to have at least one, and usually many, nutritional deficits it is not surprising that immunologic dysfunction in the chronic alcoholic is frequently described [13, 65]. Furthermore, a relationship of diverse impaired immunologic events to the development of cancer in these patients serves to compound the complexity of ethanol-cancer interaction.

It is usual for the alcohol abuser to consume one third to one half of his/her caloric intake as ethanol daily or at various time intervals throughout the year. Consequently, these individuals have marginal to greatly impaired nutritional status. The alcohol abuser is frequently protein-deficient. Folate, ascorbate, pantothenate, pyridoxine, thiamine and vitamin A deficiencies are common, as are deficiencies of magnesium, zinc, iron, copper and molybdenum [92]. Consequently, the alcohol abuser presenting with cancer of the head or neck with the added nutritional restrictions imposed by these diseases would invariably be nutritionally depleted when evaluated clinically and by laboratory tests. Such are the findings when these patients are compared to an equivalent control group [39, 40]. Specimens of esophageal tissue, serum and hair from esophageal cancer patients were lower in zinc than in control populations [51]. When nutritional intake was evaluated in US blacks with esophageal cancer, *Ziegler* et al. [105] noted that alcoholic beverage consumption was the major risk factor for esophageal cancer. However, nutritional intake was poorer among cases than controls but no specific nutrient deficiencies were identified. It is not unusual for nutrient intake to vary inversely with ethanol intake in the alcohol abuser. Consequently, it is difficult to put into perspective whether ethanol per se is causal in the development of cancer of the head and neck or whether a major etiologic factor in these diseases is nutritional inadequacy imposed by alcoholism, or both.

Malnutrition alone, in the absence of alcoholism and cigarette smoking, is associated frequently with individuals with esophageal cancer [16, 39]. Along the Caspian Littoral in Iran, the mortality rate for esophageal cancer is among the highest in the world – 206 and 262/100,000 (age-adjusted population) for men and women, respectively. *Kmet and Mahboubi* [41] and *Hormozdiari* et al. [29], in characterizing this area pointed out the association of malnutrition in this population with the high incidence of esophageal cancer. In other countries as well, for example Sweden [31] and Puerto Rico [56], esophageal cancer is more frequent in malnourished populations. An association between Plummer-Vinson (Patterson-Kelly) syndrome – iron deficiency anemia, postcricoid webs and dysphagia – and esophageal cancer in Swedish women is well appreciated [100]. It is not clear whether the associated dysphagia compounds the malnutrition in these patients or whether iron deficiency alone is key in the association of this syndrome with esophageal cancer. Nevertheless, dietary supplementation with iron and vitamins since the early 1950s have markedly reduced the incidence of Plummer-Vinson syndrome as well as esophageal cancer [47].

Thus, a common denominator for esophageal cancer throughout many parts of the world – whether related to alcohol abuse or not – appears to be nutritional inadequacy. Cooperativity of cigarette smoking in alcohol abusers in the development of esophageal cancer but not in other populations suggests that impaired nutritional status may increase the susceptibility of target tissues in some manner to the action of carcinogens – introduced by cigarette smoking, from the external environment or inherent in the food and/or water supplies.

Newberne and McConnell [60], in considering the relationship of nutrient deficiencies to cancer, stated that experimental evidence currently available indicates that protein, fat, carbohydrate, vitamin A and zinc have effects on the development of cancer. They suggest that activation of carcinogens and detoxification are both influenced by nutrients or deficiencies thereof. In addition, nutritional status may also influence the immunocompetence of the host. Thus, the relationship of alcohol as a risk factor in cancer of the head and neck must be viewed from the feedback of 'alcohol-related' nutritional disorders to the carcinogenic process.

References

1 Alcohol and Health, 1971. First special report to the US Congress. United States Department of Health, Education and Welfare, Public Health Service, No. (HSM) 72-9099 (Government Printing Office, Washington 1971).
2 Alcohol and Health, 1981. Fourth special report to the US Congress. United States Department of Health and Human Services, Public Health Service (National Institute on Alcohol Abuse and Alcoholism, Rockville 1981).

3 Anonymous: Heavy drinking and smoking, linked with oral cancer. J. Am. med. Ass. *236:* 435 (1976).

4 Beisel, W.R.; Edelman, R.; Nauss, K.; Suskind, R.: Single-nutrient effects on immunologic function. J. Am. med. Ass. *245:* 53–58 (1981).

5 Bignon, J.; Bientz, M.; Bonnaud, G.; Sebastien, P.: Evaluation numérique des fibres d'amiente dans des échantillons de vins. Nouv. Presse méd. *6:* 1148–1149 (1977).

6 Biles, B.; Emerson, T.: Examination of fibers in beer. Nature, Lond. *219:* 93–94 (1968).

7 Bjelke, E.: Case-control study of the stomach, colon, and rectum; in Clark, Cumley, McCoy, Copeland, Oncology 1970. Proc. 10th Int. Cancer Congr., pp. 320–334 (Yearbook, Chicago 1971).

8 Bjelke, E.: Epidemiologic studies of cancer of the stomach, colon, and rectum, with special emphasis on the role of diet, vol. I–IV; PhD thesis, Minneapolis (1973).

9 Brayton, R.G.; Stokes, P.E.; Schwartz, M.S.; Lourie, D.B.: Effect of alcohol and various diseases on leucocyte mobilization, phagocytosis and intracellular bacterial killing. New Engl. J. Med. *282:* 123–128 (1970).

10 Breslow, N.E.; Enstrom, J.E.: Geographic correlations between cancer mortality rates and alcohol-tobacco consumption in the United States. J. natn. Cancer Inst. *53:* 631–639 (1974).

11 Bross, I.J.; Coombs, J.: Early onset of oral cancer among women who drink and smoke. Oncology *23:* 136–139 (1976).

12 Chilvers, C.; Fraser, P.; Beral, V.: Alcohol and oesophageal cancer: an assessment of the evidence from routinely collected data. J. Epidem. Community Hlth *33:* 127–133 (1979).

13 Chirigo, M.A.; Schultz, R.M.: Animal models in cancer research which could be useful in studies of the effect of alcohol on cellular immunity. Cancer Res. *39:* 2894–2898 (1979).

14 Cook, P.: Cancer of the oesophagus in Africa: a summary and evaluation of the evidence for the frequency of occurrence, and a preliminary indication of the possible association with the consumption of alcoholic drinks made from maize. Br. J. Cancer *25:* 853–880 (1971).

15 Cook, P.; Collis, C.H.: Cancer of the oesophagus and alcoholic drinks in East Africa. Lancet *i:* 1014 (1972).

16 Day, N.E.: Some aspects of the epidemiology of esophageal cancer. Cancer Res. *35:* 3304–3307 (1975).

17 Dean, G.; MacLenna, R.; McLoughlin, H.; Sheeley, E.: Causes of death of blue-collar workers at a Dublin brewery, 1954–1973. Br. J. Cancer *40:* 581–589 (1979).

18 Diet, Nutrition and Cancer: Committee on Diet, Nutrition and Cancer, Assembly of Life Sciences, National Research Council (Natn. Academy Press, Washington 1982).

19 Enstrom, J.E.: Colorectal cancer and beer drinking. Br. J. Cancer *35:* 674–683 (1977).

20 Flamant, R.; Lasserre, O.; Lazar, P.; Leuerinais, J.; Denoix, P.; Schwartz, D.: Differences in sex ratio according to cancer site and possible relationship with use of tobacco and alcohol: review of 65,000 cases. J. natn. Cancer Inst. *32:* 1309–1316 (1964).

21 Freund, G.: Possible relationships of alcohol in membranes to cancer. Cancer Res. *39:* 2899–2901 (1979).

22 Garro, A.J.; Seitz, H.K.; Lieber, C.S.: Enhancement of dimethylnitrosamine metabolism and activation to a mutagen following chronic ethanol consumption. Cancer Res. *41:* 120–124 (1981).

23 Gaudichet, A.; Sebastien, P.; Dufour, G.; Bonnaud, G.; Bientz, M.; Bignon, J.; Puisais, J.: Asbestos fibers in wines: relation to filtration process. J. Envir. Path. Toxicol. *2:* 417–425 (1978).

24 Gibel, W.; Wildner, G.P.; Lohs, K.: Untersuchungen zur Frage einer kanzerogenen und hepatotoxischen Wirkung von Fuselöl. Arch. Geschwulstforsch. *32:* 115–125 (1968).

25 Goff, E.U.; Fine, D.H.: Analysis of volatile *N*-nitrosamines in alcoholic beverages. Fd Cosmet. Toxicol. *17:* 569–573 (1979).

26 Graham, S.; Dayal, H.; Rohrer, T.; Swanson, M.; Sultz, H.; Shedd, D.; Fischman, S.: Dentition, diet, tobacco, and alcohol in the epidemiology of oral cancer. J. natn. Cancer Inst. *59:* 1183–1189 (1977).

27 Higginson, J.: Etiological factors in gastrointestinal cancer in man. J. natn. Cancer Inst. *37:* 527–545 (1966).

28 Hinds, M.W.; Kolonel, L.N.; Lee, J.; Hirohata, T.: Associations between cancer incidence and alcohol/cigarette consumption among five ethnic groups in Hawaii. Br. J. Cancer *41:* 929–940 (1980).

29 Hormozdiari, H.; Day, N.E.; Aramesh, B.; Mahboubi, E.: Dietary factors and esophageal cancer in the Caspian Littoral of Iran. Cancer Res. *35:* 3493–3498 (1975).

30 Hyman, M.M.; Zimmerman, M.A.; Gurioli, C.; Helrich, A.: Drinkers, drinking and alcohol-related mortality and hospitalizations: a statistical compendium (Center of Alcohol Studies, Rutgers University, New Brunswick 1980).

31 Jacobsson, F.: The Patterson-Kelly syndrome and carcinoma of the cervical esophagus, in Tanner, Smithers, Tumors of the esophagus, vol. 4, pp. 53–60 (Williams & Wilkins, Baltimore 1961).

32 Johnston, W.D.; Ballantyne, A.J.: Prognostic effect of tobacco and alcohol use in patients with oral tongue cancer. Am. J. Surg. *134:* 144 (1977).

33 Kamionkowski, M.D.; Fleshler, B.: The role of alcoholic intake in esophageal carcinoma. Am. J. med. Sci. *249:* 696–699 (1965).

34 Keen, P.; Martin, P.: Is aflatoxin carcinogenic in man? The evidence in Swaziland. Trop. Geogr. Med. *23:* 44–53 (1971).

35 Keller, M. (ed.): Some consequences of alcohol use. I. Alcohol and cancer; in Alcohol and Health, Second Special Report to the US Congress. United States Department of Health, Education, and Welfare (National Institute on Alcohol Abuse and Alcoholism, Rockville 1974).

36 Keller, A.Z.: Liver cirrhosis, tobacco, alcohol and cancer among Blacks. J. Am. med. Ass. *70:* 575–589 (1978).

37 Keller, A.Z.; Terris, M.: The association of alcohol and tobacco with cancer of the mouth and pharynx. Am. J. publ. Hlth *55:* 1578–1585 (1965).

38 Kissin, B.: Epidemiologic investigations of possible biological interactions of alcohol and cancer of the head and neck. Ann. N.Y. Acad. Sci. *252:* 374–377 (1975).

39 Kissin, B.; Kaley, M.M.: Alcohol and cancer; in Kissin, Begleiter, The biology of alcoholism, vol. 3, pp. 481–511 (Plenum Publishing, New York 1974).

40 Kissin, B.; Kaley, M.M.; Su, W.H.; Lerner, R.: Head and neck cancer in alcoholics.

The relationship to drinking, smoking and dietary patterns. J. Am. med. Ass. *224:* 1174–1175 (1973).

41 Kmet, J.; Mahboubi, E.: Esophageal cancer in the Caspian of Iran: initial studies. Science *175:* 846–853 (1972).

42 Kolonel, L.N.; Hinds, M.W.; Hankin, J.H.: Cancer patterns among migrant and native-born Japanese in Hawaii in relation to smoking, drinking, and dietary habits; in Gelboin, MacMahon, Matsushima, Sugimura, Takayama, Takebe, Genetic and environmental factors in experimental and human cancer, pp. 327–340 (Japan Scientific Societies Press, Tokyo 1980).

43 Kono, S.; Ikeda, M.: Correlation between cancer mortality and alcoholic beverage in Japan. Br. J. Cancer *40:* 449–455 (1979).

44 Korsten, M.A.; Matsuzaki, S.; Feinman, L.; Lieber, C.S.: High blood acetaldehyde levels after ethanol administration. Differences between alcoholic and non-alcoholic subjects. New Engl. J. Med. *292:* 386–389 (1975).

45 Kwan, K.W.: Carcinoma of the esophagus: a statistical study. China med. J. *5:* 237–254 (1937).

46 Lamy, L.: Etude de statistique clinique de 131 cas de cancer de l'oesophage et du cardia. Archs Mal. Appar. dig. Mal. Nutr. *4:* 451–475 (1910).

47 Larsson, L.G.; Sandström, A.; Uestling, P.: Relationship of Plummer-Vinson disease to cancer of the upper respiratory tract in Sweden. Cancer Res. *35:* 3308–3316 (1975).

48 Leevy, C.M.; Zetterman, R.: Malnutrition and alcoholism: an overview; in Rothschild, Oratz, Schrieber, Alcohol and abnormal protein synthesis (Pergamon Press, New York 1974).

49 Lieber, C.S.; Seitz, H.K.; Garro, A.J.; Worner, T.M.: Alcohol-related diseases and carcinogenesis. Cancer Res. *39:* 2863–2886 (1979).

50 Lijinsky, U.; Epstein, S.S.: Nitrosamines as environmental carcinogens. Nature, Lond. *225:* 21–23 (1970).

51 Lin, H.J.; Chan, A.C.; Fong, Y.Y.; Newberne, P.: Zinc levels in serum, hair and tumors from patients with esophageal cancer. Nutr. Rep. int. *15:* 635–643 (1977).

52 Lipworth, L.L.; Rice, C.A.: Correlations in mortality data involving cancers of the colorectum and esophagus. Cancer *43:* 1927–1933 (1979).

53 Lyon, J.L.; Gardner, J.W.; West, D.W.: Cancer risk and life-style: cancer among Mormons (1967–1975); in Gelboin, MacMahon, Matsushima, Sugimura, Takayama, Takebe, Genetic and environmental factors in experimental and human cancer, pp. 273–290 (Japan Scientific Societies Press, Tokyo 1980).

54 Lyon, J.L.; Gardner, J.W.; West, D.W.: Cancer risk and life-style: cancer among Mormons from 1967–1975; in Cairns, Lyon, Skolnick, Cancer incidence in defined populations, Banbury report 4, pp. 3–28 (Cold Spring Harbor Laboratory, New York 1980).

55 MacDonald, R.A.: Cirrhosis and primary carcinomas of the liver: changes in their occurrence at the Boston City Hospital, 1897–1954. New Engl. J. Med. *255:* 1179–1182 (1956).

56 Martinez, I.: Retrospective and prospective study of carcinoma of the esophagus, mouth, and pharynx in Puerto Rico. Biol. Ass. Med. Puerto Rico *62:* 170–178 (1970).

57 Masuda, Y.; Mori, K.; Hirohata, T.; Kuratsune, M.: Carcinogenesis in the esophagus.

3. Polycyclic aromatic hydrocarbons and phenols in whiskey. Gann *57:* 549–557 (1966).

58 McCoy, G.D.; Wynder, E.L.: Etiological and preventive implications in alcohol carcinogenesis. Cancer Res. *39:* 2844–2850 (1979).

59 Moore, C.: Cigarette smoking and cancer of the mouth, pharynx and larynx. J. Am. med. Ass. *191:* 104–110 (1965).

60 Newberne, P.M.; McConnell, R.G.: Nutrient deficiencies in cancer causation. J. envir. Path. Toxicol. *3:* 323–356 (1980).

61 Obe, G.; Beek, B.: Mutagenic activity of aldehydes. Drug Alc. Dep. *4:* 91–94 (1979).

62 Obe, G.; Ristow, H.: Mutagenic, carcinogenic and teratogenic effects of alcohol. Mutation Res. *65:* 229–259 (1979).

63 Obe, G.; Ristow, H.; Herha, J.: Chromosomal damage by alcohol in vitro and in vivo; in Gross, Alcohol intoxication and withdrawals, vol. IIIa, pp. 47–70 (Plenum Publishing, New York 1977).

64 Omerovi'o, V.H.: Chronic alcoholism: its correlation with oropharyngeal carcinoma. Med. Arch. *30:* 19–21 (1976).

65 Palmer, D.L.: Alcohol consumption and cellular immunocompetence. Laryngoscope, St. Louis *88:* 13–17 (1978).

66 Pernu, J.: An epidemiological study on cancer of the digestive organs and respiratory tract. Ann. Med. intern. Fenn *49:* suppl. 33, pp. 1–117 (1960).

67 Piquet, J.; Tison: Alcohol et cancer de l'oesophage. Bull. Acad. Méd. *117:* 236–239 (1937).

68 Pothe, H.; Voigtsberger, P.: Zur Epidemiologie und Diagnostik des Ösophaguskarzinoms. Dt. GesundhWes. *31:* 2148–2152 (1976).

69 Purtilo, D.T.; Gottlieb, L.S.: Cirrhosis and hepatoma occurring at the Boston City Hospital, 1917–1968. Cancer, Philad. *32:* 458–462 (1973).

70 Ristow, H.; Obe, G.: Acetaldehyde induces crosslinks in DNA and causes sister chromatid exchanges in human cells. Mutation Res. *58:* 115–119 (1978).

71 Rothman, K.J.: The estimation of synergy or antagonism. Am. J. Epidem. *103:* 506–511 (1976).

72 Rothman, K.J.; Keller, A.: The effect of joint exposure to alcohol and tobacco on risk of cancer of the mouth and pharynx. J. chron. Dis. *25:* 711–716 (1972).

73 Sadeghi, A.; Behmard, S.; Shafiepoor, H.; Zeighmani, E.: Cancer of the esophagus in Southern Iran. Cancer *40:* 841–845 (1977).

74 Schoenberg, B.S.; Bailar, J.C., III; Fraumeni, J.F., Jr.: Certain mortality patterns of esophageal cancer in the United States, 1930–67. J. natn. Cancer Inst. *46:* 63–73 (1971).

75 Schottenfeld, D.: Alcohol as a co-factor in the etiology of cancer. Cancer *43:* 1962–1966 (1979).

76 Schottenfeld, D.; Gant, R.C.; Wynder, E.L.: The role of alcohol and tobacco in multiple primary cancers of the upper digestive system, larynx and lung: a prospective study. Prev. Med. *3:* 277–293 (1974).

77 Schwartz, D.: Alcohol and cancer. Study of pathologic geography. Cancro *19:* 200–209 (1966).

78 Schwartz, D.; Lasserre, O.; Flamant, F.; Lellouch, J.: Alcohol and cancer. A study of geographic pathology concerning 19 countries. Eur. J. Cancer *2:* 367–372 (1966).

79 Schwartz, D.; Lellouch, J.; Flamant, R.; Denoix, P.F.: Alcool et cancer. Résultats d'une enquête rétrospective. Revue fr. Etud. clin. biol. 7: 590–604 (1962).

80 Seitz, H.K.; Garro, A.J.; Lieber, C.S.: Effect of chronic ethanol ingestion on intestinal metabolism and of mutagenicity of benzo[α]pyrene. Biochem. biophys. Res. Commun. 85: 1061–1066 (1978).

81 Sherlock, S.; Fox, R.A.: Niazi, S.P.; Scheuer, P.J.: Chronic liver disease and primary liver cell cancer with hepatitis-associated (Australian) antigen in serum. Lancet i: 1243–1247 (1970).

82 Spalajkovic, M.: Alcoholism and cancer of the larynx and hypopharynx. J. fr. Oto-rino-laryngol. 25: 49–50 (1976).

83 Steiner, P.E.: The etiology and histogenesis of carcinoma of the esophagus. Cancer 9: 436–452 (1956).

84 Stevens, M.H.: Synergistic effect of alcohol on epidermoid carcinogenesis in the larynx. Otolaryngol. Head Neck Surg. 87: 751–756 (1979).

85 Stocks, P.: Report on cancer in North Wales and Liverpool region. Br. Emp. Cancer Camp. 35th Annu. Rep., suppl. to part II (1957).

86 Tuyns, A.J.: Epidemiology of alcohol and cancer. Cancer Res. 39: 2840–2843 (1979).

87 Tuyns, A.J.; Masse, L.M.F.: Mortality from cancer of the esophagus in Brittany. Int. J. Epidemiol. 2: 242–245 (1973).

88 Tuyns, A.J.; Péquignot, G.; Abbatucci, J.S.: Oesophageal cancer and alcohol consumption: importance of type of beverage. Int. J. Cancer 23: 443–447 (1979).

89 Tuyns, A.J.; Péquignot, G.; Jensen, O.M.: Esophageal cancer in Ille-et-Vilaine in relation to levels of alcohol and tobacco consumption: risks are multiplying. Bull. Cancer 64: 45–60 (1977).

90 Vincent, R.G.; Marchetta, F.: The relationship of the use of tobacco and alcohol to cancer of the oral cavity, pharynx, or larynx. Am. J. Surg. 106: 501–505 (1963).

91 Vitale, J.J.; Broitman, S.A.; Gottlieb, L.S.: Alcohol and carcinogenesis; in Newell, Ellison, Nutrition and cancer, pp. 291–301 (Raven Press, New York 1981).

92 Vitale, J.J.; Gottlieb, L.S.: Alcohol and alcohol-related deficiencies as carcinogens. Cancer Res. 35: 3336–3338 (1975).

93 Vogel, C.L.; Anthony, P.P.; Mody, N.; Barker, L.F.: Hepatitis-associated antigen in Uganda patients with hepatocellular carcinoma. Lancet ii: 621–624 (1970).

94 Wapnick, S.; Castle, W.; Nicholle, D.; Zanamwe, L.M.; Gelfand, M.: Cigarette smoking, alcohol and cancer of the oesophagus. S. Afr. med. J. 46: 2023–2026 (1972).

95 Wehman, H.J.; Plantholt, B.A.: Asbestos fibrils in beverages. 1. Gin. Bull. env. Contam. Toxicol. 11: 267–272 (1974).

96 Williams, R.R.; Horn, J.W.: Association of cancer sites with tobacco and alcohol consumption and socioeconomic status of patients: interview study from the Third National Cancer Survey. J. natn. Cancer Inst. 58: 525–547 (1977).

97 World Health Organization: cancer agents that surround us. Wld Hlth 9: 16–17 (1964).

98 Wynder, E.L.; Bross, I.J.: A study of etiological factors in cancer of the esophagus. Cancer, Philad. 14: 389–413 (1961).

99 Wynder, E.L.; Bross, I.J.; Feldman, R.M.: A study of the etiological factors in cancer of the mouth. Cancer, Philad. 10: 1300–1323 (1957).

100 Wynder, E.L.; Fryer, J.H.: Etiologic considerations of Plummer-Vinson (Patterson-Kelly) syndrome. Ann. intern. Med. *49:* 1106–1128 (1958).
101 Wynder, E.L.; Shigematsu, T.: Environmental factors of cancer of the colon and rectum. Cancer, Philad. *20:* 1520–1561 (1967).
102 Wynder, E.L.; Stellman, S.D.: Comparative epidemiology of tobacco-related cancers. Cancer Res. *37:* 4608–4622 (1977).
103 Wu, P.C.; Lam, K.C.: Cytoplasmic hepatitis B surface antigen and the ground-glass appearance in hepatocellular carcinoma. Am. J. clin. Path. *74:* 254–258 (1979).
104 Wu, Y.K.; Loucks, H.H.: Carcinoma of the esophagus or cardia of stomach: analysis of 172 cases with 81 resections. Ann. Surg. *134:* 946–956 (1951).
105 Ziegler, R.G.; Morris, L.E.; Blot, W.J.; Pottern, L.M.; Hoover, R.; Fraumeni, J.F., Jr.: Esophageal cancer among black men in Washington, DC. II. Role of nutrition. J. natn. Cancer Inst. *67:* 1199–1206 (1981).

S.A. Broitman, PhD, Departments of Pathology and Microbiology,
Boston University School of Medicine, Boston, MA 02118 (USA)

Prasad (ed.), Vitamins, Nutrition, and Cancer, pp. 212–230 (Karger, Basel 1984)

Dietary Macronutrients and Colon Cancer

Bandaru S. Reddy

Naylor Dana Institute for Disease Prevention, American Health Foundation, Valhalla, N.Y., USA

Introduction

In the last 35 years, an understanding of some of the key events during the development of cancer has been achieved even at the molecular level. Initial observations by alert clinicians and subsequent contributions by experts in epidemiological techniques have clearly demonstrated that several types of human cancers relate to identifiable causes and some types of cancer occur more frequently in societies with certain dietary habits than among other groups of people [1–4]. About 70–90% of cancers are related to our environment and life-styles and more specifically about 40–60% of environmental cancers are related in some way to diet and nutrition [1, 5].

The incidence of colon cancer shows striking differences among countries and is associated with economic and industrial development and dietary habits. Incidence figures from the Connecticut Tumor Registry show that 15–20% of all malignancies in both males and females are located in the large bowel, and about 5% of the western population will develop this disease before the age of 75 [6]. Cancer of the colon thus represents a major public health problem in the USA.

During the past two decades, epidemiological studies have investigated the influence of environmental factors on the occurrence of colon cancer. These studies suggest that diets particularly high in total fat and low in certain fibers, vegetables, and micronutrients are generally associated with an increased incidence of colon cancer in man [6–10]. Dietary fat may be a risk factor in the absence of factors that are protective, such as use of high fibrous foods and fiber [7, 11, 12]. In these situations, the high-fat diet appears to enhance carcinogenesis via the elevation of agents that are considered to be tumor promoters. No exogenous chemicals (genotoxic agents) have thus far been proven to induce colon cancer in humans.

Cancer researchers are striving toward the prevention of cancer. Those of us engaged in cancer control have as our first interest the primary and secondary prevention of neoplastic diseases. In relation to the prevention of colon cancer, there is an adequate, sound basis of facts of causative and modifying factors that are related to nutrition, and underlying relevant mechanisms to begin making recommendations to the public as well as to the patients aimed at a reduction of the risk for this neoplasm [4, 5].

Discussed here is the current research on the relation between dietary factors and colon cancer and on the mechanisms whereby dietary factors modulate the incidence of colon cancer. This review also presents dietary recommendations based on our current knowledge.

Epidemiology

Several reviews on cancer of the colon have appeared recently [6, 8, 13]. The rarity of colon cancer noted in the societies of developing countries indicates that cancer of the colon is not an inevitable consequence of aging. While the diagnosis of colon cancer in such societies may not always be adequately made, careful autopsy studies from certain populations do support the uncommoness of this disease in these populations. There are, in addition, industrialized societies where colon cancer is also relatively rare, such as Japan, where clinical diagnosis and vital statistics are at least on par with those of western countries where the incidence of colon cancer is high.

Age and Sex Differences

Cancer of the colon increases exponentially with age in both high-risk and low-risk countries, which suggests that this relationship is likely to be the result of continuous action of weak carcinogen(s) and promoters. The age incidence curves for males and females are the same for colon cancer.

In the past, the rectal cancer was often considered together with colon cancer as colorectal or large bowel cancer. Current evidence indicates that a distinction needs to be made between colon cancer and rectal cancer [14]. The male/female ratio for colon cancer is about 1, whereas it is around 1:4 for rectal cancer. The difference in incidence of colon cancer between a high-risk country like the USA and a low-risk country like Japan is about 4:1, but for rectal cancer, this difference is merely 1.1:1, thus suggesting that the etiological factors of colon and rectum may in part be different [13].

Inter- and Intracountry Differences

In general, with few exceptions, cancer of the colon is primarily a disease of the economically developed countries, although not necessarily cancer of the rectum [6, 8, 13]. The highest incidence rates are observed in North America, New Zealand, Australia and Western Europe, with the exception of Finland, where the incidence is one of the lowest in the developed countries and much lower rates are found in Eastern Europe, Asia, Africa and South America (the exception being Uruguay and Argentina, where the mortality rates are slightly lower than those found in North America). Marked differences in incidence rates are observed among the four Scandinavian countries [15].

Migrant studies indicate that colon cancer incidence is higher in the first and second generation Japanese immigrants to the USA and in Polish immigrants to Australia and the USA than in native Japanese in Japan and in the native Poles from Poland, respectively [16, 17].

The fact that the increase in this incidence of colon cancer is noted in the first generation of immigrants suggests that the dietary factor is primarily that of tumor promotion. Genetic differences cannot explain these ethnic and migrant variations in colon cancer rates, since migrants show dramatic shifts in their cancer incidence rates compared not only with those in their country of origin but also with those in their offspring who are born in their adopted country. Further support for environmental dietary factors in the development of colon cancer is derived from the time-trend in Japan where the colon cancer seems to be increasing, a finding consistent with the increasing westernization of Japanese food habits [18].

Further support for life-styles and dietary factors in colon cancer risk is derived from studies of special religious groups within a small geographical area [6, 8, 19, 20]. The incidence of colon cancer in Mormons and Seventh-Day Adventists (SDA) in the USA and in Maoris in New Zealand is lower than the rest of the population groups in their respective countries. The results of a case-control study of colon cancer among SDA and in Mormons have been supportive of the hypothesis that saturated fat or total fat in general are related to colon cancer [21].

Etiological Factors

Wynder and Shigematsu [22] were the first to suggest that differences in fat intake may be responsible for the international variation in colon cancer. Since then, considerable interest has been generated related to various dietary factors and colon cancer and several hypotheses developed [4, 5]. *Wynder* [13] and *Wynder and Reddy* [23] proposed that colon cancer incidence is mainly associated with total dietary fat. A worldwide correlation between colon cancer incidence and total fat consumption has been established [24]. *Gregor* et al. [25] found a high correlation between colon cancer mortality and the intake of animal protein. This association has later been demonstrated in similar studies of internationally available data on food consumption and incidence of mortality [26–28].

Studies attempting to explain the frequency of large bowel cancer have used case-control studies [29]. *Wynder* et al. [10] conducted a large-scale retrospective study on large bowel cancer patients in Japan, which suggested a correlation between the Westernization of the Japanese diet and colon cancer. *Haenszel* et al. [16] demonstrated an association between colon cancer and dietary beef in Hawaiian Japanese cases and Hawaiian Japanese controls. A case-control study of cancer of the colon in Utah (Mormons) indicated an elevated risk for those with an increased intake of calories, total fat and saturated fat [21]. A recent study by *Williams* et al. [30] using few cases of colon cancer indicated an inverse relationship between colon cancer and serum cholesterol in man.

Burkitt [7] recognized the rarity of large bowel cancer in most African populations and suggested that people consuming a diet rich in fiber have a low incidence of large bowel cancer. An interesting epidemiological outline is Finland. In spite of a high dietary fat intake and a parallel high incidence of coronary heart disease, the incidence of colon cancer is relatively low in Finland. A recent study comparing populations in rural and urban Finland, Denmark, Sweden and in New York indicated that one of the factors contributing to the low risk of colon cancer in rural Scandinavia appears to be high dietary fiber intake, although all populations are on a high-fat diet [11, 12, 31, 32]. In Finland, the fat consumed is largely saturated fat, but importantly, the Finns also consume diets high in fiber. Inconclusive results of early correlation studies in relation to dietary fiber could be explained by the fact that in early studies [5] the statistics of dietary fiber were based on estimates of crude fiber intake, and these calculations underestimate the intake of total dietary fiber.

In case-control studies in the San Francisco area American blacks, it was found that among a large variety of dietary constituents investigated, those that were lowest in the diets of patients with colon cancer as compared with controls were those containing fiber [33]. It is interesting that these studies have shown an increased risk of colon cancer to be associated with high-fat/low-fiber intake. *Bjelke* [34] found less frequent use of vegetables among colorectal cancer patients. Another case-control study from Roswell Park Memorial Institute in Buffalo, New York, showed a lower risk of colon cancer for individuals ingesting vegetables such as cabbage, broccoli and Brussels sprouts [9].

The bulk of epidemiological evidence suggests that diets high in total fat and low in fiber are associated with an increased incidence of colon cancer in man. In several populations consuming a high amount of total fat, dietary fiber acts as a protective factor. Moreover, laboratory animal studies discussed elsewhere have clearly demonstrated that high-fat intake promotes and high-fiber intake inhibits the development of colon cancer. Concurrence between the epidemiological and laboratory evidence offered the strength to the concept that diet is a major etiologic factor in colon cancer.

Mechanisms of Dietary Factors in Colon Cancer

The possible mechanism of the effect of dietary fat in colon carcinogenesis has been the subject of a recent workshop [35]. It has been shown that the amount of dietary fat determines the levels of intestinal bile acids as well as the composition of the gut microflora which, in turn, metabolize these sterols to tumorigenic compounds in the colon [36]. *Reddy* [37] demonstrated that high dietary fat increases the excretion of bile acids into the gut as well as modifying the metabolic activity of gut microflora which increases the secondary bile acid formation in the colon. These secondary bile acids – deoxycholic acid and lithocholic acid – have been shown to act as colon tumor promoters.

The mechanism of protective effect of dietary fiber in colon cancer has been discussed in a recent workshop [38]. Dietary fiber comprises a heterogenous group of carbohydrates, including cellulose, hemicellulose and pectin and a non-carbohydrate substance, lignin. The protective effect of dietary fiber may be due to adsorption, dilution, or metabolism of cocarcinogens, promoters and yet-to-be-identified carcinogens by the components of the fiber [39]. Different types of non-nutritive fibers possess specific binding properties. Dietary fiber could also affect the enterohepatic circulation of bile salts. Fiber not only influences bile acid metabolism, thereby reducing the formation of tumor promoters in the colon, but also dilutes potential carcinogens and cocarcinogens by its bulking effect and is able to bind bile acids and certain carcinogenic compounds.

Food contains a large number of inhibitors of carcinogenesis, including phenols, indoles, aromatic isothiocyanates, plant sterols, selenium salts, ascorbic acid, tocopherols and carotenes [40]. Since the principal sources of these compounds in the diet are plant constituents, the type and quantity of the plant material in the diet will be of importance in determining the activity of the protective system [40]. Epidemiological studies suggest an inverse relationship between consumption of vegetables and fruits containing the above inhibitors and occurrence of cancer [9]. Thus, the humans consuming relatively large amounts of vegetables and fruits would have greater defenses against carcinogenic compounds than do individuals consuming a lesser amount of these foods.

Until recently, there were no concepts on the nature of genotoxic carcinogens associated with the etiology of colon cancer. Several investigators proposed that cooking process (frying and broiling) produces powerful mutagens on the surface of meat and fish [41] and that these mutagens may be carcinogens responsible for colon cancer [42]. *Weisburger* et al. [42] also demonstrated that any form of cooking led to the formation of mutagenic activity. The fat content of food may also play a role in the mutagen formation. However, the carcinogenic activity of fried meat mutagens for the colon remains to be determined.

Thus, we can conclude that: (a) the extent of the carcinogenic stress from the exogenous source is probably rather weak; (b) high-fat diet alters concentration of bile acids and the activity of gut microflora which in turn produce tumor-promoting substances in the lumen of the colon; (c) certain dietary fibers not only enhance binding of tumorigenic compounds in the

Table I. Modifying factors in colon cancer

Dietary fat[1]	Dietary fibers[1,2]	Micronutrients[3]
1 Increases bile acid secretion into gut	1 Certain fibers increase fecal bulk and dilute carcinogens and promoters	1 Modify carcinogenesis at activation and detoxification level
2 Increases metabolic activity of gut bacteria	2 Modify metabolic activity of gut bacteria	2 Act also at promotional phase of carcinogenesis
3 Increases secondary bile acids in colon	3 Modify the metabolism of carcinogens and/or promoters	
4 Alters immune system	4 Bind the carcinogens and/or promoters and excrete them	
5 Stimulation of mixed function oxidase system		

[1] Dietary factors, particularly high total dietary fat and a relative lack of certain dietary fibers and vegetables have a role.
[2] High dietary fiber or fibrous foods may be a protective factor even in the high dietary fat intake.
[3] Include vitamins, minerals, anti-oxidants, etc.

gut, but also dilute them so that their effect on the colonic mucosa is minimal, and (d) dietary fat, fiber and certain vegetables and fruits modify the intestinal mucosal as well as hepatic enzyme inhibitors or inducers that alter the capacity of the animal to metabolize the tumorigenic compounds (table I).

Two-Stage Carcinogenesis in Human Colon Cancer: Effect of Diet

Currently, much of our knowledge of the stages of carcinogenesis is based on experiments concerning the genesis of epidermoid carcinoma in the mouse skin. The major significance of this type of observation is that carcinogenesis occurs as a multistep process in which the first step is possibly mutational and the other(s) can be promoted by a variety of compounds which are not necessarily carcinogenic. With the two-stage system of mouse skin carcinogenesis, the first tumors to be observed are papillomas. After continued promoter treatment, malignant tumors appear on the skin. Several other model systems that also demonstrate the two distinct stages of carcinogenesis, initiation and promotion, have been reviewed recently [43]. Although for some of the models, however, it is not clear whether the initiator and promoter are acting in the true sense, this model system is not limited to skin but can be extended to many other species and tissues. The fact that a large number and diversity of experimental models proceed through promotion strongly suggest that diet-induced human colon cancer involves similar stages in the development. For example, epidemiologic and metabolic epidemiologic investigations have indicated the importance of diet in human colon cancer, and the changes in incidence of colon cancer reflecting migration from low-risk regions to regions of high-risk, within the same generation. This suggests that (a) the initiating insult for colon cancer is similar in populations in low- and high-risk areas, and (b) when the population from low-risk countries migrate to high-risk regions, they follow the dietary practices of adopted countries which often lead to increased levels of promoters in the colon. Another example is the transformation of colon adenomatous polyps into carcinomas in humans, although there has been considerable controversy over the years regarding the cancer risk of adenomas (villous, tubular and tubulovillous type). From an epidemiologic point of view, the association between adenomatous polyps and colon cancer has been reinforced by the following characteristics: (a) the incidence of adenomatous polyps closely parallels the prevalence of colon cancer in all populations so far studied; (b) in the populations studied, the risk of colon cancer increases with size and multiplicity of polyps, thus suggesting a dose effect; (c) prospective studies in the USA and Sweden have shown persons with adenomatous polyps to be at higher risk to colon cancer; (d) whites, blacks and orientals have a lower prevalence of adenomatous polyps while living in areas of low colon cancer frequency, but display high polyp prevalence if they migrate to areas of high colon cancer risk, and (e) there is an inverse socioeconomic gradient found for both conditions (colon cancer and adenomatous polyps) in Cali, Columbia, a city in a developing country that has large social class differences in diet [8].

The above epidemiologic and clinical observations point to the possibility that there are two stages in human colon cancer. The extent of carcinogenic stress is rather weak and whether or not a given individual is at high risk for colon cancer may depend more on the rather important promoting stimulus from the nutritional factors.

Metabolic Epidemiology of Colon Cancer

The concept that dietary fat and certain fibers distinct from chemical contaminants of diet and from other environmental and genetic factors are important determinants of colon cancer risk is reinforced by metabolic epidemiological studies and laboratory animal studies. A key insight gained from studies in man is that the populations who are at high risk for colon cancer development appear to excrete high levels of fecal bile acids and mutagens compared to low-risk populations. Animal model studies suggest that the influence of dietary fat appears to be exerted primarily on the later, promotional phase of colon carcinogenesis.

Studies were carried out in our laboratory and elsewhere on the excretion of fecal bile acids in high- and low-risk populations for colon cancer development and to determine whether changes in the diet in terms of fat and fiber can alter the concentration of colonic bile acids. This subject has been reviewed recently [37, 44]. Briefly, the population at a high risk for colon cancer has an increased amount of colonic secondary bile acids, namely deoxycholic acid and lithocholic acid, and metabolic activity of gut microflora. In addition, people on a high-fat diet appear to have higher levels of fecal secondary bile acids and gut microbial activity compared to those on a low-fat diet. In a recent study, comparison of fecal bile acids was carried out between SDAs who are lacto-ovo-vegetarians, and age- and sex-matched non-SDAs consuming a high-fat, mixed western diet. The fat intake was 28% lower and fiber intake was 2.5-fold higher in SDAs, but the total protein and calorie consumption was similar between the two groups. The fecal excretion of deoxycholic acid and lithocholic acid was lower in SDAs as compared with non-SDAs.

Table II. Dietary intake in healthy volunteers from Kuopio (Finland), Malmö and Umeå (Sweden) and Metropolitan New York Area

Dietary constituent	Dietary intake, g/day			
	Malmö	Umeå	Kuopio	New York
Total protein	104	102	93	101
Total fat	112	132	110	112
Total carbohydrate	225	235	320	272
Total fiber	17	26	32	14

The effect of dietary fiber on fecal bile acids has been studied in many laboratories. *Reddy* et al. [11] and *Domellof* et al. [31] studied the fecal bile acid excretion in healthy controls in Kuopio (Finland) and Umeå (Sweden), low-risk and intermediate-risk populations for colon cancer development, respectively, and in Malmö (Sweden) and New York, high risk for colon cancer. The dietary histories indicate that the total fat and protein consumption in Kuopio, Umeå and Malmö is quite similar to the New York and Malmö populations, but the consumption of fiber, mainly cereal type, is 2.5-fold higher in Kuopio and 2-fold higher in Umeå, compared to the New York population (table II). The daily output of feces is 3 times higher in Kuopio and 2 times higher in Umeå than in the healthy individuals in the USA. The concentration of fecal secondary bile acids – deoxycholic acid and lithocholic acid – is lower in Kuopio and in Umeå due to high fecal bulk, than in Malmö and New York (table III). However, the daily output remained the same in the four groups because the dietary intake of fat is the same in these areas. Similar results were obtained by *Jensen* et al. [12] who showed that people in rural Parikkala, Finland, with a low risk for cancer of the colon, have a high intake of total fat and fiber yielding to low concentration of fecal secondary bile acids.

Table III. Fecal bile acids of healthy subjects from Malmö (Sweden), Umeå, Sweden, and Metropolitan New York [from ref. 32]

Bile acids	mg/g dry feces			
	Malmö (n = 23)	New York (n = 44)	Umeå (n = 22)	New York (n = 40)
Cholic acid	0.24 ± 0.15[1]	0.25 ± 0.10	0.3 ± 0.13	0.2 ± 0.04
Chenodeoxycholic acid	0.22 ± 0.05	0.12 ± 0.10	0.2 ± 0.05	0.2 ± 0.03
Deoxycholic acid	4.02 ± 0.42	4.65 ± 0.38	2.2 ± 0.55	4.5 ± 0.30[2]
Lithocholic acid	3.94 ± 0.32	4.18 ± 0.41	2.3 ± 0.38	4.0 ± 0.20[2]
Ursodeoxycholic acid	0.53 ± 0.13	0.32 ± 0.04	0.4 ± 0.13	0.3 ± 0.04
3α,7β,11α-Trihydroxy-5β-cholanic acid	0.25 ± 0.09	0.34 ± 0.05	0.3 ± 0.12	0.2 ± 0.04
12-Ketolithocholic acid	0.41 ± 0.10	0.45 ± 0.06	0.3 ± 0.08	0.4 ± 0.02[2]
Other bile acids	1.42 ± 0.18	2.96 ± 0.31	1.7 ± 0.31	3.3 ± 0.40
Total bile acids	11.02 ± 1.90	13.28 ± 2.20	7.7 ± 1.10	13.1 ± 0.60[2]

[1] Values are means ± SE.
[2] Significantly different from Umeå, $p > 0.05$.

Table IV. Colon tumor incidence in rats fed diets high in fat and treated with colon carcinogens

Experiment No.	% dietary fat	Carcinogen	% rats with colon tumors
I	Lard		
	5	DMH[1]	17
	20	DMH	67
	Corn oil		
	5	DMH[1]	36
	20	DMH	64
II	Beef fat		
	5	DMH[2]	27
	20	DMH	60
	5	MNU[3]	33
	20	MNU	73
	5	MAM acetate[4]	45
	20	MAM acetate	80
III	Beef fat		
	5	DMAB[5]	26
	20	DMAB	74
IV	Corn oil		
	5	AOM[6]	17
	20	AOM	46
	Safflower oil		
	5	AOM	13
	20	AOM	36
	Olive oil		
	5	AOM	10
	20	AOM	13
	Coconut oil		
	20	AOM	13

[1] Female F344 rats, at 7 weeks of age, were given DMH s.c. at a weekly dose rate of 10 mg/kg body wt for 20 weeks and autopsied 10 weeks later.

[2] Male F344 rats, at 7 weeks of age, were given a single s.c. dose of DMH, 150 mg/kg body weight, and autopsied 30 weeks later.

[3] Male F344 rats, at 7 weeks of age, were given MNU i.r., 2.5 mg per rat, twice a week for 2 weeks and autopsied 30 weeks later.

[4] Male F344 rats, at 7 weeks of age, were given a single i.p. dose of MAM acetate, 35 mg/kg body wt and autopsied 30 weeks later.

[5] Male F344 rats, at 7 weeks of age, were given DMAB s.c. at a weekly dose rate of 50 mg/kg body wt for 20 weeks, and autopsied 20 weeks later.

[6] Female F344 rats, at 5 weeks of age, were fed low-fat diets. At 7 weeks of age, they were given a single dose os AOM, 20 mg/kg body wt, s.c. 1 week later, they were transferred to their respective high-fat diet, and autopsied 48 weeks later.

Because of the potential importance of fecal mutagens in the genesis of colon cancer and of the possible role of dietary factors in the production of these mutagens, the fecal mutagenic activity of various population groups with distinct dietary habits and varied colon cancer incidences was determined by several investigators [45–48]. These populations included South African urban whites and blacks, high-risk Canadians, New York and Hawaiian Japanese populations and low-risk SDAs in the USA, the Finnish population and Japanese in Japan. These studies demonstrate not only that the populations who are at high risk for colon cancer excrete increased amounts of fecal mutagens compared to low-risk populations, but also the presence of several kinds of fecal mutagens.

Animal Model Studies

Studies on the mechanisms of colon carcinogenesis have been assisted by the discovery of several animal models that show the type of lesions observed in man [49]. These animals are now being used effectively to study the multiple environmental factors involved in the pathogenesis of colon cancer. The combined results obtained through human studies and animal models have provided a powerful, convincing argument for modification of risk factors so as to lower the colon cancer incidence in the human setting.

Dietary Fat and Colon Carcinogenesis
Studies were carried out by several investigators to test the effect of type and amount of dietary fat on colon tumors induced by a variety of carcinogens – 1,2-dimethylhydrazine (DMH), azoxymethane (AOM), methylazoxymethanol (MAM) acetate, 3,2′-dimethyl-4-aminobiphenyl (DMAB) and methylnitrosourea (MNU) [50–54]. The types of fat used in these studies were lard, beef tallow, corn oil, safflower oil and coconut oil. Animals fed the diets containing 20% lard, corn oil or beef tallow were more susceptible to chemically induced colon tumors than those fed the diets containing 5% lard, corn oil or beef tallow (table IV). The type of fat appears to be immaterial at the 20%, although at the 5% fat level, there is a suggestion that unsaturated fat (corn oil) predisposes to more colon tumors than the saturated fat (lard). In another study, rats fed a 20% safflower oil diet had more colon tumors than the animals fed either the 5 or 20% coconut oil diets [54]. A recent study from our laboratory indicates that the diets

Table V. Colon tumor incidence in F344 male rats fed diets containing wheat bran or citrus fiber and treated with azoxymethane

Diet	% Animals with colon tumors			Colon tumors per tumor-bearing rat		
	total[1]	adenoma	adeno-carcinoma	total	adenoma	adeno-carcinoma
Control	90	86	63	3.45 ± 0.16[2]	2.37 ± 0.16	1.08 ± 0.18
Wheat bran	71[3]	47[3]	39[3]	1.55 ± 0.12[4]	0.94 ± 0.13[4]	0.61 ± 0.11[4]
Citrus pulp	63[3]	41[3]	39[3]	1.78 ± 0.18[4]	0.90 ± 0.14[4]	0.88 ± 0.16

[1] Total represents animals with adenomas and/or adenocarcinomas.
[2] Mean $\pm$ SEM.
[3] Significantly different from the group fed the control diet by χ^2 test (p <0.05).
[4] Significantly different from the group fed the control diet by Student's t test (p < 0.05).

containing 20% olive oil or 20% coconut oil had no promoting effect in colon carcinogenesis. These studies provide evidence that not only the amount of dietary fat but also the fatty acid composition (type) of fat are important factors in determining the promoting effect in colon carcinogenesis.

The suggestion that promotion may be involved in intestinal cancer has been supported by the observation that the carcinogenic response to a variety of intestinal carcinogens is enhanced by the dietary fat which in itself is not carcinogenic. Recent studies indicate that the enhanced tumorigenesis in the animals fed the high-fat diet is due to promotional effect [55]. Ingestion of high-fat diet increased the intestinal tumor incidence when fed after AOM (carcinogen) administration, but not during or before AOM treatment.

The carcinogenic process in the human may have similar characteristics since there is a good correlation between the findings in a variety of animal studies and those done in humans [43]. The fact that ubiquitous environmental carcinogens are present at very low concentrations suggests that promoting factors may have a preponderant influence on the eventual outcome of the neoplastic process in humans. Due to the wide variety of initiating agents and the possible difficulties in removing them from the environment, the promotional phase of carcinogenesis may be a more promising area for development of preventive measures.

Dietary Fiber and Colon Carcinogenesis

The relation between the type of dietary fiber and colon cancer has been studied in experiments with animals [39, 56] (table V). Rats fed diets containing high levels of wheat bran, citrus fiber, citrus pectin, cellulose or lignin had fewer chemically induced colon tumors than did the animals not fed fiber or fed low levels of fibers (table V), whereas feeding of alfalfa or corn bran had no effect on colon tumor incidence. These studies indicate that the protection against colon cancer afforded by dietary fibers depends on the source of fiber. Several observations also suggest that dietary fiber protects against tumorigenesis during the promotional phase.

Conclusions and Interdisciplinary Approach for
Colon Cancer Prevention

During the last decade, a substantial amount of progress has been made in the understanding of the role played by the dietary constituents in general and specifically the role of lipids, fibers and micronutrients in colon cancer [4, 5]. The population with high incidences of colon cancer is characterized by consumption of high dietary fat. Furthermore, dietary fat may be a risk factor for colon cancer in the absence of factors that are protective, such as use of high fibrous foods, fiber, vegetables and fruits.

The suggestion that promotion may be involved in colon cancer has been supported by the observation that the carcinogenic response to a variety of colon carcinogens is enhanced by the dietary fat (which in itself is not carcinogenic) and inhibited by several dietary fibers. The carcinogenic process in humans may have similar characteristics. The fact that ubiquitous environmental carcinogens are present at very low concentrations suggests that promoting factors may have a preponderant influence on the eventual outcome of the neoplastic process in humans. Because promotion is a reversible process, in contrast to the rapid irreversible process of initiation by carcinogens, manipulation of promotion would seem to be the best method of colon cancer prevention. However, in prevention, it makes little difference by what mechanism an agent operates, providing that its elimination or reduction can be shown to lead to a decline in cancer incidence. Fundamental to any decision on diet, nutrition and colon cancer are timely measures to reduce the risk of cancer, including advice to the public at large. Such advice assumes particular importance since several decades may span the gap between initiating and clinical manifestation of cancer and, therefore, steps taken today may have a major impact on the nature of future events [57].

We believe that these prudent measures for the general population are imperative when evidence from various lines of investigation is concordant and associates current dietary patterns with an elevated risk for colon cancer. In terms of prevention of colon cancer, a decision to alter dietary habits leading to a lower intake of dietary fat and higher intake of certain dietary fibers has potential beneficial effects and no apparent negative effects. Such measures are unlikely to be hazardous and can be advocated with a strong hope for benefits in the population. The beneficial effects go beyond colon cancer in that a reduction in fat intake might also influence the risk for other diet-related cancers and, in particular, could reduce the rate of the leading cause of early death, coronary heart disease.

If the hypothesis that the same factors that affect tumor induction also influence the recurrence of adenomatous polyps after polypectomy, transformation of adenomas into carcinomas, and recurrence of colon carcinomas after surgical intervention in cancer patients is correct, then a reduction in dietary fat intake and increase in fiber intake in these patients should result in objective increase in disease-free survival and overall survival in these patients. The overall goal is to reduce the incidence of colon cancer in this high-risk group. We suggest that randomized prospective clinical trials be performed in patients at high risk for carcinomas of the colon with the aim of reducing the incidence of new polyps or carcinomas. On a practical basis, patient compliance with the necessary degree of dietary modification that is acceptable to patients on a continuing basis throughout lifetime is feasible in our society and might accomplish our preventive goal.

We, therefore, recommend to the public at large and to the patients with colon cancer and adenomatous polyps to reduce the fat intake and increase fiber consumption. The significance of the proposed dietary recommendation lies in its ability to provide information relevant to the use of dietary intervention as a form of totally effective non-toxic therapy for patients with colon cancer and adenomatous polyps.

The modified dietary regimen consists of (a) a reduction of dietary fat to 20–25% of fat calories with a polyunsaturated, saturated and monounsaturated fatty acid ratio of 1:1:1 and (b) an increase in complex carbohydrate intake. Total dietary fiber intake per day should be increased to 32 g. In order to achieve this objective, we recommend eating less foods high in saturated and unsaturated fats, and to increase the consumption of fruits, vegetables and whole-grain cereal products daily. These fruits and vegetables should include oranges, grapefruit, apples, dark-green leafy vegetables, carrots, winter squash, tomatoes, cabbage, cauliflower and Brussels sprouts. This is not a diet, which we generally adopt as an emergency measure after we have indulged in nutritional excesses, but rather a continuing life-long, low-risk, yet pleasant, tasteful and nutritious diet from the public health point of view.

References

1   Wynder, E.L.; Gori, G.B.: Contribution of the environment to cancer incidence: an epidemiologic exercise. J. natn. Cancer Inst. *58:* 825–832 (1977).
2   Doll, R.; Peto, R.: The causes of cancer: quantitative estimates of avoidable risks of cancer in the United States today. J. natn. Cancer Inst. *66:* 1191–1308 (1981).
3   Higginson, J.L.; Muir, C.S.: in Holland, Frei, Cancer medicine; 2nd ed., pp. 257–328 (Lea & Febiger, Philadelphia 1982).
4   National Research Council: Diet, nutrition and cancer. Assembly of Life Sciences, National Research Council (Natn. Academy Press, Washington 1982).
5   Reddy, B.S.; Cohen, L.A.; McCoy, G.D.; Hill, P.; Weisburger, J.H.; Wynder, E.L.: Nutrition and its relationship to cancer. Adv. Cancer Res. *32:* 237–345 (1980).
6   Jensen, O.M.: Colon cancer epidemiology; in Autrup, Williams, Experimental colon carcinogenesis, pp. 3–23 (CRC Press, Boca Raton 1983).
7   Burkitt, D.P.: Fiber in the etiology of colorectal cancer; in Winawer, Schottenfeld, Sherlock, Colorectal cancer: prevention, epidemiology and screening, pp. 13–18 (Raven Press, New York 1980).
8   Correa, P.; Haenszel, W.: The epidemiology of large bowel cancer. Adv. Cancer Res. *26:* 1–141 (1978).
9   Graham, S.; Dayal, H.; Swanson, M.; Mittleman, A.; Wilkinson, G.: Diet in the epidemiology of cancer of the colon and rectum. J. natn. Cancer Inst. *61:* 709–714 (1978).
10 Wynder, E.L.; Kajitani, T.; Ishekawa, S.; Dodo, H.; Takano, A.: Environmental factors of cancer of the colon and rectum. II. Japanese epidemiological data. Cancer *23:* 1210–1220 (1969).
11 Reddy, B.S.; Hedges, A.R.; Laakso, K.; Wynder, E.L.: Metabolic epidemiology of large bowel cancer. Fecal bulk and constituents of high-risk North American and low-risk Finnish population. Cancer *42:* 2382–2838 (1978).
12 Jensen, O.M.; MacLennan, R.; Wahrendorf, J.: Diet, bowel function, fecal characteristics and large bowel cancer in Denmark and Finland. Nutr. Cancer *4:* 5–19 (1982).
13 Wynder, E.L.: The epidemiology of large bowel cancer. Cancer Res. *35:* 3388–3394 (1975).
14 Weisburger, J.H.; Reddy, B.S.; Joftes, D. (eds): Colorectal cancer. UICC Tech. Rep. Ser., vol. 19 (UICC, Genève 1975).
15 Teppo, L.; Saxen, E.: Epidemiology of colon cancer in Scandinavia. Israel J. med. Scis *15:* 322–328 (1979).

16 Haenszel, W.; Berg, J.W.; Segi, M.; Kurihara, M.; Locke, F.B.: Large bowel cancer in Hawaiian Japanese. J. natn. Cancer Inst. *51:* 1765–1799 (1973).

17 Staszewski, J.; McCall, M.G.; Stenhouse, N.S.: Cancer mortality in 1962–66 among Polish migrants to Australia. Br. J. Cancer *25:* 599–618 (1971).

18 Hirayama, T.: Diet and cancer. Nutr. Cancer *1:* 67–81 (1979).

19 West, D.K.: in Cairns, Lyon, Skolnick, Banbury report No. 4: cancer incidence in defined populations, p. 31 (Cold Spring Harbor Laboratory, New York 1980).

20 Phillips, R.L.; Garfinkel, L.; Kuzma, J.W.; Beeson, W.L.; Lotz, T.; Brin, B.: Mortality among California Seventh-Day Adventists for selected cancer sites. J. natn. Cancer Inst. *65:* 1097–1107 (1980).

21 West, D.W.; Lyon, J.L.; Gardner, J.W.; Schwan, K.; Stanish, W.; Mahoney, A.; Sorenson, A.; Avlon, E.: Epidemiology of colon cancer in Utah. 1983 Workshop: A Decade of Achievements and Challenges in Large Bowel Carcinogenesis, pp. 3–5 (National Large Bowel Cancer Project, Houston 1983).

22 Wynder, E.L.; Shigematsu, T.: Environmental factors of cancers of the colon and rectum. Cancer *20:* 1520–1561 (1967).

23 Wynder, E.L.; Reddy, B.S.: Etiology of cancer of the colon; in Grundmann, Colon cancer, cancer campaign, vol. 2, pp. 1–14 (Fischer, Stuttgart 1978).

24 Carroll, K.K.; Khor, H.T.: Dietary fat in relation to tumorigenesis. Prog. biochem. Pharmacol., vol. 10, pp. 308–353 (Karger, Basel 1975).

25 Gregor, O.; Toma, R.; Prasova, F.: Gastrointestinal cancer and nutrition. Gut *10:* 1031–1034 (1969).

26 Armstrong, B.; Doll, R.: Environmental factors and cancer incidence and mortality in different countries with special reference to dietary practices. Int. J. Cancer *15:* 617–631 (1975).

27 Drasar, B.S.; Irving, D.: Environmental factors and cancer of the colon and breast. Br. J. Cancer *27:* 167–172 (1973).

28 Howell, M.A.: Diet as an etiological factor in the development of cancers of the colon and rectum. J. chron. Dis. *28:* 67–80 (1975).

29 Jain, M.; Cook, G.M.; Davis, F.G.; Grace, M.G.; Howe, G.R.; Miller, A.B.: A case control study of diet and colorectal cancer. Int. J. Cancer *26:* 757–768 (1980).

30 Williams, R.R.; Sorlie, P.D.; Feinleib, M.; McNamara, P.M.; Kannel, W.B.; Dawber, T.P.: Cancer incidence by levels of cholesterol. J. Am. med. Ass. *245:* 247–252 (1981).

31 Domellof, L.; Darby, L.; Hanson, D.; Mathews, L.; Simi, B.; Reddy, B.S.: Fecal sterols and bacterial β-glucuronidase activity: a preliminary study of healthy volunteers from Umeå, Sweden, and metropolitan New York. Nutr. Cancer *4:* 120–127 (1982).

32 Reddy, B.S.; Ekelund, G.; Bohe, M.; Engle, A.; Domellof, L.: Metabolic epidemiology of colon cancer: dietary pattern and fecal sterol concentration of three populations. Nutr. Cancer (in press).

33 Dales, L.G.; Friedman, G.D.; Wry, H.K.; Grossman, S.; Williams, S.R.: Case-control study of relationships of diet and other traits to colorectal cancer in American blacks. Am. J. Epidem. *109:* 132–144 (1979).

34 Bjelke, E.: Epidemiological studies of cancer of the stomach, colon and rectum. Scand. J. Gastroent. *9:* suppl. 31, pp. 1–253 (1974).

35 Fink, D.J.; Kritchevsky, D. (eds): Workshop on fat and cancer. Cancer Res. *41:* 3684–3825 (1981).

36 Aries, V.; Crowther, J.S.; Drasar, B.S.; Hill, M.J.; Williams, R.E.O.: Bacteria and etiology of cancer of the large bowel. Gut *10:* 334–335 (1969).

37 Reddy, B.S.: Dietary fat and its relationship to large bowel cancer. Cancer Res. *41:* 3700–3705 (1981).

38 Vahouny, G.V.; Kritchevsky, D. (eds): Dietary fiber in health and disease (Plenum Publishing, New York 1982).

39 Reddy, B.S.: Dietary fiber and colon carcinogenesis: a critical review; in Vahouny, Kritchevsky, Dietary fiber in health and disease, pp. 265–285 (Plenum Publishing, New York 1982).

40 Wattenberg, L.W.: Inhibition of neoplasia by minor dietary constituents. Cancer Res. *43:* 2448S–2453S (1983).

41 Sugimura, T.; Sato, S.: Mutagens-carcinogens in foods. Cancer Res. *43:* 2415S–2421S (1983).

42 Weisburger, J.W.; Reddy, B.S.; Spingarn, N.E.; Wynder, E.L.: Current views on the mechanisms involved in the etiology of colorectal cancer; in Winawer, Schottenfeld, Sherlock, Colorectal cancer: prevention, epidemiology and screening, pp. 19–41 (Raven Press, New York 1980).

43 Diamond, L.; O'Brien, T.G.; Baird, W.M.: Tumor promoters and the mechanisms of tumor promotion. Adv. Cancer Res. *32:* 1–74 (1980).

44 Reddy, B.S.: Diet and bile acids. Cancer Res. *41:* 3766–3768 (1981).

45 Reddy, B.S.; Sharma, C.; Darby, L.; Laakso, K.; Wynder, E.L.: Metabolic epidemiology of large bowel cancer: fecal mutagens in high- and low-risk population for colon cancer, a preliminary report. Mutation Res. *72:* 511–522 (1980).

46 Ehrich, M.; Ashell, J.E.; Van Tassell, R.L.; Wilkins, T.D.; Walker, A.R.P.; Richardson, N.J.: Mutagens in the feces of 3 South African populations at different levels of risk for colon cancer. Mutation Res. *64:* 231–240 (1979).

47 Kuhnlein, U.; Bergstrom, D.; Kuhnlein, H.: Mutations in feces from vegetarians and non-vegetarians. Mutation Res. *45:* 1–12 (1981).

48 Mower, H.F.; Ichinotsubo, D.; Wang, L.W.; Mandel, M.; Stemmerman, A.; Nomura, A.; Heilbrun, L.; Kamiyama, S.; Shimada, A.: Fecal mutagens in two Japanese populations with different colon cancer risks. Cancer Res. *42:* 1164–1169 (1982).

49 Shamsuddin, A.K.M.: Comparative pathology – human large intestinal cancer and animal models; in Autrup, Williams, Experimental colon carcinogenesis, pp. 125–128 (CRC Press, Boca Raton 1983).

50 Nigro, N.D.; Singh, D.V.; Campbell, R.L.; Pak, M.S.: Effect of dietary beef fat on intestinal tumor formation by azoxymethane in rats. J. natn. Cancer Inst. *54:* 429–442 (1975).

51 Bansal, B.R.; Rhoads, J.E., Jr.; Bansal, S.C.: Effects of diet on colon carcinogenesis and the immune system in rats treated with 1,2-dimethylhydrazine. Cancer Res. *38:* 3293–3303 (1978).

52 Rogers, A.E.; Newberne, P.M.: Dietary effects of chemical carcinogenesis in animal models for colon and liver tumors. Cancer Res. *35:* 3427–3431 (1975).

53 Reddy, B.S.; Narisawa, T.; Vukusich, D.; Weisburger, J.H.; Wynder, E.L.: Effect of quality and quantity of dietary fat and dimethylhydrazine in colon carcinogenesis in rats. Proc. Soc. exp. Biol. Med. *151:* 237–239 (1976).

54   Broitman, S.A.; Vitale, J.J.; Vavrousek-Jakuba, E.; Gottlieb, L.S.: Polyunsaturated
     fat, cholesterol and large bowel tumorigenesis. Cancer 40: 2455–2463 (1977).
55   Bull, A.W.; Soullier, B.K.; Wilson, P.S.; Haydon, M.T.; Nigro, N.D.: Promotion of
     azoxymethane-induced intestinal cancer by high-fat diets in rats. Cancer Res. 39:
     4956–4959 (1979).
56   Freeman, H.J.: Dietary fibers and colon cancer; in Autrup, Williams, Experimental
     colon carcinogenesis, pp. 267–282 (CRC Press, Boca Raton 1983).
57   Palmer, S.: Diet, nutrition and cancer: the future of dietary policy. Cancer Res. 3:
     2509S–2514S (1983).

B.S. Reddy, PhD, Naylor Dana Institute for Disease Prevention,
American Health Foundation, Valhalla, NY 10595 (USA)

Prasad (ed.), Vitamins, Nutrition, and Cancer, pp. 231–239 (Karger, Basel 1984)

Proteins of the Metabolism of Iron, Cells of the Immune System and Malignancy

Maria de Sousa, Daniel Potaznik [1]

Cell Ecology, Sloan-Kettering Institute for Cancer Research, New York, N.Y., USA

Introduction

A number of recent studies have identified significant functional inter-actions between iron and proteins classically associated with the metabolism of iron and the lymphomyeloid system [1–20]. This is perhaps not too surprising when one remembers that the lymphomyeloid system has, as one of its obligatory tasks, the function of clearing an estimated 1.9×10^{11} senescent red cells and recycling daily 90% of the 38 mg of iron associated with that number of red cells [21] for delivery to the major iron-dependent systems in the body which include erythropoiesis [22], prostaglandin synthesis [23], collagen synthesis [24] and corticoid synthesis [25]. The nutritional requirements for iron are widely documented and publicized.

Iron, however, is also recognized as a determining factor of microbial cell growth in vitro and in vivo [26] and, recently, a number of investigations have demonstrated that transformed cells acquire the capacity to bind iron through the production of small molecular weight siderophore-like products [27] and expression of surface receptors for transferrin in vitro [28–35] and in vivo [36–38].

The question we wish to consider in this review is this: In countries with adequate iron intake, where the incidence of bacterial infections is low,

[1] Work by the authors was supported by grant No. R01-AM 32363 from the NIH, the Cancer Research Institute (New York), the Jamieson Fund and the Cardinal Fund.

do malignant cells that develop effective mechanisms of iron uptake have a survival advantage? If they do, could this be simply the result of a direct interaction between iron and the malignant cell population or, in addition, can tumor cell growth be favored by the suppressive action of iron and some proteins of iron metabolism on the immune system?

Transferrin Receptors and Malignant Transformation

Transferrin receptor expression has been established as a surface marker of cell proliferation in vitro [28–35]. For the purpose of discussing the question to be considered in this paper, the more relevant data relate to the demonstration that some tumor cells express transferrin receptors in vivo. This has been done in breast cancer [36, 37] and in non-Hodgkin's lymphoma [38].

Transferrin receptors have been identified in breast cancer by immunofluorescence of tissue sections [36] and by the analysis of specific transferrin binding to microsomal preparations of tumor tissue [37]. The data from the specific binding study has been summarized in table I. In an analysis of transferrin binding to 11 primary breast tumors, non-neoplastic breast tissue and normal kidney and placental preparations, *Shindelman* et al. [37] found high levels of specific transferrin binding to the tumors (11–35%) compared to a range of 2–3% in normal tissue and 4.5% in the tissue from dysplastic disease.

Table I. Binding of transferrin to normal and tumor breast tissue [37]

Tissue	Number of cases	Specific % bound range
Infiltrating ductal carcinoma	9	11.2–35
Undifferentiated carcinoma	1	17
Stromal sarcoma	1	30
Male breast (gynecomastia)	1	2.3
Normal female breast	1	2.4
Dysplastic breast	1	4.5
Kidney	1	3.4
Placental brush border membrane	1	44.0

In the non-Hodgkin's lymphoma study, expression of the transferrin receptor was examined by immunofluorescence using the OKT9 monoclonal antibody [32] in lymph node cell suspensions [38]. The frequency of OKT9-positive cells, signifying transferrin receptor expression, correlated significantly with the histological class of the tumor. High-grade lymphomas contained an average of 22.5% positive cells (range 3–57%), low-grade lymphomas contained 2–5% positive cells (range 1–22%). Furthermore, the appearance of high percentages of cells expressing the transferrin receptor was related to poor survival [38]. Based on these observations, *Habeshaw* et al. [38] suggested that 'there is a relation between transferrin receptor and either the growth fraction, or factors affecting the growth fraction of the tumor'.

One host factor that could favor the growth of a malignant cell population expressing transferrin receptors is the degree of transferrin saturation itself. In a preliminary study designed to examine this point, we analyzed the serum iron, transferrin saturation and serum ferritin in 22 children with leukemia. In all cases with a level of bone marrow leukemic blasts higher than 90%, the transferrin saturation was higher than 50%; of the 5 relapses seen in this group (table II) 4 had serum iron levels higher than 100 (range 148–251), transferrin saturation higher than 50% (50–100%) and serum ferritins higher than 1,000 (range 1,370–6,250); only 1 case had the serum iron lower than 100 (75 µg/dl), a transferrin saturation of 23%, and a serum ferritin level of 35 ng/ml. Of the 5 relapses, this is the only child that went into remission and is alive 1 year later; the other 4 never went into remission and died.

Table II. Serum iron, transferrin saturation, serum ferritin levels in 5 childhood leukemia cases in relapse

Diagnosis	BM (%) blasts	Fe, µg/dl	% sat	Ferritin ng/ml	Clinical course
ALL	40	75	23	35	alive
ALL	76	251	86	5,625	dead
AML	90	195	91	1,635	dead
ALL	95	148	50	6,250	dead
ALL	97	206	100	1,370	dead

ALL = Acute lymphoblastic leukemia; AML = acute myeloblastic leukemia.

Ferritin and Cancer

Ferritin represents one other example of a protein classically associated with the metabolism of iron [39] whose appearance in the serum in abnormally high levels has been correlated with poor clinical course in numerous forms of cancer. The impetus for the studies of serum ferritin in malignancy derived from a paper published by *Hazard and Drysdale* [40] in 1977, in which serum ferritin levels were determined by different malignancies using antiferritin antibodies raised against liver (L, basic) ferritin and Hela (H, acidic) type ferritins. The authors suggested from the results of this study that the acidic type of ferritin might be a marker of malignancy [40]. This has not been confirmed in later studies of isoferritins in leukemia [41, 42], lymphoma [43] and solid tumors [44]. We have demonstrated that the relative subunit composition of the ferritin synthesized by all normal cell sets of the immune system is indistinguishable from the subunit composition of the ferritin synthesized by lymphoid cell lines or by selected T cells from lymphoma spleens [45, 46].

The association of ferritin with malignant and not with benign tissue has been documented recently in a study of breast cancer [47]. Ferritin concentration was measured in 44 mammary carcinomas and 14 benign breast tissues. A 6-fold difference was observed in malignant tissue (mean: 364.0 ± 223.3 ng/mcp) versus the benign tissue (mean: $60.2-42.1$ ng/mcp). Direct evidence for the release of ferritin from tumors derives mostly from studies of human serum ferritin levels in nude mice with human tumor implants [48]. In man much greater caution has to be taken in analyzing data from cancer patients who may have received repeated blood transfusions, which contribute to increasing serum ferritin levels [49]. We have been faced recently with this problem, in an analysis of serum ferritin as a marker of clinical course in neuroblastoma [*Potaznik, de Sousa, Groshen, Bhalla, Helson,* in preparation].

Previous studies from *Hann* et al. [50–52] have clearly established high serum ferritin as an indicator of poor clinical course in this childhood malignancy. In our own study of 36 patients with neuroblastoma, we confirmed these conclusions, but in addition we found in all cases a highly significant correlation between number of blood transfusions and serum ferritin. Nevertheless, when the patients were subdivided according to extent of disease in 'bulky', 'minimal' and 'free of disease' groups, the slope of the curve in the bulky disease group was significantly different from the slopes of the curves in the other two groups, suggesting a contribution of the tumor itself to the increasing serum ferritin levels well above the response to the blood transfusions.

Ferritin, Iron and Immunosuppression

The reasons why high serum ferritin levels are associated with poor prognosis in neuroblastoma and in other forms of cancer are not clear. One possible explanation resides in its immunosuppressive action on T cell responses in vitro [18, 19]. In vivo, *Dupont* et al. [53] have also reported a significant correlation between abnormal T4/T8 ratios and serum ferritin levels in multiple-transfused patients; in thalassemia intermedia patients, we have also observed diminished T cell mitogen responses in the group with serum iron higher than 200 µg/dl and serum ferritin higher than 600 ng/ml [8].

Inhibition of E-rosette formation has been demonstrated in vitro, after exposure of human peripheral blood mononuclear cells to ferritin [54] and to increasing concentrations of iron presented to the cells in the form of ferric citrate [5, 6] or fully saturated transferrin [6]. Iron and ferritin have also been shown to inhibit responder cells in the mixed lymphocyte reaction [7, 18].

Conclusion

Neoplastic growth is a complex process dictated in part by cellular sequences which have come to be known as oncogenes [55], and are known to play a role in non-neoplastic growth processes [56]. Once the neoplastic growth process starts, the speed and the degree of malignancy with which it progresses results from a complex network of interactions between host and tumor, whose balance in favor of the host is believed to depend on the cells of the immune system. Therapy strategies of immunotherapy and chemotherapy have taken into account these two elements, ignoring by and large the vast ecology within which their interplay is taking place.

In answer to the question considered at the beginning of this paper, we presented evidence indicating that indeed malignant cells that develop effective mechanisms of iron uptake have a survival advantage to the detriment of the survival of the host [38], and that hosts with high serum iron, high serum transferrin saturations and high serum ferritin may provide a more favorable environment for neoplastic growth (table II). Finally, both iron and ferritin have been shown to have immunosuppressive actions [5–7, 18, 19, 53, 54].

We recognize that a great deal more needs to be done, that evidence from much larger numbers of cases, and much more data from different types of cancer needs to be sought. However, further indirect evidence from population studies is already available: (1) from the known high incidence of cancer in patients with idiopathic hemochromatosis [52]; (2) from the increasing incidence of cancer in countries with low incidence of bacterial infections in which iron fortification programs have been implemented [58, 59].

In Sweden, between 1944 and 1963, the iron fortification of flour was 30 mg/kg; it increased to 50 mg/kg in 1963, and to 65 mg/kg in 1970 [58]. Iron deficiency anemia among Swedish women of child-bearing age dropped from 25–30% in 1963–1964 to 6–7% in 1974–1975 [60]. At approximately the same time, the highest increase in age-standardized cancer incidence rate in Swedish women (per 100,000) observed was in primary liver cancer from 0.9 in 1960 to 3.2 in 1977 [59], an increase by a factor of 3.5, in contrast with the increases in lung and breast cancer by factors of 1.9 and 1.38, respectively.

Thus, based on the small constellation of pieces of direct and indirect evidence presented above, we conclude that the iron store status of the host can be a critical determining ecological influence on neoplastic growth.

References

1   Sousa, M. de: Lymphoid cell positioning: a new proposal for the mechanism of control of lymphoid cell migration. Symp. Soc. exp. Biol. *32:* 393–409 (1983).
2   Nishiya, K.; Chiao, J.W.; Sousa, M. de: Iron binding proteins in selected human peripheral blood cell sets: immunofluorescence. Br. J. Haematol. *46:* 235–245 (1980).
3   Sousa, M. de; Martins da Silva, B.; Dörner, M.; Munn, G.; Nishiya, K.; Grady, R.W.; Silverstone, A.: Iron and the lymphomyeloid system: rationale for considering iron as a target for immune surveillance; in Saltman, Hegenauer, The biochemistry and physiology of iron, pp. 687–698 (Elsevier Biomedical, Amsterdam 1982).
4   Martins da Silva, B.; Pollack, M.S.; Dupont, B.; Sousa, M. de: A study of ferritin secretion by human peripheral blood mononuclear cells in HLA-typed donors; in Saltman, Hegenauer, The biochemistry and physiology of iron, pp. 733–737 (Elsevier Biomedical, Amsterdam 1982).
5   Sousa, M. de; Nishiya, K.: Inhibition of E-rosette formation by two iron salts. Cell. Immunol. *38:* 203–208 (1978).
6   Nishiya, K.; Sousa, M. de; Tsoi, E.; Bognacki, J.; Harven, E. de: Regulation of expression of a human lymphoid cell surface marker by iron. Cell. Immunol. *53:* 71–83 (1980).

7   Bryan, C.F.; Nishiya, K.; Pollack, M.S.; Dupont, B.; Sousa, M. de: Differential inhi-
     bition of the MLR by iron: association with HLA phenotype. Immunogenetics 12:
     129–140 (1981).
8   Munn, C.G.; Markenson, A.L.; Kapadia, A.; Sousa, M. de: Impaired T cell mitogen
     responses in some patients with thalassemia intermedia. Thymus 3: 119–128 (1981).
9   Broxmeyer, H.E.; Smithyman, A.; Eger, R.R.; Meyers, P.A.; Sousa, M. de: Identifi-
     cation of lactoferrin as the granulocyte-derived inhibitor of colony stimulating activ-
     ity production. J. exp. Med. 148: 1052–1067 (1978).
10   Bagby, G.C.; Rigas, V.D.; Bennett, R.M.; Vandenbark, A.A.; Garewal, H.S.: Interac-
     tion of lactoferrin, monocytes and T lymphocyte subsets in the regulation of steady-
     state granulopoiesis in vitro. J. clin. Invest. 68: 56–63 (1981).
11   Duncan, R.L.; McArthur, W.P.: Lactoferrin mediated modulation of mononuclear
     cell activities. Cell. Immunol. 63: 308–320 (1981).
12   Nishiya, K.; Horwitz, D.A.: Contrasting effects of lactoferrin on human lymphocyte
     and monocyte natural killer activity and antibody-dependent cell-mediated cytotox-
     icity. J. Immun. 129: 2519–2523 (1982).
13   Galbraith, R.M.; Werner, P.; Arnaud, P.; Galbraith, G.M.P.: Transferrin binding to
     peripheral blood lymphocytes activated by phytohemagglutinin involves a specific
     receptor. J. clin. Invest. 66: 1135–1143 (1980).
14   Larrick, J.W.; Cresswell, P.: Modulation of cell surface iron transferrin receptors by
     cellular density and state of activation. J. supramol. Struct. 11: 579–586 (1979).
15   Brock, J.H.: The effect of iron and transferrin on the response of serum free cultures
     of mouse lymphocytes to concanavalin A and lipopolysaccharide. Immunology 43:
     387–392 (1981).
16   Brock, J.H.; Rankin, M.C.: Transferrin binding and iron uptake by mouse lymph
     node cells during transformation in response to concanavalin A. Immunology 43:
     393–398 (1981).
17   Tanno, Y.; Arai, S.; Takishima, T.: Iron-containing proteins augment responses of
     human lymphocytes to phytohemagglutinin and pokeweed mitogen in serum free
     medium. Tohoku J. exp. Med. 137: 335–343 (1982).
18   Matzner, Y.; Hershko, C.; Polliack, A.; Konijn, A.M.; Zak, G.: Suppressive effect of
     ferritin on in vitro lymphocyte function. Br. J. Haematol. 42: 345–353 (1979).
19   Hancock, B.W.; Bruce, L.; May, K.; Richmond, J.: Ferritin, a sensitizing substance in
     leukocyte migration inhibition test in patients with malignant lymphoma. Br. J. Hae-
     matol. 43: 223–233 (1979).
20   Bryan, C.F.; Leech, S.H.: The immunoregulatory nature of iron. 1. Lymphocyte pro-
     liferation. Cell. Immunol. 75: 71–79 (1983).
21   Kay, M.M.B.: Cells, signals and receptors; in Aging phenomena: relationships among
     different levels of organization, pp. 171–200 (Plenum Publishing, New York 1980).
22   Jandl, J.H.; Katz, J.H.: The plasma to cell cycle of transferrin. J. clin. Invest. 42:
     314–326 (1963).
23   Rao, G.H.R.; Gerrard, J.M.; Eaton, J.W.; White, J.G.: The role of iron in prostaglan-
     din synthesis: ferrous iron-mediated oxidation of arachidonic acid. Prostaglandins
     Med. 1: 55–70 (1978).
24   Hunt, J.; Richards, R.J.; Harwood, R.; Jacobs, A.: The effect of desferrioxamine on
     fibroblasts and collagen formation in cell cultures. Br. J. Haematol. 41: 69–76
     (1979).

25 Williams Smith, D.L.; Cammack, R.: Oxidation-reduction potentials of cytochromes P-450 and ferredoxin in the bovine adrenal: their modification by substrates and inhibitors. Biochim. biophys. Acta *499:* 432–442 (1977).

26 Weinberg, E.D.: Iron and infection. Microbiol. Rev. *42:* 45–66 (1978).

27 Fernandez-Pol, J.A.: Isolation and characterization of a siderophore-like growth factor from mutants of SV40 transformed cells adapted to picolinic acid. Cell *14:* 489–499 (1978).

28 Hu, H.Y.Y.; Gardner, J.; Aisen, P.; Skoultchi, A.I.: Inducibility of transferrin receptors on Friend erythroleukemic cells. Science *197:* 559–561 (1977).

29 Hamilton, T.A.; Wada, H.G.; Sussman, H.H.: Identification of transferrin receptors on the surface of human cultured cells. Proc. natn. Acad. Sci. USA *76:* 6406–6410 (1979).

30 Larrick, J.W.; Cresswell, P.: Transferrin receptors on human B and T lymphoblastoid cell lines. Biochim. biophys. Acta *583:* 483–490 (1979).

31 Karin, M.; Mintz, B.: Receptor mediated endocytosis of transferrin in developmentally totipotent mouse teratocarcinoma stem cells. J. biol. Chem. *256:* 3245–3252 (1981).

32 Sutherland, R.; Delia, D.; Schneider, C.; Newman, R.; Kemshead, J.; Greaves, M.: Ubiquitous, cell surface glycoprotein on tumor cells is proliferation-associated receptor for transferrin. Proc. natn. Acad. Sci. USA *78:* 4515–4519 (1981).

33 Trowbridge, I.S.; Omary, M.B.: Human cell surface glycoprotein related to cell proliferation is the receptor for transferrin. Proc. natn. Acad. Sci. USA *75:* 3039–3043 (1981).

34 Testa, U.; Thomopoulos, P.; Vinci, G.; Titeux, M.; Bettaieb, A.; Vainchenker, W.; Rochant, H.: Transferrin binding to K562 cell line. Expl Cell Res. *140:* 251–260 (1982).

35 Ward, J.H.; Kushner, J.P.; Kaplan, J.: Regulation of HeLa cell transferrin receptors. J. biol. Chem. *257:* 10317–10323 (1982).

36 Faulk, W.P.; Hsi, B.L.; Stevens, P.J.: Transferrin and transferrin receptors in carcinoma of the breast. Lancet *ii:* 390–392 (1980).

37 Shindelman, J.E.; Ortmeyer, A.E.; Sussman, H.H.: Demonstration of the transferrin receptor in human breast cancer tissue. Potential marker for identifying dividing cells. Int. J. Cancer *27:* 329–334 (1981).

38 Habeshaw, J.A.; Lister, T.A.; Stansfeld, A.G.; Greaves, M.F.: Correlation of transferrin receptor expression with histological class and outcome in non-Hodgkin lymphoma. Lancet *i:* 498–501 (1983).

39 Harrison, P.M.: Ferritin: an iron-storage molecule. Semin. Hematol. *14:* 55–70 (1977).

40 Hazard, J.T.; Drysdale, J.W.: Ferritinaemia in cancer. Nature, Lond. *265:* 755–756 (1977).

41 Cragg, S.J.; Jacobs, A.; Parry, D.H.; Wagstaff, M.; Worwood, M.: Isoferritins in acute leukemia. Br. J. Cancer *35:* 635–642 (1977).

42 Wagstaff, M.; Worwood, M.; Jacobs, A.: Biochemical and immunological characterization of ferritin from leukaemic cells. Br. J. Haematol. *45:* 263–274 (1980).

43 Grail, A.; Hancock, B.W.; Harrison, P.M.: Serum ferritin in normal individuals and in patients with malignant lymphomas and chronic renal failure measured with seven different commercial immunoassay techniques. J. clin. Path. *35:* 1204–1212 (1982).

44   Linder, M.C.; Wright, K.; Madara, F.: Concentration, structure and iron saturation of ferritins from normal human lung and lung tumors with graded histopathology. Enzyme 27: 189–198 (1982).

45   Dörner, M.; Silverstone, A.; Nishiya, K.; Sostoa, A. de; Munn, C.G.; Sousa, M. de: Ferritin synthesis by human T lymphocytes. Science 209: 1019–1021 (1980).

46   Dörner, M.H.; Silverstone, A.E.; Sostoa, A. de; Munn, C.G.; Sousa, M. de: Relative subunit composition of the ferritin synthesized by selected human lymphomyeloid cell populations. Exp. Hematol. 11: 866–872 (1983).

47   Weinstein, R.E.; Bond, B.H.; Silberberg, B.K.: Tissue ferritin concentration in carcinoma of the breast. Cancer 50: 2406–2409 (1982).

48   Watanabe, N.; Niitsu, Y.; Koseki, J.; Oikawa, J.; Kadono, Y.; Ishii, T.; Goto, Y.; Onodera, Y.; Urushizaki, I.: Ferritinemia in nude mice bearing various human carcinomas; in Lehmann, Carcino-embryonic proteins, vol. 1, pp. 273–278 (Elsevier/North-Holland Biomedical Press, Amsterdam 1979).

49   Letsky, E.A.; Miller, F.; Worwood, M.; Flynn, D.M.: Serum ferritin in children with thalassemia regularly transfused. J. clin. Path. 27: 652–655 (1974).

50   Hann, H.L.; Levy, H.M.; Evans, A.E.: Serum ferritin as a guide to therapy in neuroblastoma. Cancer Res. 40: 1411–1413 (1980).

51   Hann, H.L.; Evans, A.E.; Cohen, I.J.; Leitmeyer, J.E.: Biologic differences between neuroblastoma stages IV-S and IV. Measurement of serum ferritin and E-rosette inhibition in 30 children. New Engl. J. Med. 305: 425–428 (1981).

52   Hann, H.L.; Levy, H.M.; Evans, A.E.: Ferritin and cancer: study of isoferritins in patients with neuroblastoma; in Evans, Adv. Neuroblastoma Res., pp. 43–48 (Raven Press, New York 1980).

53   Dupont, E.; Vereerstraeten, P.; Espinosa, O.; Tielemans, C.; Dhaene, M.; Wybran, J.: Multiple transfusions and T cell subsets: a role for ferritin? Transplantation 35: 508–510 (1983).

54   Moroz, C.; Lahat, N.; Biniaminov, M.; Ramot, B.: Ferritin on the surface of lymphocytes in Hodgkin's disease patients. A possible blocking substance removed by levamisole. Clin. exp. Immunol. 29: 30–35 (1977).

55   Cooper, G.M.: Cellular transforming genes. Science 217: 801–806 (1982).

56   Goyette, M.; Petropoulos, C.J.; Shank, P.R.; Fausto, N.: Expression of a cellular oncogene during liver regeneration. Science 219: 510–512 (1983).

57   Bomford, A.; Williams, R.: Long-term venesection therapy in idiopathic hemochromatosis. Q. Jl Med. 45: 611–623 (1976).

58   Bothwell, T.H.; Charlton, R.W.: Nutritional aspects of iron deficiency; in Saltmann, Hegenauer, The biochemistry and physiology of iron, pp. 749–766 (Elsevier/North-Holland, Amsterdam 1981).

59   Cancer Incidence in Sweden 1977. National Board of Health and Welfare. The Cancer Registry, Stockholm (1981).

60   Hallberg, L.; Bengtsson, C.; Ciarby, L.; Lennartsson, J.; Rossander, L.; Tibblin, E.: An analysis of factors leading to a reduction in iron deficiency in Swedish women. Bull. Wld Hlth Org. (1979).

M. de Sousa, MD, Cell Ecology, Sloan-Kettering Institute for Cancer Research, New York, NY 10021 (USA)

Prasad (ed.), Vitamins, Nutrition, and Cancer, pp. 240–250 (Karger, Basel 1984)

Selenium in Nutritional Cancer Prophylaxis: An Update

Gerhard N. Schrauzer

Department of Chemistry, University of California at San Diego, La Jolla, Calif., USA

Introduction

Recent research has drawn attention to the roles of dietary trace elements as inhibitors or promoters of carcinogenesis. The essential trace element *selenium* in particular has gained recognition as a nutritional anticancer agent and is expected to play a major role in future programs of *nutritional cancer prophylaxis*. Before describing some of the advances in this field it is necessary, however, to define the scope of 'nutritional cancer prophylaxis'. It aims, by definition, at establishing dietary guidelines for the protection of individuals or population groups against cancer by nutritional means. Because of the different regulations governing foods, food additives and drugs, nutritional cancer prophylaxis must be distinguished from *cancer chemoprevention*. Research in this area attempts to identify anticancer agents among synthetic antioxidants, food additives and drugs. Selenium has been sometimes included among the chemopreventive agents. However, for the applications which I have in mind, it should be regarded as a nutritional prophylactic rather than chemopreventive agent. Nutritional cancer prophylaxis aims to protect the healthy and thus must be clearly distinguished from any form of *nutritional cancer therapy*. To be relevant for nutritional prophylaxis, experimental designs should reflect the nutritional rather than therapeutic approach to the problem. Our research during the past 15 years has followed that direction.

Selenium: Essential Element and 'Resistance Factor'

Essentiality of Selenium

Selenium was considered to be an environmental poison until it was shown in 1957 to prevent dietary liver necrosis in rats [1]. Subsequently, selenium deficiency was associated with previously widespread diseases of farm animals such as white muscle disease in lambs and goats, 'ill thrift' and reproductive failure in cattle, and exudative diathesis in chicks [2]. Human selenium deficiency syndromes were for long believed to be nonexistent. Recent reports from China, however, provided striking evidence to the contrary and produced an upsurge of interest in nutritional selenium research.

Keshan disease, a cardiomyopathy for long claimed thousands of victims each year until it was found to be limited to areas extremely low in selenium. Although the disease is not caused by selenium deficiency alone (a Coxsackie-type virus has been implicated as the agent causing the myocardial lesions), selenium supplementation of the population at risk led to the virtual eradication of the disease [3]. In other low-selenium regions of central China, a condition known as *Kaschin-Beck syndrome* or 'big joint disease', characterized by inflammation, swelling and degenerative changes of the joints, was linked to selenium deficiency [4]. Selenium supplementation is effective in the prevention of this disease. A lack of selenium has also been associated with accelerated aging, the increased deposition of lipofuscin, the formation of cataracts and other degenerative conditions in old age [5].

Glutathione Peroxidase

Selenium deficiency diseases in animals are mainly caused by a lack of the enzyme glutathione peroxidase (GSH/Px), which was shown to be selenium-dependent [6]. This enzyme protects cell membranes and tissues against the destructive effects of OH radicals generated as by-products of lipid peroxidation. There is a synergistic association of selenium with vitamin E.

Selenium as a Resistance Factor

Apart from its functions as an essential micronutrient, selenium also appears to have other physiological functions in which it acts as a physiological *resistance factor.* Its cancer protecting effects fall into this category.

In addition, selenium protects against free radicals, mutagens, toxic heavy metals and certain bacterial, fungal and viral pathogens. The selenium requirement increases under stress, just as the requirements for certain vitamins increase during infections.

Anticarcinogenic Effects of Selenium

Experiments with C3H/St Mice

To demonstrate a protecting effect of selenium on mammary tumorigenesis we used female C3H/St mice infected with the 'Bittner milk factor', a b-type RNA tumor virus. Animals of this strain develop mammary adenocarcinoma with 80–100% incidence under normal maintenance conditions. This tumor model system is particularly relevant for human breast as antigenic components identical to those against the murine mammary tumor virus have been detected in a significant percentage of human breast cancer tissues [7].

Mammary tumors develop in female C3H/St mice with the expected high incidence if they are maintained on standard laboratory diets. These usually contain no more than 0.2 ppm selenium, sufficient only to prevent nutritional selenium deficiency. The average American diet usually contains only 0.1–0.15 ppm selenium and thus would also not be expected to protect against the carcinogenic effects of tumor viruses.

In a series of initial life-term experiments, 0.1–2 ppm of additional selenium was supplied in the drinking water in the form of selenite. A significant reduction of the tumor incidence was observed, optimally at selenium concentrations of 1–2 ppm [8–11]. Since selenite is not a normal dietary form of selenium, experiments were also performed in which nutritional organic forms of the element, such as present in specially grown yeast, were added to the diet. These natural organic forms of selenium also caused significant reductions of the mammary tumor incidence. At concentrations of up to 2 ppm of selenium the tumor incidence was reduced without causing adverse effects on weight gains, reproductive performance and survival [12]. For maximum protective effect, selenium supplementation must be introduced as early in the life of the animals as possible. This is because malignant transformation may occur even in very young animals and selenium exerts its protective effects only prior to this event.

Selenium supplementation must be maintained over the entire life span. Midlife cessation of selenium supplementation resulted in a subsequent rapid increase of the number of tumors; the tumor incidence ultimately became the same as that of the unsupplemented controls [12]. This experiment shows that selenium exerts no long-term protecting effects against virally induced cancer, consistent with its role as a water-soluble micronutrient.

Effect of Selenium on Tumors

Selenium supplementation of the diet of animals with established spontaneous or transplanted mammary tumors produced a diminution of tumor growth rates [8]; however, genuine remissions were not observed. Certain malignant cell lines are susceptible to selenium preparations at pharmacological dosage. However, detailed discussion of these therapeutic experiments is outside the scope of this review [see ref. 13–15].

Mechanisms of Anticarcinogenic Action

Effects of Selenium on Cell Division

In chemical carcinogenesis, selenium inhibits activation and accelerates detoxification of the carcinogenic substances. It also protects against carcinogen-induced chromosomal damage, inhibits the mutagenicity of direct and indirect acting carcinogens and appears to stimulate DNA repair processes. Selenium in various forms of administration (not necessarily nutritional) has by now been shown to prevent or retard tumorigenesis induced by virtually all of the major known chemical carcinogens.

Several years ago, I proposed that selenium exerts its anticarcinogenic effects by modulating the rate of cell division [16]. In cells infected with tumor virus, a modulation of the rate of mitosis could prevent the integration of cellular with viral DNA and thus prevent malignant transformation. In chemical carcinogenesis, diminution of the rates of certain phases of cell division could prevent the expression of cancer genes, create conditions favorable for DNA repair and carcinogen detoxification.

Inhibitory effects of selenite on cell division and growth have been observed for example in cultures of HeLa S3 and Galeati-Lieberkuehn cells. With HeLa S3 cells, the threshold of inhibition of protein biosynthesis was observed at intracellular selenium concentrations of 0.5 ppm; DNA and RNA biosynthesis is inhibited at higher selenium levels. Although the cells eventually become completely nonviable they are not damaged by selenite even at intracellular concentrations of 130 ppm; normal growth resumes on transfer into low-selenium media [17, 18].

Reactions with GSH and Other Intracellular SH Compounds

Selenium is a catalyst of oxidation-reduction reactions involving thiols and disulfides. In these reactions, selenotrisulfides (RSSeSR) are the reactive intermediates. Since selenodiglutathione (GSSeSG) inhibits protein biosynthesis of rat liver polyribosomes [19], it is reasonable to assume that GSSeSG could be formed and that it possibly plays a role in controlling the rate of cell division. That dietary selenium interacts with intracellular reduced glutathione (GSH) and other SH compounds follows from recent work with rats exposed to 6 ppm of dietary selenium in form of selenite [20]. Hepatic oxidized glutathione (GSSG) and nonprotein SH levels increased in the selenium-exposed rats. However, the question as to which specific enzyme, protein or other cellular component is reacting with selenium and is ultimately responsible for its protective effect cannot be answered and is probably unanswerable in view of the complexity of the process of malignant transformation and because of the strong interdependence of the processes associated with mitosis and malignant transformation.

Alteration of Carcinogen Metabolism

In rats exposed to s-dimethylhydrazine (DMH), selenium pretreatment slowed down DNA biosynthesis in cells of large intestine [21], consistent with the proposed modulating effect of selenium on mitosis. In addition, DMH metabolism was altered as well, providing an example for the possible role of selenium in the detoxification of carcinogens.

Immunopotentiation

Other mechanisms of anticarcinogenic action to be mentioned in this context include the *stimulation of the immune system*. Immunopotentiation by selenium has been demonstrated in several animal model systems [22]. Selenium-mediated immunopotentiation may increase natural tumor resistance and could thus become important both for cancer therapy and prophylaxis. In one pertinent experiment with tumor-bearing mice, infection with *Corynebacterium parvum* did not improve survival except in animals pretreated with selenium [23].

Selenium Antagonists

Many elements and compounds with high chemical affinities for selenium possess selenium-antagonistic properties. This includes elements such as Pb, Cd, Hg, Sn, Ag, whose adventitious presence in foods and in the environment thus is not only of toxicological significance but must now also be viewed in relation to the cancer problem.

Experiments with female C3H/St mice showed that the cancer-protecting effects of selenium are abolished for example by arsenite and Pb^{2+} at comparatively low dosage levels [24, 25]. Both elements also increased tumor growth rates. Even zinc, itself an essential element, is a selenium antagonist. In experiments with C3H/St mice, zinc abolished the anticarcinogenic effects of selenium and stimulated tumor growth [9]. In vitro, addition of selenite to the medium caused a significant inhibition of RNA-dependent DNA polymerase activity in Rauscher leukemia cells [26]. DNA polymerases are zinc-dependent enzymes but could be envisaged to be susceptible to inhibition by selenium. It should also be noted that a variety of heavy metals are usually detected in DNA and RNA preparations whose biological significance is not yet understood [27]. Some of the metals which have been detected are known to increase the frequency of misincorporation and other errors in replication. Intracellular selenium could inactivate these metals by forming stable complexes. The observed interactions of zinc with selenium suggested that diets too rich in zinc increase the human cancer risk; this hypothesis is supported by epidemiological studies [28].

As casein-rich diets are known to prevent selenium toxicity in rats [29], it is possible that the ingestion of protein-rich diets may increase the selenium requirement for cancer protection. The same is true for unsaturated fats which are known to increase the selenium requirement. Conversely, by selecting diets low in selenium-antagonistic metals, adequate but not excessive in zinc and proteins and low in unsaturated fats, it should be possible to achieve protection of experimental animals against cancer with less than the presently considered optimal amounts of selenium.

Epidemiological Evidence

Several epidemiological studies have demonstrated inverse associations between human cancer mortalities and regional availabilities of selenium, dietary selenium intakes and blood selenium levels [30–32]. In the following, only the results of some of the most recent studies will be discussed.

Lung Cancer in China [33]

Serum selenium levels of residents in areas with high and low incidence of lung cancer were found to differ substantially. The serum selenium levels of healthy subjects and of lung cancer patients in the high lung cancer region were 0.088 ± 0.001 and 0.070 ± 0.013 ppm, respectively. In a low lung cancer region they were 0.123 ± 0.002 ppm. The selenium levels are similar to those reported previously, for example, for healthy adults (0.102 ± 0.018 ppm), hospitalized patients (0.088 ± 0.021 ppm) and hospitalized cancer cases (0.070 ± 0.013 ppm), in San Diego, Calif., collected in 1972 [34].

Skin Cancer in North Carolina [35]

Although several previous studies indicated lower serum or plasma selenium levels in cancer patients than in noncancer patients or healthy subjects, these are not necessarily conclusive as cancer patients may be low in selenium for reasons unrelated to diet. One case-control study which does not suffer from this potential shortcoming involved 240 cancer patients examined at the Wilson Dermatology Clinic in Wilson, North Carolina, between 1974 and 1980. The odds ratio for the lowest versus the highest decile of plasma selenium versus current or past clinic controls was 4.39 or 5.81, respectively. Since all patients in this study were light ambulatory cases, the disease itself could not have had any major effect on plasma selenium concentrations. In the range of plasma selenium concentrations from 0.22 to 0.08 ppm, the skin cancer odds ratio, corrected for variations in age, sun damage, etc., increased monotonously 4- to 6-fold with decreasing plasma selenium.

Gastrointestinal and Other Cancers in the USA [36]

In 1973–1974, participants of the Hypertension Detection and Follow-up Program collected serum samples of 10,940 hypertensive, otherwise healthy, men and women from various parts of the USA and stored for later analyses. During the subsequent 5 years, 111 of the subjects developed cancer, mainly of the gastrointestinal tract. Serum selenium levels of the cancer cases were significantly lower than those of 210 controls from the same set, matched for age, race, sex and smoking history. The relative cancer risk in the lowest quintile of serum selenium (0.107 μg/ml) was twice that of subjects in the highest quintile (0.172 μg/ml). The risk associated with low selenium was even greater if serum vitamin E and retinol were also low.

Selenium Supplementation

The studies in the preceding section indicate that plasma selenium levels below 0.10 ppm are associated with increased cancer risks, while significantly lower cancer risks are observed for plasma selenium levels of 0.2 ppm or more. *Schrauzer* et al. [28] suggested that the doubling of the current US per capita selenium intakes to about 250–300 µg/day would be required to more fully utilize the cancer-protecting potential of selenium. The epidemiological observations discussed above support this proposal.

Dietary selenium intakes of about 250–300 µg/day could be reached in the selenium-adequate region by a modifications of the diet, i.e. through the increased consumption of whole grain cereals, organ meats and seafoods at the expense of animal fats and refined carbohydrates. However, in low selenium regions this would not work unless selenium-rich foods were specifically transported into these areas or foods were fortified with appropriate forms of selenium. Since none of this can be expected to happen within the forseeable future, extradietary supplementation is the only available means for the improvement of selenium status.

Extradietary selenium supplementation can be recommended for humans only if the supplements contain the element in the same forms as found in common foods [37]. Selenium-rich yeast preparations were first developed and introduced commercially for human supplementation around 1976 [38]. They consist of Brewer's yeast *(Saccharomyces cerevisiae)* grown in selenium-containing media and contain selenium mainly form of seleno-amino acids such as selenomethionine. The bioavailability of yeast selenium is high and comparable to that of high selenium wheat [39]. In addition, however, various artificially selenized supplements containing inorganic selenium compounds are also marketed, which are of little or no value. The daily administration of 150 µg of selenium as present in such supplements failed to raise blood selenium levels of healthy human subjects during a 5-week loading test, in contrast to the significant increase of the blood selenium concentrations on administration of same amount of selenium in form of high selenium yeast [37].

Working with healthy adults we previously observed a linear association between the whole blood selenium concentrations and the dietary selenium intakes in terms of equation 1 [40]:

$$[Se]_{Blood} = 0.0009057 \times [Se]_{intake} + 0.0595, \tag{1}$$

wherein $[Se]_{Blood}$ is the selenium concentration in whole blood in µg/ml and $[Se]_{intake}$ is the mean daily total dietary selenium intake in µg/day.

At selenium intakes of 250–300 µg/day, adult blood selenium concentrations are expected to increase to, and become stationary at, about 0.25–0.33 ppm. The serum selenium concentrations would reach approximately 0.15–0.18 ppm, which would place the selenium-supplemented subjects into the highest quintiles or deciles of baseline serum selenium levels of references 35 and 36. Dietary intakes of selenium of this order thus would lower the cancer risk, are safe and reasonably far removed from the lower limit of chronic selenium toxicity that they can be recommended as a general means of nutritional cancer prophylaxis.

Concluding Remarks

Still only few years ago it was almost generally accepted that the dietary selenium supply of Americans is fully adequate and extradietary supplementation was considered unnecessary. This view is now changing as an increasing number of studies reaffirm the cancer-protecting effects of selenium. Several large-scale intervention studies are presently being planned which should provide the ultimate proof of the value of selenium in nutritional cancer prophylaxis.

References

1 Schwarz, K.; Foltz, C.M.: Selenium as an integral part of factor 3 against dietary necrotic liver degeneration. J. Am. chem. Soc. 79: 3292–3293 (1957).
2 Spallholz, J.E.; Martin, J.L.; Ganther, H.E.: Selenium in biology and medicine (Avi Publishing, Westport 1981).
3 Chen, X.; Yang, G.; Chen, J.; Chen, X.; Wen, Z.; Ge, K.: Studies on the relations of selenium and Keshan disease. Biol. Trace Element Res. 2: 91–107 (1980).
4 Li, J.; Ren, S.; Chen, D.: A study of Kaschin-Beck disease associated with environmental selenium in Shanxi area. Huanjing Kexue Xuebao 2: 91–101 (1982).
5 Shamberger, R.J.: Biochemistry of selenium, pp. 254–257, and references cited therein (Plenum Publishing, New York 1983).
6 Rotruck, J.T.; Pope, A.L.; Ganther, H.E.; Swanson, A.B.; Hafeman, D.G.; Hoekstra, W.G.: Selenium: biochemical role as a component of glutathione peroxidase. Science 179: 588–590 (1973).
7 Mesa-Tejada, R.; Keydar, I.; Ramanarayanan, M.; Ohno, T.; Fenoglio, C.; Spiegelman, S.: Immunohistochemical evidence for RNA virus related components in human breast cancer. Ann. clin. Lab. Sci. 9: 202–211 (1979).

8   Schrauzer, G.N.; Ishmael, D.: Effects of selenium and of arsenic on the genesis of spontaneous mammary tumors in inbred C3H/St mice. Ann. clin. Lab. Sci. *4:* 441–447 (1974).

9   Schrauzer, G.N.; White, D.A.; Schneider, C.J.: Inhibition of the genesis of spontaneous mammary tumors in C3H mice. Effects of selenium and of selenium antagonistic elements and their possible role in human breast cancer. Bioinorg. Chem. *6:* 265–270 (1976).

10   Schrauzer, G.N.; White, D.A.; Schneider, C.J.: Selenium and cancer. Effects of selenium and of the diet on the genesis of spontaneous mammary tumors in virgin inbred female C3H/St mice. Bioinorg. Chem. *8:* 387–396 (1978).

11   Medina, D.; Shepherd, F.: Selenium-mediated inhibition of mouse mammary tumorigenesis. Cancer Lett. *8:* 241–245 (1980).

12   Schrauzer, G.N.; McGinness, J.E.; Kuehn, K.: Effects of temporary selenium supplementation on the genesis of spontaneous mammary tumors in inbred female C3H/St mice. Carcinogenesis *1:* 199–201 (1980).

13   Greeder, G.A.; Milner, J.A.: Factors influencing the inhibitory effect of selenium on mice inoculated with Ehrlich ascites tumor cells. Science *209:* 825–827 (1980).

14   Ip, C.: Factors influencing the anticarcinogenic efficacy of selenium in DMBA-induced mammary tumorigenesis in rats. Cancer Res. *41:* 2683–2686 (1981).

15   Jacobs, M.M.; Jansson, B.; Griffin, A.C.: Inhibitory effects of selenium on 1,2-dimethylhydrazine and methylmethoxyazomethanol acetate induction of colon tumors. Cancer Lett. *2:* 133–138 (1977).

16   Schrauzer, G.N.: Trace elements in carcinogenesis; in Draper, Adv. Nutr. Res., vol. 2, pp. 219–244 (1979).

17   Vallini, R.; Faveri, P.; Sarto, G.: Activity of sodium selenate on intestinal mitosis in mice. Ann. Univ. Ferrara *11:* 17–33 (1972).

18   Gruenwedel, D.W.; Cruishank, M.K.: The influence of sodium selenite on the viability and intracellular synthetic activity (DNA, RNA and protein synthesis) of HeLa S3 cells. Toxicol. appl. Pharmacol. *50:* 1–7 (1979).

19   Vernie, L.N.; Collard, J.G.; Eker, A.P.M.; De Wildt, A.; Wilders, I.T.: Studies on the inhibition of protein synthesis by selenodiglutathione. Biochem. J. *180:* 213–218 (1979).

20   LeBoeuf, R.A.; Hoekstra, W.G.: Adaptive changes in hepatic glutathione metabolism in response to excess selenium in rats. J. Nutr. *113:* 845–854 (1983).

21   Harbach, P.R.; Swenberg, J.A.: Effects of selenium on 1,2-dimethylhydrazine metabolism and DNA alkylation. Carcinogenesis *2:* 575–580 (1981).

22   Martin, J.L.; Spallholz, J.S.: Selenium in the immune response. Proc. Symp. Selenium-Tellurium in the Environment, Notre Dame 1976, pp. 204–209 (Industrial Health Foundation, Pittsburgh 1976).

23   Howells, J.M.; Crounse, R.G.; Thomas, J.M.; Whitly, T.K.; Finn, M.; Bray, J.T.; Smith, A.M.; Jones, C.: Prolonged survival of Balb/c mice with a transplanted tumor (MOPC 467) induced by oral selenium plus immunoactivation with *C. parvum.* Abstr., 1st Ann. Scient. Meet., SEGH, East Carolina U., Greenville 1982.

24   Schrauzer, G.N.; White, D.A.; McGinness, J.E.; Schneider, C.J.; Bell, L.J.: Arsenic and cancer: effects of the joint administration of arsenic and of selenium on the genesis of spontaneous mammary tumors in mice. Bioinorg. Chem. *9:* 245–253 (1978).

25 Schrauzer, G.N.; Kuehn, K.; Hamm, D.: Effects of dietary selenium and of lead on the genesis of spontaneous mammary tumors in mice. Biol. Trace Element Res. *3:* 185–196 (1981).

26 Balansky, R.M.; Argirova, R.M.: Sodium selenite inhibition of the reproduction of some oncogenic RNA-viruses. Experientia *37:* 1194 (1981).

27 Guille, E.; Grisvard, J.; Sissoeff, I.: Implications of reiterative DNA-metal ion complexes in the induction and development of neoplastic cells. Biol. Trace Element Res. *1:* 299–311 (1979).

28 Schrauzer, G.N.; White, D.A.; Schneider, C.J.: Cancer mortality correlation studies. IV. Association of dietary intakes and blood levels of certain trace elements, notably selenium antagonists. Bioinorg. Chem. *7:* 35–56 (1977).

29 Moxon, A.L.; Rhian, M.: Selenium toxicity. Physiol. Rev. *23:* 305 (1943).

30 Schrauzer, G.N.: Selenium and cancer. A Review. Bioinorg. Chem. *5:* 275–291 (1975).

31 Shamberger, R.J.; Willis, C.E.: Selenium distribution and human cancer mortality. Crit. Rev. clin. Lab. Sci. *2:* 211–221 (1971).

32 Schrauzer, G.N.; White, D.A.; Schneider, C.J.: Cancer mortality correlation studies. III. Statistical associations with dietary selenium intakes. Bioinorg. Chem. *6:* 265–270 (1977).

33 Zhu, Y.; Liu, Q.; Hou, C.; Yu, S.: Serum selenium concentrations in high and low lung CA regions of China. Zhongua Zhonglia Zazhi *4:* 158 (1982).

34 Schrauzer, G.N.; Rhead, W.J.; Evans, J.A.: Selenium and cancer. Chemical interpretation of a plasma cancer test. Bioinorg. Chem. *2:* 329–340 (1973).

35 Clark, L.C.; Graham, G.F.; Crounse, R.G.; Grimson, R.; Hulka, B.; Shy, C.M.: Plasma selenium and skin neoplasms: a case control study. Abstr., 1st Ann. Sci. Meet., SEGH, Greenville 1982.

36 Willett, W.C.; Morris, J.S.; Pressel, S.; Taylor, J.O.; Polk, B.F.; Stampfer, M.J.; Rosner, B.; Schneider, K.; Hames, C.G.: Prediagnostic serum selenium and risk of cancer. Lancet *July 6:* 130–134 (1983).

37 Schrauzer, G.N.; McGinness, J.E.: Observations on human selenium supplementation. Trace Subst. in Environm. Health XIII, pp. 64–67 (1979).

38 Boynton, H.: Nutrition 21, San Diego, Calif.

39 Levander, O.A.; Alfthan, G.; Arvilommi, H.; Gref, C.G.; Huttunen, J.K.; Kataja, M.; Koivistoinen, P.; Pikkarainen, J.: Bioavailability of selenium to Finnish men as assessed by platelet glutathione peroxidase activity. Abstracts, Int. Symp. Hlth Eff. and Interact. of Ess. and Tox. Elements, Lund 1983, p. 134.

40 Schrauzer, G.N.; White, D.A.: Selenium in human nutrition. Dietary intakes and effects of supplementation. Bioinorg. Chem. *8:* 303–318 (1978).

Prof. G.N. Schrauzer, PhD, Department of Chemistry,
University of California at San Diego, La Jolla, CA 92093 (USA)

Prasad (ed.), Vitamins, Nutrition, and Cancer, pp. 251–265 (Karger, Basel 1984)

Vitamin B$_6$ Metabolism in Relation to Morris Hepatomas

John W. Thanassi

Department of Biochemistry, University of Vermont, College of Medicine, Burlington, Vt., USA

Introduction

Pyridoxal-5′-phosphate, the coenzymatically active form of vitamin B$_6$, is essential for the action of a large number of enzymes involved in the intermediary metabolism of amino acids [1, 2]. The mechanistic aspects of its catalytic roles in such enzymes have been studied extensively [3, 4]. Other roles for pyridoxal-5′-phosphate also have been suggested, for example, in lymphoid and immune system function [5], blood coagulation [6] and, most recently, in steroid receptor function [7, 8]. In addition, pyridoxal-5′-phosphate has been used widely in various kinds of biological studies as a labelling reagent and chromophoric reporter group because of its ability to bind to reactive ε-amino groups of lysine residues in proteins [9, 10]. Thus, the versatile nature of this particular form of vitamin B$_6$ makes it unique among the essential micronutrients.

Because pyridoxal-5′-phosphate is the vitamer form of interest, it is apparent that other vitamer forms, such as pyridoxine, must undergo transformation in vivo. The conversion of precursor vitamer forms to pyridoxal-5′-phosphate involves the actions of an oxidase and kinase as shown in figure 1 [11]. Pyridoxal-5′-phosphate also can be formed from pyridoxamine-5′-phosphate via transamination reactions as indicated in figure 1 but these reactions do not lead to the net synthesis of pyridoxal-5′-phosphate.

If one assumes that pyridoxal-5′-phosphate is a micronutrient essential for the growth of tumors as it is for growth in normal tissues, then it is rather

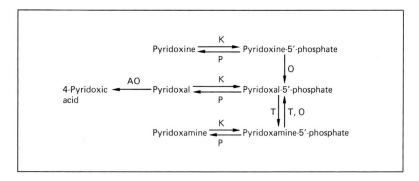

Fig. 1. Major routes of vitamin B$_6$ metabolism in mammalian cells. K = Pyridoxine (pyridoxal, pyridoxamine) kinase; O = pyridoxine (pyridoxamine)-5'-phosphate oxidase; P = pyridoxine (pyridoxal, pyridoxamine)-5'-phosphate phosphatase; T = amino acid transaminases; AO = aldehyde oxidase [19].

surprising that there was essentially no information on vitamin B$_6$ metabolism in tumors prior to the initiation of our own investigations several years ago. Certainly, there had been reports on the effects of vitamin B$_6$ nutriture [12, 13] and vitamin B$_6$ antagonists [14] in neoplasia but virtually nothing was known about how tumors might deal with coenzymatically inactive B$_6$ vitamer forms.

Accordingly, we chose to study vitamin B$_6$ metabolism in Morris hepatomas. The rationale for the choice of these tumors follows. First, liver is the organ having the key role in the conversion of B$_6$ vitamer forms to pyridoxal-5'-phosphate and its subsequent export as a complex with albumin [15]. It follows that the transplantable liver-derived Morris hepatomas are particularly attractive tumors in which to study vitamin B$_6$ metabolism. Second, rapidly growing, normal hepatic tissue, i.e. regenerating rat liver after subtotal hepatectomy, can serve as a reference tissue for rapidly growing neoplastic hepatic tissue in the form of Morris hepatomas. Third, the available spectrum of Morris hepatomas [16] which ranges from highly differentiated, slowly growing, e.g. 9618A, to poorly differentiated, rapidly growing, e.g. 7777, might allow one to establish if there are correlations between the patterns of vitamin B$_6$ metabolism and the differentiation and growth characteristics of the hepatomas. Studies of this kind reveal that there can be 'progression-linked' alterations of enzyme activity patterns and have been performed most extensively by *Weber* [17]. Fourth, fetal, neonatal and adult rat liver provide normal controls for hepatic tissue at various stages of differentiation. It is within this general frame of reference that we carried out our studies on vitamin B$_6$ metabolism in Morris hepatomas.

Materials and Methods

The details of the experimental procedures employed have been described elsewhere. These include methods for the determination of pyridoxal-5'-phosphate and the activities of pyridoxine kinase, pyridoxine-5'-phosphate oxidase, pyridoxine-5'-phosphate phosphatase [18] and ornithine decarboxylase [19]. Purification of rat liver pyridoxine-5'-phosphate oxidase and preparation of rabbit antibodies to it have also been described [20]. Morris hepatomas were grown in the hind legs of Buffalo rats [19, 21] which, depending on the experiments, were fed either Purina laboratory chow [21] or a defined diet [19].

Results and Discussion

Effects of Vitamin B$_6$ Nutriture on the Pyridoxal-5'-Phosphate Content of Morris Hepatoma 7777

Morris hepatoma 7777 is a rapidly growing, poorly differentiated tumor. We have determined the amount of pyridoxal-5'-phosphate in this hepatoma, in host liver from hepatoma-bearing animals, and in control liver from Buffalo rats fed pyridoxine-sufficient and pyridoxine-deficient diets [19]. The results are provided in figure 2. From the data presented in figure 2, one can conclude that the presence of the hepatoma has relatively little effect on the pyridoxal phosphate content of host liver when compared to liver from control animals. Particularly evident is the fact that the hepatomas have markedly lower levels of pyridoxal phosphate than either host or control livers, amounting to approximately 40% of the host liver values in animals fed the pyridoxine-sufficient diet and only 15% of the host liver values in animals fed the deficient diet. The difference in hepatoma pyridoxal phosphate content between the two diets is approximately 80% whereas the corresponding difference in host liver is only about 40%. Thus, the hepatoma appears to lose its pyridoxal phosphate about twice as readily as host liver when animals are fed a pyridoxine-deficient diet. These data and the data displayed in figure 3 are similar in kind to those reported by *Reynolds and Morris* [22] who found that the pyridoxal phosphate contents of six different hepatoma lines were markedly less than those found in host livers, ranging from a low of 9% to a high of 57% of the values in host livers.

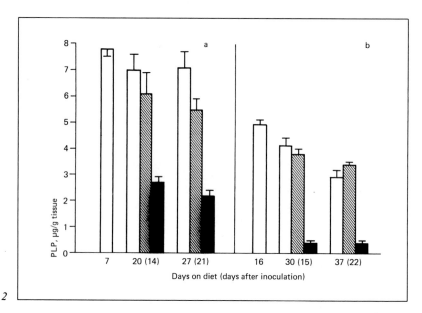

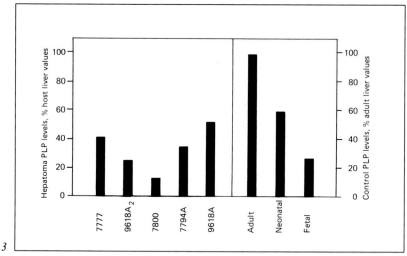

Fig. 2. Pyridoxal-5′-phosphate (PLP) levels in livers and Morris hepatoma 7777 of rats maintained on pyridoxine-sufficient and pyridoxine-deficient diets (panels a and b, respectively). Open bars = livers from control animals; striped bars = host livers from hepatoma-bearing animals; solid bars = Morris hepatoma 7777. Each group was comprised of 3 or 4 animals [19].

Fig. 3. Pyridoxal-5′-phosphate (PLP) levels in Morris hepatomas and rat liver at various stages of development.

Table I. PLP content (µg/g liver) of rat liver[1]

Hours after surgery	Control diet		Pyridoxine-deficient diet	
	sham-operated	hepatectomized	sham-operated	hepatectomized
0	6.3 ± 0.4	–	2.0 ± 0.2	–
4	7.0 ± 0.5	6.5 ± 0.7	2.1 ± 0.4	2.2 ± 0.2
12	7.6 ± 0.6	5.2 ± 0.5	2.2 ± 0.3	2.5 ± 0.2
24	7.7 ± 0.6	6.2 ± 1.0	2.8 ± 0.3	2.8 ± 0.4
72	7.6 ± 0.6	7.1 ± 0.7	2.4 ± 0.2	2.1 ± 0.3

[1] Values are expressed as the means ± standard deviation of the data obtained from 4 animals (sham-operated) or 6 animals (partially hepatectomized) [24].

Vitamin B$_6$ Metabolism in Morris Hepatomas

After obtaining the results shown in figure 2, we decided to investigate vitamin B$_6$ metabolism in a limited spectrum of Morris hepatomas [19, 21]. Five hepatomas were examined: 7777 and 9618A$_2$ (fast growth rate, poorly differentiated), 7800 and 7794A (intermediate growth rate, well differentiated) and 9618A (very slow growth rate, highly differentiated). Animals employed were Buffalo rats maintained on laboratory chow. Fetal, neonatal and adult rat livers were used as controls. The results of these experiments are provided in figures 3–5.

It is apparent that the concentration of pyridoxal phosphate increases during normal hepatic ontogeny and development. Similar findings have been reported by others [23]. All of the hepatomas had pyridoxal phosphate concentrations that fell in the fetal to neonatal range, with the highest concentration of pyridoxal phosphate being found in 9618A. The lower concentrations in the hepatomas are not a result of rapid growth per se since we have determined that the pyridoxal-5'-phosphate concentrations in regenerating rat liver following partial hepatectomy are maintained at levels found in sham-operated controls (table I) [24]. Developmental correlations also are found for the activities of hepatic pyridoxine kinase (fig. 4) and pyridoxine-5'-phosphate oxidase (fig. 5). As shown in figure 1, these two enzymes are essential for the conversion of precursor vitamer forms to coenzymatically active pyridoxal-5'-phosphate. Marked increases in the activities of these two enzymes occur during liver ontogeny and development. Hepatoma pyridoxine kinase activities, with the exception of 9618A, all fall within the range found for fetal and neonatal rat liver (fig. 4). Similarly, pyridoxine-5'-phosphate oxidase activities in the hepatomas are in the fetal to neonatal range (fig. 5). Thus, the 5 Morris hepatomas we have examined display oncodevelopmental characteristics [25] with respect to vitamin B_6 metabolism in that they closely resemble fetal and neonatal rat liver and not adult liver. The most highly differentiated hepatoma, 9618A, is most like adult rat liver in relation to vitamin B_6 metabolism.

One should note that the values for the activity of pyridoxine-5'-phosphate oxidase in hepatomas 7777, $9618A_2$ and 7800 are very near zero and may fall within the detection limits of the assay method. Missing or low oxidase activity would indicate that these hepatomas are completely or nearly completely dependent on the acquisition of pyridoxal-5'-phosphate. Alternatively, pyridoxal could be taken up and then phosphorylated by pyridoxine kinase, the activity of which is low but nevertheless present in these hepatomas (fig. 4). It follows that *only* pyridoxal-5'-phosphate or pyridoxal can be classified as B_6 vitamins for hepatomas which lack pyridoxine-5'-phosphate oxidase activity.

In light of this, we decided to investigate further the reasons for the absent or low activity of pyridoxine-5'-phosphate oxidase in Morris hepatoma 7777. We rendered unlikely by various methods the following possible causes for low or missing oxidase activity in Morris hepatoma 7777: an alternate pathway involving initial oxidation of pyridoxine to pyridoxal followed by a phosphorylation, low or missing cofactor (FMN) for pyridoxine-5'-phosphate oxidase, the presence of an inhibitor in the hepatomas, and subcellular relocation of the enzyme [19, 20, 26]. It then became necessary to determine if the pyridoxine-5'-phosphate oxidase enzyme was absent in Morris hepatoma 7777 or if it was present but enzymatically inactive. These experiments required an immunological approach. To this end, we purified rat liver pyridoxine-5'-phosphate oxidase for the purpose of raising antibodies to it in rabbits.

Purification of Rat Liver Pyridoxine-5'-Phosphate Oxidase [20]

The purification of rat liver pyridoxine-5'-phosphate oxidase generally followed the procedure developed by *Kazarinoff and McCormick* [27] for the purification of the rabbit liver enzyme. In addition, an affinity chromatography step using *N*-5'-phosphopyridoxyl-aminohexyl Sepharose 4B [28] was employed as a final step. The results of the purification of the rat liver

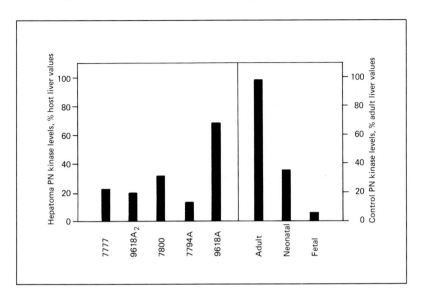

Fig. 4. Pyridoxine (PN) kinase activity in Morris hepatomas and rat liver at various stages of development.

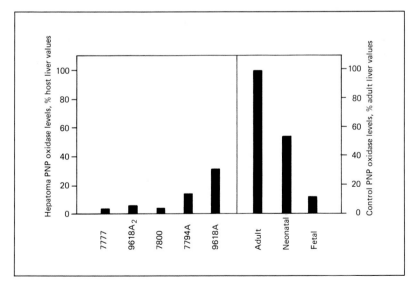

Fig. 5. Pyridoxine-5'-phosphate (PNP) oxidase activity in Morris hepatomas and rat liver at various stages of development.

enzyme are presented in table II. The highest specific activity for purified rat liver pyridoxine-5'-phosphate oxidase that we obtained was 11,400 U/mg protein which is about half of the highest specific activities reported for purified rabbit liver oxidase [27, 29]. The Coomassie blue staining patterns obtained after sodium dodecyl sulfate/polyacrylamide gel electrophoresis of the fractions designated 1–6 in table II are provided in lanes 1–6 of figure 6. In addition, an immunoblot, described below, of affinity chromatography-purified oxidase, is shown in lane I. Both the Coomassie and immunoblot detection methods reveal the presence of two bands having molecular weights in the range of 25,000–28,000 daltons, corresponding to subunit-molecular weights reported for the rabbit liver enzyme [30]. We have evidence which suggests that the faster moving band may arise from the slower moving band, presumably by proteolysis, but do not have definitive data on this matter.

For the purpose of obtaining purified rat liver oxidase for use as an antigen to immunize rabbits, 200 µg of affinity chromatography-purified oxidase was subjected to polyacrylamide gel electrophoresis under non-denaturing conditions using a 4–12% linear gradient. The position of the enzyme on the gel was determined by staining marker lanes on either side, one with Coomassie blue and one with an oxidase-specific activity stain [27, 31]. The corresponding area of the untreated lane was excised, homogenized with saline and Freund's adjuvant, and injected into the footpads of a rabbit [32, 33]. This procedure was repeated 3 times at weekly intervals followed by an injection, without Freund's adjuvant, directly into an ear vein of the rabbit. The IgG fractions of immune and preimmune serum from the same rabbit were partially purified by the method of *Fahey* [34].

Figure 7 provides the results of polyacrylamide gel electrophoresis of affinity chromatography-purified rat liver pyridoxine-5'-phosphate oxidase under non-denaturing conditions and its detection after transfer to nitrocellulose paper by an immunoblot procedure.

The electroelution and immunoblot analyses were performed essentially as described by *Towbin* et al. [35]. The immunoblot detection method is an enzyme-linked immunosorbent assay (ELISA) procedure adapted for use on nitrocellulose paper. It involves incubation of the antigen-containing nitrocellulose paper with antibodies specific for the antigen, followed by addition of horseradish peroxidase conjugated to goat antirabbit IgG. Addition of a suitable substrate for horseradish peroxidase, e.g. diaminobenzidine and hydrogen peroxide, produces a precipitating stain which allows one

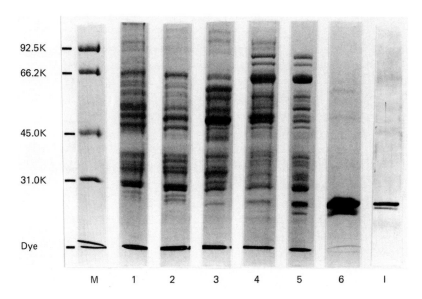

Fig. 6. Sodium dodecyl sulfate-polyacrylamide gel electrophoresis of pyridoxine (pyridoxamine)-5'-phosphate oxidase fractions at various stages of purification. Lanes 1–6 correspond to the fractions obtained from steps 1–6 in table II and were stained with Coomassie blue; 35 µg of protein was applied to each well. Lane M contains marker proteins of known molecular weights. Lane I is an immunoblot of enzyme purified through step 6 in table II [20].

Table II. Purification of rat liver pyridoxine (pyridoxamine)-5'-phosphate oxidase

	Step	Vol ml	U/ml	Total units	Protein mg/ml	Specific activity	Yield %	Purification
Extract	1	1,800	181.7	327,060	27.7	6.6	100	–
Acid supernatant	2	2,000	122.0	243,980	11.6	10.5	75	1.6
Ethanol precipitation	3	112	1,710	191,543	39.1	43.7	59	6.7
Chromatography								
DEAE-A50	4	203	438.9	89,089	0.72	610	27	93
G-100	5	51	868.6	52,114	0.34	2,555	14	389
Affinity	6	1.3	11,702	15,213	1.29	9,072	4.7	1,375

1 unit is defined as that amount of enzyme that catalyzes the formation of 1 nmol of pyridoxal-5'-phosphate/h under the conditions used; specific activity is units/mg protein [20].

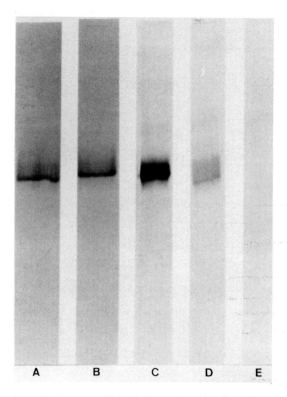

Fig. 7. Polyacrylamide gel electrophoresis of affinity chromatography purified rat liver pyridoxine (pyridoxamine)-5′-phosphate oxidase under non-denaturing conditions: Lane A = stained with Coomassie blue; lane B = stained for activity. Amido black and immunoblot detection of oxidase after horizontal electroelution from polyacrylamide gels to nitrocellulose paper: lane C = stained with amido black; lane D = stained by immunoblot method; lane E = same as lane D but the IgG fraction from preimmune rabbit serum was used as the first antibody [20].

to visualize the oxidase on the nitrocellulose paper. It is apparent from figure 7 that affinity chromatography-purified rat liver pyridoxine-5′-phosphate oxidase runs as a single band on non-denaturing gels (lanes A and B), that it can be transferred to nitrocellulose paper (lane C) and that immunization of rabbits with the oxidase produces antiserum containing antibodies specific for the enzyme (lanes D and E).

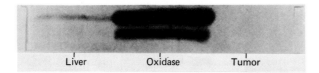

Fig. 8. Immunoblot analysis for pyridoxine (pyridoxamine)-5′-phosphate oxidase in cytosolic extracts of normal rat liver and Morris hepatoma 7777. Affinity chromatography purified oxidase was run as an authentic marker [20].

Lack of Antigenically Reactive Pyridoxine-5′-Phosphate Oxidase in Cytosolic Extracts of Morris Hepatoma 7777

Immunoblot analysis for pyridoxine-5′-phosphate oxidase in cytosolic extracts of normal adult rat liver and Morris hepatoma 7777 was carried out as described above using heavily loaded (500 μg protein/lane) denaturing gels. Under these conditions, it was possible to detect in cytosolic extracts of normal rat liver an immunologically reactive band corresponding to authentic oxidase (fig. 8). However, there was no such band apparent in cytosolic extracts of Morris hepatoma 7777. As a confirmation of these results, we performed conventional microtiter plate ELISA analyses [36] using *o*-phenylenediamine as the chromogenic substrate for second antibody-linked horseradish peroxidase. The results of these experiments are provided in figure 9. The upper curve is obtained when cytosolic extracts of normal rat liver are tested for immunologically reactive pyridoxine-5′-phosphate oxidase by the ELISA method. In a control experiment, the IgG fraction of preimmune serum reacts with cytosolic extracts of normal rat liver in the expected non-specific manner (lower curve, triangles). Cytosolic extracts of Morris hepatoma 7777 (squares), matched for protein concentration with normal liver extracts, react with the IgG fraction of immune serum in a fashion indistinguishable from the control. Thus, within the limits of detection, there is no immunologically reactive pyridoxine-5′-phosphate oxidase in this hepatoma.

Implications for Tumor Nutrition

Our data indicate that the absence of pyridoxine-5′-phosphate oxidase activity in Morris hepatoma 7777 results from missing rather than inactive enzyme. The genetic capability to make this enzyme evidently has been

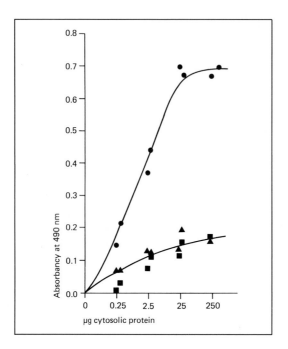

Fig. 9. Enzyme-linked immunosorbent assay for pyridoxine (pyridoxamine)-5′-phosphate oxidase in cytosolic extracts: normal rat liver (●) and Morris hepatoma 7777 (■). The control (▲) was run with liver cytosolic extracts and the IgG fraction from preimmune serum [20].

shed or rendered inactive in this tumor. Its metabolic requirements for pyridoxal phosphate apparently cannot be met by metabolism of a precursor vitamer form such as pyridoxine. Thus, in contrast to normal rat liver, which is very active in the metabolism of B_6 vitamer forms and which is a net exporter of pyridoxal-5′-phosphate [15], Morris hepatoma 7777 must acquire specific forms of vitamin B_6.

The Morris hepatomas more resemble fetal and neonatal rat liver than adult rat liver with respect to pyridoxal phosphate levels and vitamin B_6 metabolism. In light of the fact that alterations in transport for nutrients such as amino acids are found in transformed hepatocytes [37, 38], it seems reasonable to suppose that metabolites derived from the actions of pyridoxal-5′-phosphate-dependent enzymes may be acquired by less differentiated tissues by transport processes rather than by mechanisms operating in terminally differentiated normal tissues. It seems equally reasonable to suppose that less differentiated tissues may be much more restrictive or selective in their use of a micronutrient such as pyridoxal-5'-phosphate. For example, there is invariably an increase in the activity of pyridoxal-5'-phosphate-dependent ornithine decarboxylase in rapidly growing normal and neoplastic tissue [39] even in the face of a vitamin B$_6$ deficiency [19, 24], suggesting that there is selective utilization of pyridoxal-5'-phosphate in such tissues.

The manner of the acquisition and use of essential micronutrients by tumors is an important question in tumor biology. Recently, monoclonal antibodies to vitamin B$_6$ have been developed [40]. The availability of such antibodies may be of considerable help in elucidating how tumors acquire and utilize specific B$_6$ vitamer forms [41].

Acknowledgements

Much of this research was performed by *Louise M. Nutter,* in partial fulfillment of the requirements for the PhD degree from the University of Vermont, and by Dr. *Natalie T. Meisler.* We gratefully acknowledge the support of PHS Grant Number AM-25490 and BRSG Grant Number 2-32908 from the University of Vermont College of Medicine. L.M.N. acknowledges the support of PHS Training Grant Number CA-T32-09826 und tuition fellowships provided by a benefactor of the University of Vermont.

References

1   Meister, A.: Biochemistry of the amino acids; 2nd ed., pp. 375–413 (Academic Press, New York 1965).
2   Snell, E.E.: Chemical structure in relation to biological activities of vitamin B$_6$. Vitams Horm. *16:* 77–113 (1958).
3   Bruice, T.C.; Benkovic, S.J.: Bioorganic mechanisms; vol. 2, pp. 227–300 (Benjamin, New York 1966).
4   Jencks, W.P.: Catalysis in chemistry and enzymology, pp. 133–146 (McGraw-Hill, New York 1969).
5   Robson, L.C.; Schwartz, M.R.: The effects of vitamin B$_6$ deficiency on the lymphoid system and immune responses; in Tryfiates, Vitamin B$_6$ metabolism and role in growth, pp. 205–222 (Food & Nutrition Press, Westport 1980).
6   Subbarao, K.; Kuchibhotla, J.; Kakkar, V.V.: Pyridoxal-5'-phosphate – a new physiological inhibitor of blood coagulation and platelet function. Biochem. Pharmacol. *28:* 531–534 (1979).
7   Cidlowski, J.A.; Thanassi, J.W.: Pyridoxal phosphate: a possible cofactor in steroid hormone action. J. Steroid Biochem. *15:* 11–16 (1981).

8   Schmidt, T.J.; Litwack, G.: Activation of the glucocorticoid receptor complex. Phys-
     iol. Rev. *62:* 1131–1192 (1982).

9   Cabantchik, I.Z.; Balshin, M.; Breuer, W.; Rothstein, A.: Pyridoxal phosphate: an
     anionic probe for protein amino groups exposed on the outer and inner surfaces of
     intact human red blood cells. J. biol. Chem. *250:* 5130–5136 (1975).

10   Gould, K.G.; Engel, P.C.: The reactions of pyridoxal-5'-phosphate with the M_4 and
     H_4 isoenzymes of pig lactate dehydrogenase. Archs Biochem. Biophys. *215:* 498–507
     (1982).

11   Snell, E.E.; Haskell, B.E.: The metabolism of vitamin B_6. Compr. Biochem. *21:* 47–71
     (1971).

12   Tryfiates, G.P.: Vitamin B_6 effects on the growth of Morris hepatomas and the devel-
     opment of enzymatic activity; in Morris, Criss, Morris hepatomas: mechanisms of
     regulation, pp. 607–642 (Plenum Publishing, New York 1978).

13   Tryfiates, G.P.; Morris, H.P.: Vitamin B_6 and neoplasia; in Tryfiates, Vitamin B_6
     metabolism and role in growth, pp. 173–186 (Food & Nutrition Press, Westport
     1980).

14   Rosen, F.; Mihich, E.; Nichol, C.E.: Selective metabolic and chemotherapeutic effects
     of vitamin B_6 antimetabolites. Vitams Horm. *22:* 609–641 (1964).

15   Lumeng, L.; Li, T.-K.: Mammalian vitamin B_6 metabolism: regulatory role of pro-
     tein-binding and the hydrolysis of pyridoxal-5'-phosphate in storage and transport; in
     Tryfiates, Vitamin B_6 metabolism and role in growth, pp. 27–51 (Food & Nutrition
     Press, Westport 1980).

16   Sell, S.; Morris, H.P.: Relationship of rat α-fetoprotein to growth rate and chromo-
     some composition of Morris hepatomas. Cancer Res. *34:* 1413–1417 (1974).

17   Weber, G.: Enzymology of cancer cells. New Engl. J. Med. *296:* 486–493, 541–551
     (1977).

18   Meisler, N.T.; Thanassi, J.W.: Pyridoxine kinase, pyridoxine phosphate phosphatase
     and pyridoxine phosphate oxidase activities in control and B_6-deficient rat liver and
     brain. J. Nutr. *110:* 1965–1975 (1980).

19   Thanassi, J.W.; Nutter, L.M.; Meisler, N.T.; Commers, P.; Chiu, J.-F.: Vitamin B_6
     metabolism in Morris hepatomas. J. biol. Chem. *256:* 3370–3375 (1981).

20   Nutter, L.M.; Meisler, N.T.; Thanassi, J.W.: Absence of pyridoxine (pyridoxamine)-
     5'-phosphate oxidase in Morris hepatoma 7777. Biochemistry, N.Y. *22:* 1599–1604
     (1983).

21   Meisler, N.T.; Nutter, L.M.; Thanassi, J.W.: Vitamin B_6 metabolism in liver and
     liver-derived tumors. Cancer Res. *42:* 3538–3543 (1982).

22   Reynolds, R.D.; Morris, H.P.: Effects of dietary vitamin B_6 on the in vitro inactiva-
     tion of rat tyrosine aminotransferase in host liver and Morris hepatomas. Cancer Res.
     39: 2988–2994 (1979).

23   Nakahara, I.; Morino, Y.; Morisue, T.; Sakamoto, T.: Enzymatic studies on pyridox-
     ine metabolism. J. Biochem., Tokyo *49:* 338–342 (1961).

24   Meisler, N.T.; Thanassi, J.W.: Vitamin B_6 metabolism and its relation to ornithine
     decarboxylase activity in regenerating rat liver. J. Nutr. *112:* 314–323 (1982).

25   Ibsen, K.H.; Fishman, W.H.: Developmental gene expression in cancer. Biochim.
     biophys. Acta *560:* 243–280 (1979).

26   Nutter, L.M.: Vitamin B_6 metabolism in liver and liver-derived tumors; PhD thesis,
     Burlington (1983).

27 Kazarinoff, M.N.; McCormick, D.B.: Rabbit liver pyridoxamine(pyridoxine)-5′-phosphate oxidase: purification and properties. J. biol. Chem. *250:* 3436–3442 (1975).

28 Cash, C.D.; Maitre, M.; Rumigny, J.-F.; Mandel, P.: Rapid purification by affinity chromatography of rat brain pyridoxal kinase and pyridoxamine-5′-phosphate oxidase. Biochem. biophys. Res. Commun. *96:* 1755–1760 (1980).

29 Merrill, A.H.; Kazarinoff, M.N.; Tsuge, H.; Horiike, K.; McCormick, D.B.: Pyridoxamine (pyridoxine)-5′-phosphate oxidase from rabbit liver. Meth. Enzym. *62:* 568–574 (1979).

30 Horiike, K.; Merrill, A.H.; McCormick, D.B.: Activation and inactivation of rabbit liver pyridoxamine (pyridoxine)-5′-phosphate oxidase activity by urea and other solutes. Archs Biochem. Biophys. *195:* 325–335 (1979).

31 Feinstein, R.N.; Lindahl, R.: Detection of oxidases on polyacrylamide gels. Analyt. Biochem. *56:* 353–360 (1973).

32 Hartman, B.K.; Udenfriend, S.: A method for immediate visualization of proteins in acrylamide gels and its use for preparation of antibodies to enzymes. Analyt. Biochem. *30:* 391–394 (1969).

33 Boulard, C.; Lecroisey, A.: Specific antisera produced by direct immunization with slices of polyacrylamide gels and its use for preparation of antibodies. J. immunol. Methods *50:* 221–226 (1982).

34 Fahey, J.L.: Chromatographic separation of immunoglobulins; in Williams, Chase, Methods in immunology and immunochemistry, vol. 1, pp. 321–326 (Academic Press, New York 1967).

35 Towbin, H.; Staehelin, T.; Gordon, J.: Electrophoretic transfer of proteins from polyacrylamide gels to nitrocellulose sheets: procedure and some applications. Proc. natn. Acad. Sci. USA *76:* 4350–4354 (1979).

36 Engvall, E.; Perlmann, P.: Enzyme-linked immunosorbent assay, ELISA. III. Quantitation of specific antibodies by enzyme-labeled anti-immunoglobulin in antigen-coated tubes. J. Immun. *109:* 129–135 (1972).

37 Kelly, D.S.; Potter, V.R.: Repression, derepression, transinhibition, and trans-stimulation of amino acid transport in rat hepatocytes and four rat hepatoma cell lines in culture. J. biol. Chem. *254:* 6691–6697 (1979).

38 White, M.F.; Christensen, H.N.: Cationic amino acid transport into cultured animal cells. II. Transport system barely perceptible in ordinary hepatocytes, but active in hepatoma cell lines. J. biol. Chem. *257:* 4450–4457 (1982).

39 Jänne, J.; Pösö, H.; Raina, A.: Polyamines in rapid growth and cancer. Biochim. biophys. Acta *473:* 241–293 (1978).

40 Viceps-Madore, D.; Cidlowski, J.A.; Kittler, J.M.; Thanassi, J.W.: Preparation, characterization and use of monoclonal antibodies to vitamin B$_6$. J. biol. Chem. *258:* 2689–2696 (1983).

41 Kittler, J.M.; Viceps-Madore, D.; Cidlowski, J.A.; Thanassi, J.W.: Immunoblot detection of pyridoxal phosphate-binding proteins in liver and hepatoma cytosolic extracts. Biochem. biophys. Res. Commun. *112:* 61–65 (1983).

J.W. Thanassi, MD, Department of Biochemistry, University of Vermont,
College of Medicine, Burlington, VT 05405 (USA)

Clinical Trials

Prasad (ed.), Vitamins, Nutrition, and Cancer, pp. 266–273 (Karger, Basel 1984)

Prevention and Treatment of Cancer with Vitamin A and the Retinoids

Frank L. Meyskens, Jr.

Cancer Center and Department of Internal Medicine, University of Arizona, Tucson, Ariz., USA

Introduction

Extensive laboratory investigations have documented that vitamin A and its natural and synthetic derivatives (the retinoids) can inhibit proliferation and stimulate differentiation and/or maturation in normal and many transformed cells [1, 2]. Epidemiological studies also support the general notion that vitamin A is a natural inhibitor of the development of human cancer [3–5]. These observations have prompted us to examine the role of retinoids as anticancer agents. We propose a general strategy which defines precancer and cancer as a continuum from normality to abnormality in which the modalities of prevention and treatment are blurred (fig. 1).

Three types of prevention are identified. Primary prevention seeks to abrogate or block primary exposure to carcinogens or to correct a deficiency state (e.g. vitamin A or C supplementation). Examples would include cessation of smoking and application of sunscreen. Secondary prevention involves active intervention and the use of an inhibitor of neoplasia in individuals who are at high risk for the development of a cancer because of current or prior exposure to a carcinogenic agent. Examples of such individuals include smokers, individuals with known asbestos, ultraviolet light, or other carcinogen exposure.

Intervention strategies would encompass provision of anti-initiators and/or antipromotors (such as retinoids) at low non-toxic doses. Tertiary prevention is defined as the reversal of histologically or cytologically identifiable preneoplastic lesions and/or inhibition of progression to definitive cancer. Cervical dysplasia, leukoplakia, or pulmonary metaplasia are exam-

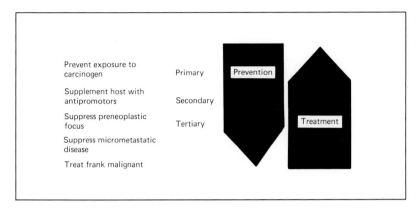

Prevent exposure to
carcinogen   Primary

Supplement host with
antipromotors   Secondary

Suppress preneoplastic
focus   Tertiary

Suppress micrometastatic
disease

Treat frank malignant

Fig. 1. Prevention and treatment of cancer represents a continuum.

ples of lesions amenable to tertiary prevention. Active intervention with
retinoids or other compounds, perhaps even at mildly toxic doses, will be
required. The dose to inhibit progression may well be different than the
amount required for reversion of preneoplastic lesions to normal. This
intent clearly represents the prevention of cancer although the strategy is
treatment-oriented. The treatment of cancer with retinoids can be either in
the adjuvant setting (? prevention of micrometastases) or with advanced
cancers. The question of toxicity and efficacy is an important issue and
clearly much greater toxicity would be acceptable as more advanced lesions
are approached.

Prevention

In southwestern Arizona the incidences of non-melanoma and melanoma skin cancer are high [6]. This has provided us with the ready availability of patients who are at various risks for skin cancer, ranging from very
low to almost 100% per year. We have therefore developed a comprehensive program to study the prevention of skin cancer (table I), which is
described below.

Primary prevention is defined as avoidance of a carcinogen or correction of a deficiency state which predisposes to the development of a malignancy. For non-melanoma skin cancer a common predisposing deficiency

Table I. Prevention of skin cancer

Type	Investigation	
	target population	intervention
Primary	individuals in high sun area (Southern Arizona)	sunscreens
Secondary		
Early	prior actinic keratoses	placebo vs 13-*cis*-retinoic acid
Late	≥ 8 squamous/basal skin cancers	placebo vs retinol vs 13-*cis*-retinoic acid
Tertiary	dysplastic nevus syndrome	local or systemic 13-*cis*-retinoic acid

or familial tendency has not been recognized. However, primary prevention of skin cancer can be achieved by avoiding the sun or blocking access of the sun to the skin. The former is not feasible and therefore the aggressive use of sunscreens has been advocated. Although sunscreens clearly block the effect of ultraviolet light in animal models, the premise that sunscreens can reduce the incidence of skin cancer has never been tested in humans. We are now planning such a trial, which will be a massive undertaking.

Secondary prevention is the prophylactic administration of an agent to individuals at risk. Such investigations should be carefully stratified, randomized, and at least single- if not double-blinded. Extensive provisions must be made to assess adherence, compliance, and other confounding issues. We have recently initiated two distinct trials to address early and late secondary prevention. In the first study patients with actinic keratoses will be randomized to receive placebo or a low dose of 13-*cis*-retinoic acid. They will be followed for the development of skin cancer. In the second study, patients at very high risk (40% new lesions/year) for the development of a new skin cancer will be eligible for entry. This will include patients with greater than 8 prior squamous/basal skin cell carcinomas. The randomization will be placebo versus vitamin A (25,000 IU/day) versus low-dose 13-*cis*-retinoic acid. The results from these two groups of patients will allow assessment of the effect of retinoids in early and late stages of skin carcinogenesis in humans.

Tertiary prevention is defined as the reversal or suppression of measurable precancerous lesions. We divide these conditions into two distinct groups, hyperproliferative and preneoplastic. Examples of the former include laryngeal papillomatosis, keratoacanthoma, epidermal dysplasia verruciformis (EDV) and of the latter, cervical dysplasia, leukoplakia, and pulmonary metaplasia. We [7, 8] and others [9] have documented the effects of retinoids on keratoacanthomas and EDV. We have recently used 13-*cis*-retinoic acid in 4 patients with severe laryngeal papillomatosis and 2 excellent and 1 good response were seen [10].

The prevention (? treatment) of cervical dysplasia has presented an interesting challenge. As the disease process is confined to a discrete area, local or regional treatment should be possible with obviation of systemic side effects. Our initial studies explored the use of a diaphragm as a delivery device and various formulations of vitamin A acid (β-*trans*-retinoic acid) as the retinoid [11, 12]. A cream preparation was the most easily applied, but the diaphragm leaked. Therefore, we subsequently have used a cervical cap as the delivery device. The present prototype consists of a self-adhering cervical cap within which is a collagen sponge impregnated with β-*trans*-retinoic acid in a cream formulation. Using this approach we have completed a phase I trial in patients with mild and moderate cervical dysplasia [13]. Vaginal side effects were dose-limiting and occurred after the application period. This suggested that the cervix was saturated and leaking of retinoic acid onto the vaginal mucosa had occurred. Systemic side effects were not dose-related. No cervical side effects were noted, although biological changes were clearly evident. Our current plans include a phase II trial in moderate cervical dysplasia using a dose of 0.37% retinoic acid. In addition to the initial 4 days of treatment, patients will be retreated for 2 days every 3 months for 1 year. Both the effect on the regression of the preneoplastic lesion to normal and the inhibition to cancer will be measured. Separate assessments of both frequency and rate will be obtained.

Treatment

We have conducted a number of trials including an adjuvant trial of retinol in phase I and II malignant melanoma [14], a phase I trial of retinol [15], a broad phase II study of 13-*cis*-retinoic acid [8], a trial of β-*trans*-retinoic acid directly applied to intracutaneous metastatic melanoma [16], and an investigation of 13-*cis*-retinoic acid and mycosis fungoides [17].

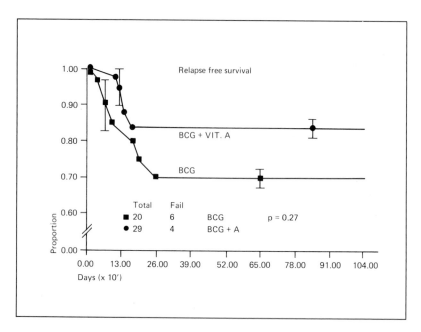

Fig. 2. Relapse-free survival of stage I and II melanoma patients treated with BCG or BCG + vitamin A [from ref. 14 with permission].

With rare exceptions malignant melanoma is an incurable cancer once metastatic disease has occurred. Considerable effort has been directed by innumerable investigators to prevent the recurrence of melanoma after surgical excision, using immunomodulation and/or chemotherapy. The attempts have been uniformly unsuccessful. Based on the favorable immunomodulatory effects of retinoids and their activity as differentiating agents for murine and human melanoma cells, we initiated in 1978 an adjuvant trial of BCG versus BCG + vitamin A (retinol) in stage I (high risk, > 1.5 mm Breslow) and stage II malignant melanoma [14]. Side effects were acceptable and the overall evaluability rate in the first 120 patients was 85%. The initial evaluation suggested a favorable trend for the vitamin A arm (fig. 2).

We have reported a broad phase II trial of 13-*cis*-retinoic acid [8]. Considerable antitumor activity was detected against several types of premalignant and malignant skin conditions, a result consistent with earlier observations of other investigators [9]. We also recorded short-term responses in skin or subcutaneous sites in patients with advanced or metastatic head and neck and lung cancers. Evaluation and confirmation of these findings in larger trials will be quite important. We had also previously treated intracutaneous metastatic deposits of retinoids with local application of β-*trans*-retinoic acid and substantial responses in 2 patients were recorded [16]. The activity of retinoids against malignant melanoma was confirmed in our phase II trial of 13-*cis*-retinoic acid as 2 of 18 patients exhibited partial responses, including 1 patient with pulmonary metastases [7; and unpublished data].

A number of laboratory investigations have suggested that retinoids and T lymphocytes interact in a positive fashion. In this context and as part of our phase II trial with 13-*cis*-retinoic acid we treated patients with the cutaneous T cell lymphoma mycosis fungoides [16]. Our overall clinical experience to date has included responses in 8 of 12 patients with 4 demonstrating nearly complete resolution of the disease. Additional experience with mycosis fungoides and other T cell malignancies should be quite informative.

Conclusions

Retinoids are clearly active against a number of proliferative, preneoplastic, and neoplastic conditions. As potential preventive agents only retinol (and the precursor β-carotene), β-*trans*-retinoic acid (for local application), and 13-*cis*-retinoic acid would appear sufficiently developed to use. A large number of retinoid derivatives have been synthesized with the expectation that an improved toxicity/efficacy ratio could be obtained. Although this goal has been achieved in animal models [18], this information has not yet been successfully translated to humans. Alternative strategies for the development of the retinoids as treatment modalities should also be considered. Growing tissues, including tumors, are clearly dependent on retinol (? and retinoic acid) delivered via an intracellular binding protein. The treatment of estrogen-dependent cancers has been considerably enhanced by the development of antiestrogens. Perhaps antiretinoids can be developed. However, such an approach has not yet been taken. The pace for use of retinoids for the prevention and treatment of cancer over the next few years should quicken as they clearly represent an alternative and complementary strategy for the management of human cancers.

Acknowledgements

We thank *L. Kimball* for secretarial assistance and acknowledge the role of many colleagues in these studies, particularly *T. Moon, N. Levine, E. Surwit, D. Alberts, M. Chvapil, R. Dorr, L. Loescher,* and *V. Graham.* Supported in part by the National Cancer Institute (CA27502, NO1-CM-17500) and a grant from Hoffmann-La Roche, Inc. (Nutley, N.J.).

References

1   Lotan, R.: Effects of vitamin A and its analogs (retinoids) on normal and neoplastic cells. Biochim. biophys. Acta *605:* 33–91 (1980).

2   Sporn, M.B.; Roberts, A.B.: Role of retinoids in differentiation and carcinogenesis. Cancer Res. *43:* 3034–3040 (1983).

3   Kummet, T.; Meyskens, F.L., Jr.: Vitamin A: a natural inhibitor of human malignancy. Semin. Oncol. *10:* 281–289 (1983).

4   Kummet, T.; Moon, T.E.; Meyskens, F.L., Jr.: Vitamin A: evidence for its preventive role in human malignancy. Nutr. Cancer *5:* 96–106 1983).

5   Peto, R.; Doll, R.; Buckley, J.D.; Sporn, M.B.: Can dietary beta-carotene materially reduce human cancer rates? Nature, Lond. *290:* 201–208 (1981).

6   Schreiber, M.M.; Bozzo, P.D.; Moon, T.E.: Malignant melanoma in southern Arizona. Archs Derm. *117:* 6–14 (1981).

7   Levine, N.; Miller, R.C.; Meyskens, F.L., Jr.: Oral 13-*cis*-retinoic acid therapy for multiple cutaneous squamous cell carcinomas and keratoacanthomas. Archs. Derm. (in press, 1983).

8   Meyskens, F.L., Jr.; Gilmartin, E.; Alberts, D.S.; Levine, N.S.; Brooks, R.; Salmon, S.E.; Surwit, E.A.: Activity of isotretinoin against squamous cell cancers and preneoplastic lesions. Cancer Treat. Rep. *66:* 1315–1319 (1982).

9   Mayer, M.; Bollag, W.; Hanni, R.; Riiegg, R.: Retinoids, a new class of compounds with prophylactic and therapeutic activities in oncology and dermatology. Experientia *34:* 1105–1119 (1978).

10 Alberts, D.S.; Coulthard, S.; Meyskens, F.L., Jr.: Regression of laryngeal papillomatosis with 13-*cis*-retinoic acid (submitted).

11 Surwit, E.A.; Graham, V.; Droegemuller, W.; Chvapil, M.; Dorr, R.T.; Davis, J.R.; Meyskens, F.L., Jr.: Evaluation of topically applied trans-retinoic acid in the treatment of cervical intraepithelial lesions. Am. J. Obstet. Gynec. *143:* 821–823 (1982).

12 Dorr, R.T.; Surwit, E.A.; Meyskens, F.L., Jr.; Droegemuller, W.; Alberts, D.S.; Chvapil, M.: In vitro retinoid binding and release from a collagen sponge material in a simulated intravaginal environment. J. biomed. Mater. Res. *16:* 839–850 (1982).

13 Meyskens, F.L., Jr.; Graham, V.; Chvapil, M.; Dorr, R.T.; Alberts, D.S.; Surwit, E.A.: A phase I trial of β-*all-trans*-retinoic acid for mild or moderate intraepithelial cervical neoplasia delivered via a collagen sponge and cervical cap. J. natn. Cancer Inst. (in press, 1983).

14 Meyskens, F.L., Jr.; Aapro, M.S.; Voakes, J.B.; Moon, T.E.; Gilmartin, E.: A stratified randomized adjuvant study of BCG ± high dose vitamin A in stage I and II

malignant melanoma; in Salmon, Jones, Adjuvant therapy of cancer, vol. III, pp. 217–224 (Grune & Stratton, New York 1981).

15   Goodman, G.E.; Alberts, D.S.; Earnest, D.L.; Meyskens, F.L., Jr.: Clinical trial of retinol in cancer patients. J. clin. Oncol. *1:* 394–399 (1983).

16   Levine, N.; Meyskens, F.L., Jr.: Topical vitamin A acid therapy for cutaneous metastatic melanoma. Lancet *ii:* 224–226 (1980).

17   Kessler, J.F.; Meyskens, F.L., Jr.; Levine, N.; Lynch, P.; Jones, S.E.: Successful treatment of cutaneous T cell lymphoma (mycosis fungoides) with 13-*cis*-retinoic acid. Lancet *i:* 1345–1347 (1983).

18   Bollag, W.: Vitamin A and vitamin A acid in the prophylaxis and therapy of epithelial tumors. Int. J. Vit. Res. *40:* 299–314 (1970).

F.L. Meyskens, Jr., MD, Cancer Center and Department of Internal Medicine, University of Arizona, Tucson, AZ 85724 (USA)

Prasad (ed.), Vitamins, Nutrition, and Cancer, pp. 274–281 (Karger, Basel 1984)

A Phase I Study of Vitamin E and Neuroblastoma

Lawrence Helson

Memorial Sloan-Kettering Cancer Center, New York, N.Y., USA

Introduction

During the last 30 years, several articles have been published concerning the effects of vitamin E on dietary pro-carcinogens, carcinogens, and in patients with cancer [1–4]. The few clinical studies of oral vitamin E effects on cancer have been complicated by the concomitant administration of radiation and lack of adequate controls.

As a precondition to initiating clinical trials in patients with cancer, we recognized certain requirements. These included the need for an intravenous preparation and preclinical in vitro and animal model evidence of antitumoral effects of the vitamin E preparation. Such data could be used to support its application in the clinical setting and to identify susceptible tumors. *Prasad* et al. [5] made the initial observations on the in vitro effects of vitamin E (RRR-α-tocopheryl acetate) on murine neuroblastoma and melanoma. Based upon these observations we focused our initial in vitro experiments on human neuroblastoma and melanoma cells.

This in vitro demonstration of antitumor effects of vitamin E required circumvention of its water-insoluble characteristics. Because the various vehicles used to solubilize the commercial vitamin E preparations are cytoxic, it was difficult to attribute an antitumor effect specific to the vitamin. This was particularly pertinent when we evaluated the parenteral preparation of vitamin E (all-rac-α-tocopherol) also called Ephynal® (Hoffmann-La Roche, Inc.). Because of its design for parenteral use and extensive previous clinical experience in infants this product appeared to be an appropriate drug for clinical trials with cancer patients. It comes formulated as a water miscible preparation and contains the emulsifier, Emulphor EL-620. Unfortunately, in in vitro studies the vehicle also exhibited cytotoxic activity against human neuroblastoma cells. We were obliged to test other preparations of vitamin E and were able to document the first in vitro evidence of human neuroblastoma cell growth inhibition and lysis following exposure to vitamin E [6]. Tumor cell lysis was noted with vitamin E acid succinate solubilized in normal saline containing 1 % ethyl alcohol. The vehicle control consisting of sodium succinate in a 1 % solution of ethyl alcohol had no effect on tumor cell growth. Another compound, vitamin E polyethylene glycol 1000 succinate (Eastman Company, Kingsport, Tenn.), is a water soluble preparation. It is equally cytotoxic to neuroblastoma cells. The polyethylene glycol-1000-succinate vehicle control was devoid of antitumor activity [7].

These data were complemented by determination of the antitumoral effect of various vitamin E preparations in nude mice bearing human neuroblastomas [8]. The toxicity of the vehicle for Ephynal in vivo in nude mice was negligible. When Ephynal with this same vehicle was administrated parenterally in nude mice it did cause lysis of heterotransplanted human tumors. This antitumor response was associated with a 10–15% weight loss [7, 8].

Based upon these studies, we initiated a phase I study of parenteral Ephynal in patients with disseminated neuroblastoma, primitive neuroectodermal tumors and retinoblastoma. These patients were refractory to conventional and other experimental therapy.

Materials and Methods

Ephynal was supplied by Hoffmann-La Roche, Nutley, N.J., in 1 ml stained glass vials. Each vial contains 50 mg of all-rac-α-tocopherol in an aqueous medium containing the emulsifier, Emulphor EL-620. The vitamin mixture was further diluted in 5 % glucose in water containing half normal saline and passaged through a 5-μm filter to exclude glass splinters from the infusion. Infusion rates were as high as 700 mg vitamin/m^2/h and schedules varied from twice weekly to daily 3-hour or 24-hour continuous infusions for 5–9 days.

The purpose of this study was to determine a maximally tolerated dose of Ephynal in neuroblastoma, primitive neuroectodermal tumor or retinoblastoma patients resistant to conventional chemotherapy or radiotherapy.

Patient ages were between 6 months and 29 years of age. Measurable or evaluable tumors were present in all patients. The patients had anticancer chemotherapy 2 or more weeks prior to treatment with the vitamin. The estimated survival time of all patients was

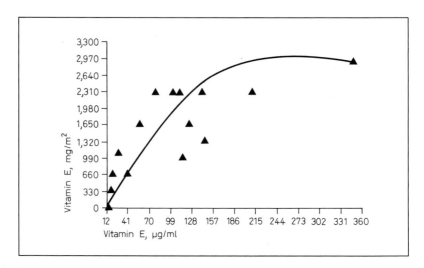

Fig. 1. Blood concentrations of vitamin E measured 24 h after injections at different dosages. The average blood concentrations at 24 h increased with the dose administered.

4 or more weeks and they or their parents were required to sign an informed consent form describing the experimental nature of the study. In the first 3 patients, dosages were initiated at 330 mg/m^2 twice weekly. In the absence of detectable toxicity, this dose was escalated using a modified Fibonnacci scheme. In succeeding patients, the maximal dosage reached was 2,300 mg/m^2/day for 9 continuous days (fig. 1). Toxicity evaluation included pretreatment and serial posttreatment complete blood counts, SMA-12, cholesterol and triglycerides. Prothrombin time and accelerated partial thromboplastin time were determined in patients receiving the highest dosage of vitamin E, i.e. 2,300 mg/m^2 daily. Plasma tocopherol levels were determined prior to treatment and following administration of the compound by Dr. *Herman Baker* of New Jersey Medical School, East Orange, N.J., and Dr. *H. Kupperman,* Roche Biomedical Labs., Raritan, N.J.

Side Effects

13 patients entered in the study were evaluable. The only side effect seen was at the highest dosage administered. 1 patient was administered the undiluted vitamin preparation through a constant infusion pump. Following an episode of extravasation into the soft tissues of his forearm, he experienced a local erythema without any ulceration or pain for a period of 36 h. In 2 patients receiving the highest dosage, i.e. 2,300 mg/m^2 decreases in factors II, VII, IX and X were observed. The most extensive depression was noted with factor VII [9]. Other than this hemorrhagic diathesis, no nausea, vomiting, diarrhea, constipation, fever, infections, appetitie changes or other side effects attributable to vitamin E were noted. No vitamin E-associated changes in the peripheral blood counts, CBC, SMA-12 profile, or serum levels or cholesterol or triglycerides could be ascertained. Although

precautionary dilution of vitamin E infusions at 50–100 mg/ml D5W-½ normal saline/h were infused in initial studies, gradually increasing concentrations were used and as much as 700 mg Ephynal in 100 ml of D5W/h were infused without undue side effects.

Although the original objectives of this study were to determine a maximal tolerated dose of intravenous vitamin E, we also recorded measurements of any antitumoral effects which occurred during the period of observation and therapy. Subjective (pain relief) and objective (tumor regression) therapeutic responses were observed in 5 of 13 evaluable patients.

Pain relief was noted in 2 patients. 1 was a 5-year-old male with neuroblastoma. He was previously treated with numerous drugs and radiation over a 4-year period. Upon referral to Memorial Hospital he had extensive bone metastases and was experiencing intractable pain requiring Levodromeran and Methadone for control. Within 24 h of the second infusion of Ephynal at 660 mg/m^2 his pain symptoms disappeared. He was continued on twice weekly injections for 2 months. During this period, he remained pain free and tumor progression ceased. During the third month of treatment, he developed further tumor regrowth, paraplegia, and his pain required narcotics for control. Although no evidence of tumor lysis was noted during vitamin E treatment, the pain relief and tumor stasis were clinically of value to the patient. During this period of time, no untoward infections or increases in blood or platelet requirements occurred.

Objective responses associated with Ephynal treatment were observed in 5 patients. Patient 1 had radiation refractory retinoblastoma treated with 330 mg/m^2 twice weekly for 4 weeks. A decrease in the size of the tumor was noted and lasted about 3 weeks. In the presence of regrowth, the parents refused additional escalated doses. In patient 2, temporary decrease in size of epidural neuroblastoma metastases was noted following 4 weeks of treatment with 660 mg/m^2 twice weekly.

Patient 3 had a recurrent disseminated primitive neuroectodermal tumor. She was treated with 660 mg/m^2 twice weekly. This was eventually escalated to daily treatments for 5 continuous days. Both pain relief and a decrease in mediastinal metastases were noted. This mediastinal lung tumor response could be partially attributable to vitamin E since the patient also received an estimated 700 rad to the same region from radiation scatter due to radiation treatment of her spinal cord at the same time. She also experienced systemic pain relief during the time of administration. Of interest was her reaction when the drug was stopped. She appeared to experience the equivalent of a withdrawal syndrome with rapid recurrence of pain and generalized discomfort. While on therapy, she developed a recurrence of pain, anasarca and died. At autopsy, the ascites appeared to be due to multiple disseminated 1- or 2-mm nodules on her peritoneal surfaces with no gross tumor. Her lungs and mediastinum did not have any tumor (fig. 2, 3).

Patient 4 had chemotherapy and radiotherapy resistant tumor metastases noted on CT scan. Following treatment with vitamin E, 660 mg/m^2 twice weekly for 4 weeks, the metastases decreased in size. The patient was also noted to have a 1.5-kg weight loss.

Patient 5 had disseminated neuroblastoma of the clavicle and scalp which developed after conventional and experimental therapy using high dosage L-phenlyalanine mustard and dianhydrogalactitol [10]. He was treated with Ephynal 2,300 mg/m^2 daily for 9 days. Toxicity was manifested as bleeding associated with inhibition of hepatic dependent procoagulant factors II, VII, IX and X. His cranial tumor masses shrunk to about 50% of their sizes after therapy. A second course of vitamin E was repeated with a lesser response. Finally the mother refused further therapy because of rapidly progressive disease.

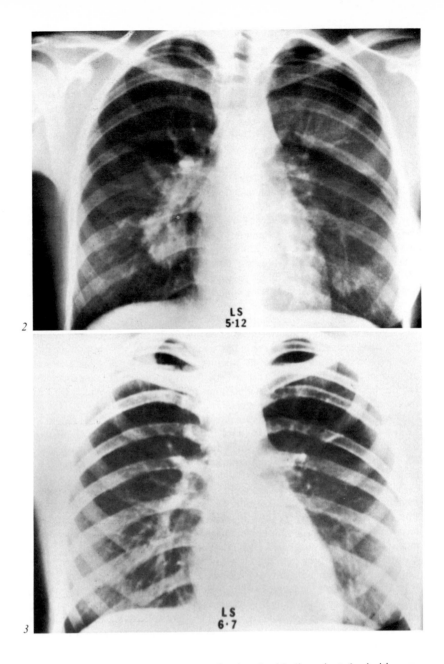

Fig. 2. Pretreatment chest radiograph of patient 3 with disseminated primitive neuroectodermal tumor.

Fig. 3. Post-treatment with intravenous vitamin E of patient 3. The previously noted metastatic tumor mass is markedly decreased.

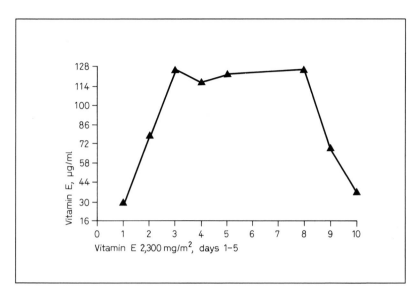

Fig. 4. Blood concentrations of vitamin E reached levels of 100 µg/ml after 3 days when 2,300 µg/m² were infused daily. These levels were sustained an additional 3 days after therapy was stopped.

Discussion

The purpose of this study was to establish a safe therapeutic level of parenteral vitamin E for use in phase II trials. Based upon in vitro data with human neuroblastomas, highly resistant to chemotherapy, adequacy was defined by cytolytic concentrations of TPGS or α-tocopheryl succinate, i.e. about 100 µg/ml × 24 h. Dosages of intravenous vitamin E which yield plasma levels of 100 µg/ml at 24 h after injection seemed to be an appropriate goal. Such levels were achieved after infusing 2,300 mg/m² daily for 2–3 days (fig. 4).

A minor inconvenience in preparing the product for administration was the large number of ampules required for larger patients. One attempt at infusion of undiluted material with a pump over 24 h was made. During this trial, extravasation of undiluted Ephynal was a minor inconvenience. This would probably be of no importance if diluted material accidentally extravasated.

The responses noted did not correlate with the dosage of drug used or the plasma levels attained. After 3 days, plasma levels of vitamin E with doses of 2,300 mg/m^2 reached between 100 and 130 µg/ml and were sustained during this period of time (fig. 1). An increased bleeding diathesis due to an inhibition of production of the procoagulant factors II, VII, IX and X was the only side effect noted. This followed the maximum dose of 2,300 mg/m^2 given daily for 5–10 days and could be circumvented by administering 10 mg of vitamin K$_3$ prior to the vitamin E infusion.

Among the mechanisms of action of vitamin E at physiologic levels, the anti-oxidant characteristic of the vitamin appears to be its major effect. The relationship between anti-oxidants and murine tumor cell lysis, or tumor cell growth inhibition has been suggested, but the mechanism has not been demonstrated [11]. The intimate relationship of vitamin E and cell membranes suggests that membranes might be the site where the major antitumoral activity of vitamin E occurs although there are no data to support this.

The most remarkable aspect of this clinical study was the virtual lack of toxicity at relatively high dosages. The intravenous administration of vitamin E led to minor objective and subjective responses in patients with neuroblastoma, primitive neuroectodermal tumor and retinoblastoma. The lack of major responses and their brief duration may be due to the heterogeneity of tumors, a recently appreciated aspect of neuroblastomas. These data suggest phase II trials with vitamin E in patients with these and other tumors. A suggested dosage level of Ephynal at 2,300 mg/m^2/day preceded by 10 mg vitamin K$_3$ for 5 days for three courses may be considered a useful baseline requirement to evaluate its antitumor activity. Even if the mechanism of the antitumor effects induced by vitamin E is unknown, the lack of clinically important toxicity noted in this phase I trial along with the limited responses obtained are suggestive that specific sensitive tumor types might be detected in broader based phase II trials. It is predicted that identification of selected subtypes of responsive tumors may result in consistent therapeutic effects.

Acknowledgements

I am indebted to Ms. *Joan Callahan* for the collection and preparation of blood samples, and to Dr. *Hemmige Bhagavan* of Hoffmann-La Roche, Inc., Nutley, N.J., for his help with the study.

References

1   Graham, J.; Graham, R.; Kallamacer, H.: Potentiation of radiotherapy by supple-
     mental agents in cancer of the uterine cervix; four-year result. Acta int. Un. ag.
     Cancer *16:* 1291–1293 (1978).
2   Mergens, W.; Kamm, J.; Newmark, H.: Alpha-tocopherol uses in preventing nitro-
     samine formation in environmental aspects of *N*-nitroso compounds. IARC Sci.-
     Publ. *19:* 199–212 (1978).
3   Kamm, J.; Dashman, T.; Newmark, H.: Inhibition of aminonitrate hepato-toxicity
     by alpha-tocopheraol. Toxicol. appl. Pharmacol. *41:* 575–583 (1977).
4   Ts'o, P.; Caspary, W.; Lorentzen, R.: The involvement of free radicals in chemical
     carcinogenesis; in Pryor, Free radicals in biology, No. 3, pp. 251–303 (Academic
     Press, New York 1977).
5   Prasad, K.; Ramanujam, S.; Gaudreau, D.: Vitamin E induces morphological differ-
     entiation and increases the effect of ionizing radiation on neuroblastoma cells in
     culture. Proc. Soc. exp. Biol. Med. *161:* 570–573 (1979).
6   Helson, L.; Verma, M.; Helson, C.: Vitamin E and neuroblastoma. N.Y. Acad. Sci.
     393: abstr. 22, p. 226 (1982).
7   Helson, L.; Verma, M.; Helson, C.: Vitamin E and human neuroblastoma. 1st Int.
     Conf. on the Modulation and Mediation of Cancer by Vitamins, Tucson 1982 (Kar-
     ger, Basel 1983).
8   Verma, M.; Helson, C.; Traganos, F.; Helson, L.: Effect of vitamin E compounds on
     human neuroblastoma in vitro and in nude mice. J. exp. Cell Biol. *52:* 379–384
     (1984).
9   Helson, L.: The effect of intravenous vitamin E and menadiol sodium diphosphate
     on vitamin K-dependent clotting factors. Thromb. Res. (in press).
10   Helson, L.; Gulati, S.; Langleben, A.; Helson, C.; Jain, K.; Yopp, J.; O'Reilly, R.;
     Jereb, B.; Clarkson, B.: Surgery, chemotherapy, radiotherapy and autologous marrow
     (SCRAM) for neuroectodermal tumors. Proc. 19th Annu. Meet. Amer. Soc. Clin.
     Oncol., San Diego 1983. Abstract C–309 (1983).
11   Ramma, B.; Prasad, K.: Study on the specificity of alpha-tocopherol (vitamin E) acid
     succinate effects on melanoma, glioma and neuroblastoma cells in culture 1,2. Proc.
     Soc. exp. Biol. Med., vol. 174, pp. 302–307 (1983).

L. Helson, MD, Head, Pediatric Cancer Research Laboratory,
Memorial Sloan-Kettering Cancer Center, 1275 York Avenue,
New York, NY 10021 (USA)

Prasad (ed.), Vitamins, Nutrition, and Cancer, pp. 282–291 (Karger, Basel 1984)

Chemoprevention Program of the National Cancer Institute

Peter Greenwald[a], *William D. DeWys*[a], *Louis M. Carrese*[b],
Barbara Murray[c]

[a] Division of Cancer Prevention and Control;
[b] Office of Program Planning and Analysis, and [c] Systems Planning Branch,
National Cancer Institute, National Institutes of Health, Bethesda, Md., USA

Research on nutrition and cancer prevention is sponsored by the National Cancer Institute (NCI) in two related programs: the Chemoprevention Program and the Diet, Nutrition, and Cancer Program. This paper will describe primarily the planning for these programs. It will also indicate briefly new human intervention trials in these areas.

Chemoprevention is the introduction into the diet of defined chemicals, such as vitamins, synthetic analogues, or other substances for the purpose of reducing cancer incidence. The agents to be used are chemically defined and can be administered in precisely specified dosages. An advantage of the chemoprevention approach is that it may be easier to add a constituent to the diet for preventive purposes than to achieve acceptance of a major modification of dietary patterns.

Whereas chemoprevention deals with micronutrients, the related Diet, Nutrition, and Cancer Program has as its chief focus macronutrients. Rather than precise dosages of one or a few defined agents, the dietary studies will examine the effects of changes in classes of foods or nutrient content of the diet in rough percentages that may be either added to or subtracted from the diet. The ultimate aim is to develop effective and acceptable ways to lower cancer incidence by means of dietary modifications.

Increased emphasis is being given to these programs in response to mounting laboratory evidence that certain chemopreventive agents or dietary modifications may halt or reverse cancer progression in animals and epidemiologic evidence that certain dietary patterns may reduce the incidence of cancer in humans. The proportion of cancers attributable in major part to diet and nutrition has been estimated to be one third or more [1], although only a very crude estimate is possible at this time.

The NCI and a number of our advisory groups recognize the importance of this expanded research effort. For example, a subcommittee on Diet, Nutrition, and Cancer of the National Cancer Advisory Board [2] asked that NCI 'give top priority to diet, nutrition and cancer research'. This committee stated that:

> Research in nutrition and cancer is at an evolutionary stage in its development. It needs to bring new sciences and scientists into the field and persuade them to apply their technologies to cancer research. It has to conceive and implement multidisciplinary research approaches and to prepare the way for community based trials of cancer prevention.

The National Cancer Advisory Board's Diet, Nutrition, and Cancer subcommittee further stated that:

> There is need for a definite diet, nutrition, and cancer research program with its outline and goals known to the scientific community so that individual research projects and additional research needs can be designed and identified in relation to the goals of the program.

The Advisory Board [2] asked that there be a plan for a comprehensive, interdisciplinary research program; that a research agenda be prepared; that the scientific community be informed of the plan and agenda; and that some sheltering of the peer review be provided until the state of the art of nutrition research stabilizes. The latter has been approached by use of the Request for Application mechanism, whereby certain funds are set aside for targeted research areas.

Basic Program Model

Program planning helps to identify what research must be done in order to achieve the purposes of the program. Plans have been developed using the technique originated by *Carrese and Baker* [3] at NCI. This technique requires the description of research judged necessary to achieve program objectives and involves the formulation of a series of flows and arrays

NCI Chemoprevention Program		
Research	Laboratory	Description of research judged necessary to achieve program objective(s) sequentially ordered, by stages, with decision points controlling movement from stage to stage.
	Human Intervention Studies	
	Epidemiology	
Methods Development	Laboratory	Identification of the methods required to conduct the research described in each of the stages for laboratory, human intervention, and epidemiological studies.
	Human Intervention Studies	
	Epidemiology	
Operations	Description of the managerial, administrative and informational requirements judged necessary for the efficient and effective operation of the program.	
Resources	Personnel	Identification of resource requirements for each stage of each flow in terms of the four resource categories.
	Facilities	
	Materials	
	Funds	

Fig. 1. Basic program model.

depicting major research program elements, or stages, sequentially ordered on the basis of research logic, with decision points controlling movement from stage to stage. Graphically the program components are represented by a matrix which relates research performance to resources required (including personnel, equipment, facilities, and funds). The completed matrix is called a basic program model (see figure 1 for major components of the chemoprevention program model).

At this time only the linear array or lead research flow has been developed for the chemoprevention and diet programs. It is the baseline of research from which all other planned activities are derived, and it is the only array based on the sequential logic of the work to be performed.

An underlying principle of the plan is that it calls for balance between investigator initiative versus research according to a preconceived strategy. Although the NCI is taking the organizational initiative, many of the projects in the program will come from the scientific community. The plan provides for wide participation by expert advisors in the critical decision-

Table I. Objectives of the NCI diet, nutrition, and cancer plan, and of the chemoprevention plan

	A. NCI diet, nutrition, and cancer prevention plan	B. NCI chemoprevention plan
1	Identifying and characterizing dietary factors with proven activity in preventing carcinogenesis in animals	Identifying and characterizing agents with proven activity in preventing carcinogenesis in animals
2	Identifying dietary factors based on epidemiologic studies	Identifying agents based on epidemiologic studies
3	Determination of acceptability and biochemical effects of dietary modifications	Pharmacologic and toxicologic testing of such agents to select the most promising agents
4	Human intervention trials of potential dietary factors	Human intervention trials of potential chemoprevention agents
5	Application of research results to the general population	Application of research results to the general population

making process and for a high degree of flexibility and an ability to adapt to new findings.

Use of the chemoprevention research plan entails several steps. These steps are usually performed in a certain sequence, but there can be some variation, e.g., each of the first three steps contains certain aspects that can be performed simultaneously. The steps are as follows:

(1) Determine the 'envelope' or boundaries of the program: that is, identify what is and what is not to be included in the program. In the diet, nutrition, and cancer plan, the emphases are on identifying food constituents, determining which are helpful and which are harmful, determining the changes and modifications to be made in the diet, taking into account bioavailability and elucidating metabolic and other interactions. Excluding certain activities from a plan is not a value judgment but simply a logistic consideration: any plan must have some limitations. In the diet plan nutritional methods used in therapy are excluded because the research logic is quite different. The chemoprevention plan does not include studies of

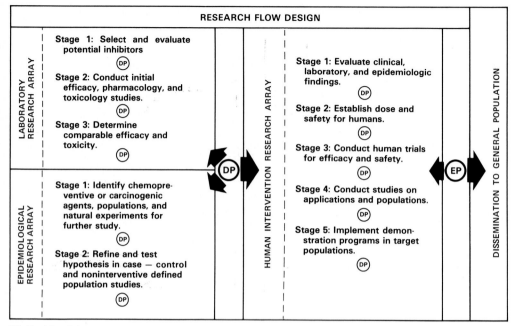

DP: Decision Point
EP: Evaluation Point

Fig. 2. NCI Chemoprevention Program.

mechanism of action which are viewed as being basic research which underlies the plan but which are not specifically encompassed in the plan. Instead the plan focuses on applied research and emphasizes agents which either can prevent carcinogenesis in the laboratory or which are suggested by epidemiologic studies. In the chemoprevention plan, pharmacology and toxicology are emphasized, followed by the consideration of large-scale intervention trials and application to the population at large.

(2) Determine the overall goal of the program and its major objectives. The objectives of the NCI diet, nutrition, and cancer plan and of the chemoprevention plan are shown in table IA and B. The two have many similarities and will be described together, with an indication of the major differences. Table 1A and B refer to randomized, controlled human intervention trials aimed at determining whether a dietary factor, or chemopre-

ventive agent is useful and acceptable to humans as a cancer preventative measure.

(3) Determine the structure of the research flow, that is, the headings for the linear, concurrent, and supplementary arrays. Only the linear array has been developed for the NCI Chemoprevention Program, and Diet and Cancer Programs.

(4) Differentiate the linear research flow into a series of arrays based on content of the program and the judgment that a particular research structure and organization provides the highest probability of achieving the objectives (fig. 2). For both plans, the overall operational flow provides for the results of laboratory and epidemiologic studies to feed into human intervention studies.

(5) Further differentiate the arrays into major stages of research sequentially ordered on the basis of research logic, and develop decision points between contiguous stages to assure that movement from one stage to the next is based on accomplishing the research objective(s) of the previous stage. Figure 2 depicts the stages for laboratory, epidemiologic and human intervention studies arrays in the Chemoprevention Program. Each array will be discussed separately. The decision points contain two elements: (1) a description of the decision to be made, e.g., 'Select Agents for Human Intervention Trials', and (2) a set of criteria which are specific requirements or standards whose satisfaction demonstrates that the research objective(s) of the stage in question has been accomplished. Only essential or 'minimally acceptable' criteria are described. Constraint conditions, e.g., risk/benefit ratio, may also be included in the decision point. This will assist in establishing an agent's priority for moving to the next stage.

Laboratory Array

The laboratory research array (fig. 2) has three stages. Stage 1 is primarily a literature search and review of ongoing research aimed at selecting potential inhibitors for further study. Laboratory and epidemiologic studies are examined in order to identify agents and to consider their inhibitory potential and safety. If a lead fulfills certain criteria, it is then moved to stage 2 where initial efficacy and pharmacology and toxicology testing is carried out in laboratory models. In the chemoprevention plan, stage 2 includes acquiring and/or producing the agent, identifying the agent, its mechanism of action, and its toxicity at levels required for inhibition of carcinogenesis. In the diet, nutrition and cancer plan, experimental and control diets are designed to accomplish the work, and a determination is made about whether the intake of these diets and their biochemical effects can be satisfactorily monitored. Efficacy is established in model systems, and toxicity, identity of the dietary factor, and the mechanism of action may be explored. If specified criteria are fulfilled, the agent or dietary factor is moved to stage 3 where studies are performed to determine comparative efficacy and toxicity. Dose-response relationships, frequency of administration, duration, and the very important issue of timing relative to stage of carcinogenesis are considered. Some agents may be particularly effective in the initiation stage of carcinogenesis, while others may be effective in the promotion stage.

This information is important for designing the relevant human trials. At this stage, long-term toxicity and teratogenicity studies are begun. (Stage 2 included the less expensive short-term toxicity testing.) Long-term toxicity information will be necessary before full-scale human studies are conducted. When both laboratory and clinical data become available, the relevance of models to the human situation will be evaluated. A large number of models will be used initially and as the assessment of their predictive value is achieved, the number of models in the panel will be reduced, based on correlation with clinical results. If an agent fulfills the decision point criteria for stage 3, it can be considered for human studies.

Epidemiology Array

Leads developing in epidemiology are structured in two stages. The initial epidemiology stage, as in the laboratory flow, includes review of the literature and ongoing research (fig. 2). Also in stage 1, appropriate populations for further study are identified by means of descriptive studies. Natural experiments are also identified, and the relationships between intake and subsequent cancer incidence and mortality examined.

Stage 2 studies refine and test hypotheses regarding agents in target populations in case-control and noninterventive defined population studies. Analytical epidemiologic methods are used to determine preventive effects in selected populations and perhaps in the population at large. Again, a set of criteria are specified, and leads fulfilling these criteria are then brought into human trials.

Plans for Human Trials

Randomized, controlled human trials provide the most direct evidence of the preventive benefits of chemopreventive agents or dietary modifications. At this point in the state of our knowledge, it is uncertain to what extent animal results apply to humans, and the best way to address that question is by design of human trials which can then be compared to animal results. In epidemiologic research, the information on specificity is often incomplete and can best be defined in a prospective human trial. In addition, the human trial, as it is formulated, will help define strategies for acceptance of diet or acceptance of a chemopreventive agent. Finally, trials will provide information on adverse affects and allow consideration of risk-benefit relationships.

The human intervention array is shown in figure 2. As with the other research arrays, stage 1 is information-gathering. Previous studies in animals or humans are reviewed, including information on effectiveness and side effects, parameters of exposure to the agent, available data bases, and end points and outcomes.

Human intervention stage 2 studies establish intake levels and safety for humans. For chemoprevention, this will involve pharmacologic studies; for nutrition, the emphasis will be on biochemical end points. The issues of acceptability are pursued and related to the intake level and the dose of the intervention. At the same time that these initial human studies are going on, the long-term toxicity studies in animals, mentioned in the laboratory flow, will be coming to completion, and long-term toxicity studies in humans will begin.

Stage 3 involves the conduct of human trials for efficacy and safety. (The terminology is analogous to phase 3 in the pharmacologic development of a new drug.) The issues here relate to selection of the appropriate study population and the development of a protocol, taking into account the information on efficacy and safety. During the conduct of the trial, ongoing analyses are performed to be sure that if side effects occur, they are detected immediately, and remedial action is taken. The analyses will also focus on terminating the study early if the benefits are established at any point during the study.

The long-range goal is application of the research leads to the population at large. With that in mind, specific research is conducted on methods of intervention for large-scale application for preventive measures in stage 4, which may involve demonstration programs. The amount of agent which may be required for demonstration programs, the availability of monitoring systems, and methods for assessing the outcome of large population studies are the kinds of factors that need to be considered before performing population-wide studies (stage 4). If an agent has shown efficacy in stage 3 and if the methods are available for applying this lead to large populations (stage 5), then sufficient amounts of the agent must be formulated, protocols developed, demonstration programs conducted, and both the acceptability and the adverse affects of this intervention must be monitored. Finally, if all of the previous steps are successful, the intervention can then be introduced to the general population.

Identifying the factors for making priority decisions, such as risk/benefit considerations, cost/benefit considerations, and trade-off studies are an integral part of the planning process. Operationally, a decision committee with subcommittees for the laboratory, epidemiology, and human trials research flows are responsible for all decision-making in the program. The subcommittees review and synthesize research results, relate these data to the decision criteria and bring the data to the decision committee for determination of whether to proceed to the next step, recycle for additional information, or drop an agent from further consideration.

The Division of Cancer Prevention and Control's Board of Scientific Counselors, the National Cancer Advisory Board, and various task forces have been used extensively during the planning process. The process described seeks advice from experts and attempts to remain flexible and able to adapt to new findings. It can be systematically applied in the present and future to all relevant new research projects.

Most of the current intervention trials were investigator-initiated, often stimulated from advisory group and workshop efforts related to the development of these plans. Many of the current studies were in response to requests for applications in these research areas. All relevant projects which were in place prior to the planning have been incorporated in the plan.

Cancer Prevention Trials

By the fall of 1983, 17 NCI-sponsored human cancer prevention trials have been funded using micronutrients or synthetic retinoids. The best known to US physicians is the study by Dr. *Charles Hennekens* and his colleagues in which approximately 22,000 physicians are the study subjects. This is a randomized, double-blind trial to test the effectiveness of alternate day use of aspirin and β-carotene in the prevention of coronary heart disease and cancer, respectively. It is jointly supported by the National Heart, Lung, and Blood Institute. Two other studies test chemopreventive agents in groups that may be roughly representative of the population at large. Finnish and NCI scientists are collaborating in a study of β-carotene in Finnish citizens who are at higher lung cancer risk than the US physicians. A pilot study of selenium and vitamins A and E is planned in which dentists will be the study population.

Four studies focus on high risk groups. Two of these involve heavy smokers; retinol and vitamin B_{12}/folate are the agents. The third, a study of asbestos workers, also uses retinol. In the fourth study, β-carotene and canthaxanthin are being tested in Africa as a means of preventing skin cancer among albinos.

Patients with precancerous lesions comprise the study groups in six projects. Two treat polyposis coli, either with 13-cis-retinoic acid or with a combination of vitamins C and E and wheat fiber. A third tests retinol for preventing transformation of adenomatous polyps. Study subjects in the other three studies have cervical dysplasia. One group is being treated with folic acid. The other studies are pharmacological phase 1 clinical trials to determine whether any local or systemic toxicity occurs when escalated dosages of a topical retinoid are applied to the uterine cervix. Prevention of new primary skin cancers in patients previously treated for nonmelanoma skin cancer is the subject of four studies. Two of these studies use β-carotene and two use 13-cis-retinoic acid.

As defined in the planning process, additional research in diet, nutrition, and cancer and in chemoprevention is being encouraged through requests for grant applications and other mechanisms. Although years will be required before the full potential benefits of this research will be known, this clearly is one of the most promising areas for cancer prevention research.

References

1   Doll, R.; Peto, R.: The causes of cancer: quantitative estimates of avoidable risks of cancer in the United States today. J. natn. Cancer Inst. 66: 1933–1308 (1981).
2   NCAB, Subcommittee on Diet, Nutrition and Cancer (Feb. 1982).
3   Carrese, L.M.; Baker, C.G.: The convergence technique: a method for the planning and programming of research efforts. Manag. Sci. 13: B420–B438 (1967).

P. Greenwald, MD, National Cancer Institute, National Institutes of Health, Building 31, Room 4A32, Bethesda, MD 20205 (USA)

Abstracts

Prasad (ed.), Vitamins, Nutrition, and Cancer, pp. 292–303 (Karger, Basel 1984)

Mechanisms of Carcinogenesis and the Role of Retinoids

R.K. Boutwell, A.K. Verma
McArdle Laboratory, University of Wisconsin, Madison, Wisc., USA

There is increasing evidence that chemically induced neoplasms originating from a number of tissues arise through a series of qualitatively different steps. Examples include tumors of the skin, liver, bladder, and mammary gland. The experimental prototype is the skin model system, pioneered by *Berenblum, Rous, Mottram,* and others, in which the stages known as initiation and promotion were defined. More recently, *Slaga* has identified two components of the promotion step in mouse skin. Furthermore, there is evidence that endogenously produced substances such as epidermal growth factor/urogastrone, sodium deoxycholate, and several hormones may accomplish one or both components of promotion.

Following the accomplishments of *Hecker and Van Duuren,* a number of phorbol esters became available and progress toward understanding the promoting component of carcinogenesis has progressed rapidly. Receptors for phorbol esters in cells from a number of mouse tissues were defined by *Blumberg.* Recently *Ashendel and Boutwell* have shown that protein kinase activity is associated with the phorbol ester receptor purified from mouse brain.

There is strong evidence that, of the many responses in mouse epidermis triggered by phorbol esters, increased polyamine biosynthesis is an essential component of promotion. A number of diverse agents have parallel effects on polyamine synthesis and tumor promotion. Of particular interest is the fact that a number of retinoids are capable of blocking the synthesis of polyamines in response to tumor promoters and, as well, prevent tumor formation by tumor promoters.

Knowledge of the mechanisms that are essential to tumor promotion provides a firm basis for devising practical measures for prophylaxis of human cancer.

Statistical Considerations in the Design of Chemoprevention Studies

Thomas E. Moon, Frank L. Meyskens, Jr.
Cancer Center, University of Arizona, Tucson, Ariz., USA

A number of differences can be identified in the design of cancer prevention trials as contrasted with therapeutic cancer clinical trials. An important difference is the choice of trial end points and selection of criteria to terminate the trial. Clinical trials commonly address a single primary end point that relates to the frequency of reduction in tumor size or duration of disease-free interval. Cancer prevention trials focus on persons who have developed a precancerous lesion and therefore two equally important end points should be addressed: (1) the frequency of developing cancer; (2) the frequency of regression of precancerous lesion.

Examples of such high-risk groups include polyposis coli, actinic keratosis, bronchial metaplasia and cervical dysplasia. Although not commonly used, statistical methods do permit the definition of a study design (including sample size) that is adequate to simultaneously address both end points. The following table illustrates the approach for cervical dysplasia and the changes that would be considered of significant medical importance:

Regression ⟵——————————— Precancer ——————————⟶ Cancer
                                      ↓
                                 No change

End point	Response frequency due to		Sample size
	placebo	prevention	
1	20	10	310
2	20	30	460

where statistical significance level = 0.05 and power = 0.80. Selecting only one trial end point may result in a study design inadequate to yield sufficient confidence in the conclusion for the other end point. Thus, the explicit consideration of both trial end point 1 and 2 is essential and is statistically feasible to adequately evaluate a cancer prevention regimen.

Putative Mechanisms in Nutrient Inhibition of Cancer

Dana F. Flavin
The Nutrition Foundation, Washington, D.C., USA

The role of nutrition in cancer prevention and treatment is best understood if the mechanism of action of specific vitamins and minerals is taken into consideration. The application of these mechanisms can then be applied to the initiation, promotion and growth changes seen in carcinogenesis, with emphasis on the molecular changes within the cell. Since the activities of these vitamins and minerals may change at pharmacological doses or in combination these factors must also be taken into consideration. Animal studies seem to indicate a difference with vitamins and minerals in prevention compared to treatment. Those substances which may prevent tumor induction may actually enhance tumor growth if given after the tumor is in situ. Excess dosage of some of these substances may enhance tumor induction in one organ while inhibiting in another. In these studies the type of carcinogen used, its metabolism and the promoter involved are all necessary to evaluate. The inhibitory effects of vitamins and minerals on tumors that are already cancerous have been noted with: ascorbic acid combined with copper, ascorbic acid with B_{12}, folic acid, α-tocopherol, riboflavin, 13-*cis*-retinoic acid, selenium, selenium and retinoic acid. More research is needed to evaluate the specific types of cancer and their molecular alterations in order to investigate which inhibitory substances may be most effective alone or in combination with other chemicals in tumor reduction. In addition, the pharmacological activities of these vitamins and minerals need further investigation in order to be applied effectively in cancer prevention and treatment.

Retinyl Palmitate and Its Effect on Enzymes in Skin Papillomas of the Egyptian Toad

N. Abdelmegid, A. Ismail, I.A. Sadek
Zoology Department, Faculty of Science and Medical Research Institute,
Alexandria University, Alexandria, Egypt

Retinyl palmitate have anticarcinogenic effect in the Egyptian Toad, *Bufo regularis* [*Sadek*, Oncology *38:* 23, 1981]. Skin papillomas were induced in *B. regularis* by skin painting with 7, 12-dimethylbenz[a]anthracene (DMBA) daily for 8 weeks, as described by *Sadek and Abdelmegid* [Oncology *39:* 399, 1982]. The activities of succinic dehydrogenase (SDH) and lactic dehydrogenase (LDH) were found to be increased in skin papillomas in comparison with the normal skin. However, its activity was found to be decreased in skin papillomas after treatment with retinyl palmitate injection in the dose of 40 mg/kg body weight daily for 8 days. This change in this enzyme may be due to decrease in the anaerobic glycolysis as a result of vitamin A effect on skin papilloma. A previous study by *Frigg and Torhost* [J. natn. Cancer Inst. *58:* 1365, 1977] on regressing skin papillomas had shown that the mechanism of action of vitamin A analog resulted in an induction of necrosis.

Vitamin A and Oral Carcinogenesis

S.V. Kandarkar, Satyavati M. Sirsat
Ultrastructure Division, Cancer Research Institute, Parel, Bombay, India

Since vitamin A is necessary for normal differentiation and maintenance of physiological function of epithelial tissue, it is of interest to investigate its effect on the pattern of induction of tumors in the hamster cheek pouch by chemical carcinogens. 64 weanling

Syrian hamsters were divided in four groups and painted 3 times a week, either with 0.5% DMBA or 15% vitamin A palmitate singly or in combination. A possible mild immune response evoked by vitamin A palmitate is considered responsible for the delayed induction of the tumors. In all animals exposed to carcinogen + vitamin A the induced tumors were small in size and histologically verified as well-differentiated epidermoid carcinomas.

Influence of Dietary Bread, Vitamins A and C, and Meat Cookery Method upon Mutagenicity of Human Fecal Extracts

D.G. Hendricks, D.P. Cornforth, D.T. Bartholomew, K. Kangsadalampai, A.W. Mahoney
Department of Nutrition and Food Sciences, Utah State University, Logan, Utah, USA

Epidemiologic studies have associated consumption of a Western type diet (relatively high in meat and fat, low in vegetables and cereals) with increased risk of large bowel cancer. Our purpose was to study the effects of boiling versus frying of beef round steaks and of fiber consumption (whole wheat bread and tossed salad versus white bread and jello) on mutagenicity of fecal samples of free-living humans.

Using a Latin square design, 4 healthy male professors consumed each of the 4 diets (wheat bread and fried meat, wheat bread and boiled meat, white bread and fried meat, white bread and boiled meat) for a 1-week period, as well as a control, free-choice diet for an additional week. Each individual consumed 135 g beef cubed steak each day, and 6 slices of wheat bread and a tossed salad, or 6 slices of white bread and no salad. The individual was free to eat any other food, in the quantity desired.

Each individual weighed every serving of all foods that he consumed. Total fecal samples were collected on the fifth and sixth days of each period. The stool sample was frozen at $-80\,°C$ for later analysis. The mutagen content of water and chloroform-methanol extracts of the samples was assayed by the forward mutation assay in *Salmonella typhimurium* using 8-azaguanine resistance as a genetic marker. As expected, total fecal weight and total daily dry matter content of the stool was significantly greater when the whole wheat bread diets were consumed, and the percent dry matter was reduced.

84% of fecal lipid extracts were mutagenic, compared to 78% mutagenicity of water-soluble fecal extracts. 23% of the assays (n = 96) of water-soluble stool extracts from individuals consuming boiled meat diets were not mutagenic, while only 12% of assays (n = 96) from fried meat diets were not mutagenic. Similarly, 16 and 20%, respectively, of the fecal assays from white and whole wheat bread diets were not mutagenic. No significant correlations were observed between dietary vitamins A or C and fecal mutagenicity.

Mechanism of Action of Vitamins A and C in Aflatoxin Demethylation in the Guinea Pig

Z.S.C. Okoye, O. Bassir, A.A. Adekunle
Department of Human Chemistry, University of Jos, Jos;
Department of Biochemistry, University of Ibadan, Ibadan, Nigeria

In view of the close association ascorbic acid has with the drug metabolizing enzyme system and the fact that its mechanism as well as that of aflatoxin B_1 (AFB_1) is influenced by an animal's tissue vitamin A level, AFB_1 demethylation by the guinea pig liver was assayed using slices of male weanling pigs deprived of vitamins A and C for 16 days. The demethylation of AFB_1 by the liver slices was significantly altered only when both vitamins were lacking thereby suggesting that the pathway is sensitive to vitamins A and C interaction. The mechanism of a possible conjugative binding of DNA, RNA and/or tissue protein with the 2'-3'-furan double bonds in vivo is explained to be based on a mesomeric effect in the unsaturated system resulting in electron displacement by a demethylation reaction occurring in the methoxy side group of AFB molecule.

Beta Carotene Prevents Dimethylbenz[a]anthracene-Induced Tumors

Giuseppe Rettura, Stanley M. Levenson, Eli Seifter
Departments of Surgery and Biochemistry, Albert Einstein College of Medicine, Bronx, N.Y., USA

We showed that supplemental β-carotene prevented tumors due to an oncogenic virus (MuSV-M) or inoculation with C3H breast adenocarcinoma cells. On this basis, we suggested that supplemental β-carotene would likely protect against lung tumors in smokers, skin tumors due to exposure to actinic rays and hydrocarbon-induced tumors. We have now investigated the role of β-carotene in DMBA-induced tumors. Groups of 40 female Sprague-Dawley rats received 20 mg of DMBA by intubation. 2 weeks later, they were begun on chow containing 15,000 IU of vitamin A plus 6.4 mg β-carotene/kg diet (control) or the chow supplemented with β-carotene, 90 mg/kg or retinyl palmitate 150,000 IU/kg diet. After 180 days, the following results were obtained: 8 control rats died while there were no deaths in the rats receiving supplements. Tumors developed in 33 control rats, in 8 β-carotene and in 7 vitamin A-supplemented rats. There were 93 total tumors in control rats, 12 in the β-carotene group and 10 in the vitamin A supplemented group. We conclude that supplemental β-carotene, like supplemental vitamin A, inhibits hydrocarbon-induced carcinogenesis. The finding that β-carotene and vitamin A supplements are effective, even when given weeks after the carcinogen, is important. Several NIH supported research groups have recently rediscovered the β-carotene-tumor prevention connection. Based on the data from these groups, officials of the Department of Health and Human Services have implied that, in view of β-carotene's tumor preventive action, toxic chemical safety standards can be safely altered. Such a conclusion is a gross misinterpretation of experimental results.

Transplantation of Retinoic Acid Differentiated Murine Embryonal Carcinomas

Wendell C. Speers, Barbara Zimmerman, Magda Altmann
Department of Pathology, University of Colorado Health Sciences Center, Denver, Colo., USA

Murine embryonal carcinoma (EC) tumors were induced to differentiate in vivo with retinoic acid. Solid areas of 7 completely differentiated tumors from long-term surviving hosts were transplanted subcutaneously. Untreated EC tumor cells were transplanted as control. All transplants of differentiated tumor cells survived. 12 transplants from 5 such tumors gave rise to benign cystic teratomas. Transplants of 2 differentiated tumors gave rise to 2 types of malignant tumors, characterized morphologically as chondrosarcoma and astrocytoma. Both grew progressively and were retransplantable. Cytogenetic analysis of these differentiated tumors demonstrated unequivocal origin from the EC stem cells, but significant karyotypic differences were present. We believe that EC differentiation is an epigenetic change which suppresses the malignant phenotype. The malignant phenotype may be regained by secondary genetic changes in differentiated cells.

Adjuvant Vitamin A Treatment in Stage I and II Malignant Melanoma – Preliminary Results

M.R. Thomas, W.A. Robinson, V.M. Peterson, T.I. Mughal, G. Perry, L. Krebs
Division of Oncology, Department of Medicine, University of Colorado, Health Sciences Center, Denver, Colo., USA

Vitamin A and other retinoids have been shown to have an inhibitory effect on the growth of human melanoma cell lines in vitro. Based upon these observations, we initiated a prospective randomized clinical trial of oral vitamin A in patients with resected stage I and stage II cutaneous malignant melanoma with high risk for recurrence. In order to initiate rapid entry into the vitamin A arm, 2 patients were randomized to receive vitamin A treatment versus 1 for no further therapy. No placebo was given. 28 patients (20 stage I and 8 stage II) were randomized to receive oral vitamin A in a dosage of 100,000 IU daily for 2 years and 13 patients (9 stage I and 4 stage II) were randomized to no further treatment. 4 patients in the vitamin A arm discontinued therapy before 2 years; 2 were due to severe dermatologic toxicity, 1 had nodular hyperplasia of the liver and 1 opted out. The majority of patients taking vitamin A had mild dryness of the skin and chelosis. Vitamin A levels in the two treatment groups were not different prior to the initiation of vitamin A but were significantly different after therapy was started. The recurrence of melanoma in the two treatment groups is shown in the table.

Treatment modality	Total patients	Stage I	Stage II	No recurrence (%)	Recurrent disease (%)
Vitamin A	28	20	8	21 (75)	3 (10.7)
No vitamin A	13	9	4	11 (85)	2 (15)

The difference in the recurrence of melanoma in the 2 groups is not statistically significant at the present time. This initial data does however appear encouraging and further patient accrual continues. Further, we have demonstrated that vitamin A in dosage of 100,000 IU is tolerable to most patients.

Antimetastatic Activity of Combined Ascorbate and Levodopa Methyl Ester-Benserazide against B16-BL6 Melanoma

Gary G. Meadows, Rokia M. Abdallah
College of Pharmacy, Washington State University, Pullman, Wash., USA

Levodopa methyl ester administered with an aromatic amino acid decarboxylase inhibitor and supplemental oral ascorbate increases survival of female $B_6D_2F_1$ mice bearing subcutaneous B16 melanoma tumors by 55% when mice are fed a nutritionally adequate crystalline amino acid diet (purified diet) and by 123% when they are fed a diet restricted in tyrosine and phenylalanine [Cancer Res. *43:* 2047–2051, 1983]. We now report the effect of this combination therapy against the highly invasive BL6 line of B16 melanoma using a quantitative lung colony assay. Mice were given sodium ascorbate (30 mg/ml) continuously in the drinking water and were given daily intraperitoneal injections of levodopa methyl ester (1,000 mg/kg) and benserazide (100 mg/kg) for 12 consecutive days beginning 1 day after inoculation of 1.25×10^4 BL6 cells into the lateral tail vein. Neither the tyrosine and phenylalanine-deficient diet nor the drug and ascorbate therapy administered to mice fed this diet affected the numbers of pulmonary metastases, but both the size and pigmentation of the lung colonies were markedly decreased. In mice fed the purified diet, the numbers of pulmonary metastases were decreased by 56% by the levodopa methyl ester-benserazide and ascorbate therapy.

Enhancement of the Effect of Hyperthermia on Neuroblastoma Cells by *DL*-Alpha-Tocopheryl Succinate

Bhola N. Rama, Kedar N. Prasad

Center for Vitamins and Cancer Research, Department of Radiology, School of Medicine, University of Colorado Health Sciences Center, Denver, Colo., USA

DL-α-Tocopheryl (vitamin E) succinate (5 µg/ml) and hyperthermia (43 and 41 °C) markedly inhibited the growth (due to cell death and the inhibition of cell division) of mouse neuroblastoma (NBP₂) cells in culture. Vitamin E enhanced the growth inhibitory effect of heat at both 43 and 41 °C. Vitamin E succinate at the same concentration and heat at 41 °C did not reduce the growth of mouse fibroblasts (L cells) in culture. However, at 43 °C vitamin E (5 µg/ml) enhanced the growth inhibitory effect of heat on L cells. The presence of vitamin E during the heat treatment and during the entire period of observation was necessary for the maximal effect. Sodium succinate (5 µg/ml) and an equivalent amount of solvent (ethanol 0.25 %) failed to modify the effect of hyperthermia on NB cells or L cells. Butylated hydroxyanisole (2 µg/ml), a lipid-soluble antioxidant, also enhanced the effect of heat on NB cells, but to a lesser degree than that produced by vitamin E succinate; however, at a lower temperature (41 °C), they were equally effective. This suggests that the effect of vitamin E in modifying the hyperthermic response may be mediated, in part, by antioxidation mechanisms. If the similar results are obtained in vivo, the addition of vitamin E in hyperthermia (41 °C) protocols may improve their effectiveness in the management of tumor. (Supported by Hoffmann-La Roche.)

Enhancement of the Effect of Gamma-Irradiation on Neuroblastoma Cells by *DL*-Alpha-Tocopheryl Succinate

Alfonso Sarria, Kedar N. Prasad

Center for Vitamins and Cancer Research, Department of Radiology, School of Medicine, University of Colorado Health Sciences Center, Denver, Colo., USA

The effect of *DL*-α-tocopheryl (vitamin E) succinate in modifying the radiation response of mouse neuroblastoma (NBP₂) and mouse fibroblast (L cells) cells in culture was studied on the criterion of growth inhibition (due to cell death and inhibition of cell division). Results show that vitamin E succinate markedly enhanced the growth inhibitory and differentiating effects of ^{60}CO-γ-irradiation on NB cells, but it did not significantly modify the effect of irradiation on mouse fibroblasts. Sodium succinate plus ethanol (0.25 % final concentration) did not modify the radiation response of NB cells or fibroblasts. Butylated hydroxyanisole, a lipid-soluble antioxidant, also enhanced the effect of irradiation on NB cells, indicating that the effect of vitamin E in modifying the radiation response may be mediated, in part, by antioxidant mechanisms. If similar results are obtained in vivo, the addition of vitamin E to radiation therapy protocol may markedly improve its effectiveness in the management of cancer. (Supported by Hoffmann-La Roche.)

The Effect of Vitamin E on Serum Steroid Concentrations in Women with Mammary Dysplasia

R.S. London, G.S. Sundaram, S. Manimekalai, L. Murphy, M. Reynolds, P.J. Goldstein
Division of Clinical Research, Department of Obstetrics and Gynecology, Sinai Hospital of Baltimore, Baltimore, Md., USA

Our preliminary investigations in women with mammary dysplasia, a group considered at increased risk for breast cancer, have demonstrated alterations in serum steroid concentrations after treatment with vitamin E (α-tocopherol). To validate these findings, we performed a double-blind randomized study on women with mammary dysplasia. 65 women in the luteal phase of the menstrual cycle were randomized into 4 groups and treated with one of the following: placebo, vitamin E 150 IU/day, vitamin E 300 IU/day, or vitamin 600 IU/day for 2 months. Plasma concentrations (see below) of dehydroepiandrosterone sulfate (DHEA-S), testosterone (T), 17β-estradiol (E), and progesterone (P) were measured by radioimmunoassay before and after treatment. The effect of tocopherol on DHEA and T concentrations were evaluated statistically using Pearsons Partial Coefficient, controlling weight, age, height, and pretreatment level. No significant dose effect on either hormone was seen ($r = 0.2$ and 0.04, respectively). E and P were similarly analyzed, additionally controlling day of menstrual cycle, and no significant dose effects were seen. These findings suggest that exogenous tocopherol does not alter circulating steroid concentrations in women with mammary dysplasia.

Treatment	DHEA-S ± SD pg/dl	T ± SD ng/dl	E ± SD ng/dl	P ± SD ng/dl
Placebo	1,977 ± 1,050	0.371 ± 0.18	100.3 ± 85	11.9 ± 12.5
Vitamin E, IU				
150	2,320 ± 1,301	0.411 ± 0.17	106 ± 86	9.5 ± 11.2
300	2,114 ± 794	0.386 ± 0.15	99.2 ± 77	11.6 ± 12.3
600	2,446 ± 1,589	0.404 ± 0.23	78.1 ± 45	10.7 ± 8.6

SD = Standard deviation.

Pharmacologic and Genetic Studies on the Modulatory Effects of Butylated Hydroxytoluene on Mouse Lung Adenoma Formation

Alvin M. Malkinson

School of Pharmacy, University of Colorado, Boulder, Colo., USA

The food additive butylated hydroxytoluene (BHT) modulates the multiplicity of mouse lung adenomas induced by the carcinogen, urethane, according to the following administration schedules: BHT presented prior to urethane treatment is prophylactic, while multiple doses of BHT following urethane promote tumor formation. Treatment with BHT alone causes lung damage in mice, but is not carcinogenic. Both an inducer of xenobiotic metabolism, cedrene, and an inhibitor, SKF-525A, prevent the lung toxicity caused by BHT, suggesting that biotransformation of BHT is required for this activity. Cedrene also prevents both types of tumor modulatory effects of BHT, which suggests that a metabolite of BHT which is probably different from the toxic metabolite is responsible for these actions.

Recombinant inbred (RI) lines of mice, derived from C57BL/6ByJ and BALB/cByJ progenitors, were used to study the genetics of tumor promotion. Few C57 mice form adenomas after urethane treatment, while most BALB mice do; C57 mice are not promoted by BHT, while BALB mice are; and most BALB mice die following repeated dosing with high BHT concentrations, while C57 mice do not. Of the 7 C×B RI lines derived from these progenitor strains, 3 lines had the C57-resistant phenotype, and 2 lines had the BALB parental phenotype. Two lines had more tumors than either progenitor, however, and this suggests that > 1 gene controls the susceptibility difference between these strains. BHT only enhanced tumor formation in the lines with BALB-like susceptibility. This means that in the two RI lines which had more urethane-induced tumors than BALB but were not promoted by BHT, susceptibility to urethane and susceptibility to BHT had assorted independently from each other. This implies that different genes regulate the sensitivity to these agents. Only one RI line was highly sensitive to the lethal effects of BHT, and this line was resistant to adenoma formation; this shows that sensitivity to the lethal and promoting effects of BHT are controlled by separate genes. (Supported by USPHS Grant ES 2370 and CA 33497.)

Caffeic and Ferulic Acid as Blockers of Nitrosamine Formation

W. Kuenzig[a], *J. Chau*[a], *E. Norkus*[a], *H. Holowaschenko*[a], *H. Newmark*[b],
W. Mergens[a], *A.H. Conney*[a]

[a] Research Division, Hoffmann-LaRoche, Nutley, N.J., USA;
[b] Ludwig Institute for Cancer Research, Toronto, Canada

Caffeic acid and ferulic acid, which are naturally occurring phenols present in a wide variety of plants, were examined for their ability to react with nitrite in vitro and to inhibit nitrosamine formation in vivo. Their activities were compared with other phenols (butylated hydroxyanisole and Trolox) and with a nonphenolic compound, glycerol guaiacolate. In simulated gastric fluid, caffeic and ferulic acids reacted rapidly and completely with an equimolar quantity of sodium nitrite. Elevated serum glutamic pyruvic transaminase levels, associated with hepatotoxicity, were induced in rats by oral administration for 3 days of 0.15 mmol aminopyrine and 0.43 mmol sodium nitrite per animal. Coadministration of 0.13 mmol caffeic acid or 0.51 mmol ferulic acid blocked the aminopyrine-nitrite hepatotoxicity. Serum levels of N-nitrosodimethylamine (NDMA) were detectable in rats 30 and 60 min after receiving 0.15 mmol of aminopyrine and 0.43 mmol of sodium nitrite, and the coadministration of 0.51 mmol of caffeic or ferulic acid effectively lowered serum NDMA levels at both time periods. Caffeic and ferulic acids had no effect on serum levels of NDMA in rats treated with NDMA. In both the in vitro (reaction with nitrite) and in vivo (inhibition of hepatotoxicity) systems, caffeic acid was more effective than ferulic acid. Butylated hydroxyanisole and Trolox were partially effective, and glycerol guaiacolate was inactive. The results of this study suggest that dietary caffeic and ferulic acids may play a role in the body's defense against carcinogenesis by inhibiting the formation of N-nitroso compounds.

Antineoplastic Anthracycline-Induced Carcinogenicity: Mechanism and Prevention

Yeu-Ming Wang, Scott K. Howell, Terri Bruin, Charles Haidle
Departments of Experimental Pediatrics and Molecular Biology, University of Texas M.D. Anderson Hospital and Tumor Institute, Houston, Tex., USA

Antineoplastic agents have been recognized as carcinogens for a number of years and secondary malignancies in cancer patients has been documented. Malignancies induced by these cytotoxic agents have also been reported in patients treated for other diseases. Daunorubicin is a widely used anticancer drug that is mutagenic and carcinogenic in laboratory animals. Daunorubicin interacts with DNA by intercalation and also produces free radicals which damage DNA. In addition, the anthracycline antibiotics are genotoxic to both animal and human cells in vitro. At therapeutic doses in man, daunomycin produces chromatid aberrations of all types in up to 90% of metaphases analyzed. The mechanism by which the anthracyclines elicit oncogenic effects is unknown; however, free radicals may play a significant role.

In two separate experiments, female Sprague-Dawley rats (~ 150 g) were infected with daunorubicin (10 mg/kg) through a tail vein. This treatment induced mammary adenocarcinomas and fibroadenomas in about 50% of the rats within 4 months. Multiple injections of high doses of α-tocopherylacetate a free radical scavenger, prior to the injection of daunorubicin, prevents or delays the onset of drug-induced tumors.

The tissue distributions of daunorubicin and α-tocopherylacetate were studied. In vitro studies of daunorubicin metabolism and uptake were performed using enzymatically isolated mammary epithelial cells and hepatocytes, the target and non-target cells, respectively. The metabolism of daunorubicin to the aglycone metabolites was substantially lower in mammary cells than in hepatocytes. There was a greater number of single strand breaks of DNA observed in mammary cells than liver cells as determined by alkaline elution.

Glutathione levels were quantitated after daunorubicin treatment in isolated mammary cells of rats fed with three levels of α-tocopherylacetate (deficient, normal and supplemented with 1,000 mg/kg). Also, alkaline elutions were performed in these cells after incubation with various concentrations of daunorubicin.

Human Breast Cancers Heterotransplanted into Vitamin B_6-Deficient Nude Mice

C. Timm[a], *H.P. Fortmeyer*[a], *H. Forster*[b], *G. Bastert*[c]

Departments of [a] Animal Experimentation, [b] Experimental Anesthesiology, and [c] Obstetrics and Gynecology, Klinikum der J.W.-Goethe-Universität, Frankfurt, FRG

Recently [1] we reported that a mouse diet poor in vitamin B_6 led to considerable diminution of growth in one human mammary carcinoma serially passaged into athymic nude mice. This finding was reason for systematic investigations on further human breast cancers transplanted and passaged into nude mice. Until now 11 tumor specimens had been studied. 4 of them showed the same response to a mouse diet poor in vitamin B_6, i.e. a diminished growth rate in comparison with such tumor transplants in normal nourished control mice. The results were reproducible. There was a tendency toward generally lowered tryptophan levels in sera of those mice which were grafted with vitamin B_6-responding breast cancers. This observation concerned both mice fed a control diet and animals in pyridoxine deficiency. Our results are of special interest in respect to clinical findings of lowered levels of plasma pyridoxal phosphate in specific types of cancer patients, especially those with breast cancers. From our above-described investigation and others [2, 3], it became obvious that the model of human malignant tumors heterotransplanted and multiplied in athymic nude mice offers new possibilities for investigations on nutritional influences on tumor tissue of human origin in vivo.

References
1   Fortmeyer, H.P.; Bastert, G.: 1st Int. Conf. Modulation and Mediation of Cancer by Vitamins, Tucson 1982.
2   Fortmeyer, H.P.; et al.: Z. Versuchstierk. *24:* 139 (1982).
3   Helson, L.: 1st Int. Conf. Modulation and Mediation of Cancer by Vitamins, Tucson 1982.

Future Perspectives

A special session was held to discuss the future perspectives of the role of vitamins in the prevention and treatment of cancer. I am presenting my views, some of which are similar to those discussed by my colleagues.

For the prevention of tumor, there is no competing models except for vitamins and nutrition. Therefore, the ongoing or the planned intervention trials of individual vitamins and nutrition among the high-risk population will provide the most useful data to develop a rational protocol for the prevention of cancer among general population. Therefore, a continued emphasis on this particular topic is essential.

Although we know a great deal about the initiating events, we know very little about the crucial biochemical events which are associated with the tumor promotion. Vitamins have been shown to inhibit a promotional stage of carcinogenesis; however, the exact biochemical mechanisms involved in such an inhibition are not known. The knowledge of promotional events and how they are affected by vitamins may help in designing a more effective protocol for the prevention of tumor in human.

The concept of a two-step hypothesis of carcinogenesis has been very useful and continued efforts must be made to identify additional tumor initiators and tumor promoters in the environment. At this time, it is not known whether the effect of more than one tumor promoter is more pronounced than the individual promoter in enhancing the initiator-induced incidence of cancer.

One of the major mechanisms of vitamins in reducing the risk of cancer involves stimulation of host's immune system. Although we have a significant amount of data on the effect of vitamins on immune system in animals, we have very limited data on humans. A dose-effect relationship for an immune response in humans must be established for each vitamin.

Therefore, the assay of immune competency during any interventional trial will be very useful in correlating the reduction of cancer incidence with the stimulation of host's immune system.

Some recent studies suggest that vitamins may reverse newly transformed cells back to normal phenotype. More data are needed to substantiate this role of vitamins using different cell systems and different transforming agents. The studies on the role of other nutrients and vitamins in modifying the incidence of cancer in experimental systems should be continued.

It is becoming apparent that vitamins (A, C, and E) could be very useful in the treatment of tumor provided they are used on a biological rationale. A given vitamin may be effective for certain tumors, but not for others. The selection for a particular form of vitamin for a given tumor is very essential. The same vitamin which may be effective in previously untreated tumors may become completely ineffective for phase I tumor cells. While making a phase I trial of vitamins, one must constantly remember that the phase I tumor cells have become very complex because of accumulation of additional mutations which have been induced by tumor therapeutic agents. Therefore, vitamins will be most useful when they are given before any other chemotherapy or radiation therapy.

The route of administration may be very important during vitamin therapy. The rapid accumulation of vitamins in tumor tissue is essential for an optimal antitumor effect. This may not be accomplished by an oral administration because of poor and variable absorption from the small intestine. Therefore, I believe that the intravenous infusion of vitamins may be necessary for a maximum effect on tumor cells.

Experimental and clinical data suggest that the tumor cells are sensitive to vitamins, whereas the normal cells are not. These data also show that the tumor cells resistant to vitamins exist in the tumor mass. The mechanisms of sensitivity or of resistance are completely unknown. In order to maximize the therapeutic effectiveness of vitamins, we must understand the mechanisms of their effects on tumor and normal cells. One of the productive ways of studying these problems would be to generate vitamin-resistant mutant tumor clones from a vitamin-sensitive clone.

Although the effect of individual vitamin is being studied on experimental and human tumor, the effect of multiple vitamins (A, C, and E) on the growth of tumor is unknown. It is possible that the effect of more than one vitamin is more pronounced than the individual vitamin. Therefore, extensive preclinical studies are needed on this topic before the above concept can be applied to human tumors. The levels of vitamins in tumor tissue must be measured in order to establish a correlation with the vitamin levels and tumor response.

In metastatic lesions, the use of multiple vitamins may not be sufficient to manage the tumor in an effective manner. Therefore, an additional approach must be developed. Recent observation that vitamins can enhance the effect of tumor therapeutic agents (most chemicals, radiation and hyperthermia) is very exciting, and may markedly improve the current management of tumor. However, extensive preclinical studies are needed on this subject before the above concept can be applied to human tumors. In all such studies, the level and distribution of vitamins in normal and tumor tissue must be determined. In addition, the immune competency of the patients must be monitored during therapy.

Kedar N. Prasad, PhD

Subject Index